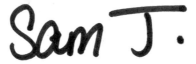

MW00575975

FREE Study Skills DVD (

Dear Customer,

Thank you for your purchase from Mometrix! We consider it an honor and privilege that you have purchased our product and want to ensure your satisfaction.

As a way of showing our appreciation and to help us better serve you, we have developed a Study Skills DVD that we would like to give you for <u>FREE</u>. **This DVD covers our "best practices" for studying for your exam, from using our study materials to preparing for the day of the test.**

All that we ask is that you email us your feedback that would describe your experience so far with our product. Good, bad or indifferent, we want to know what you think!

To get your **FREE Study Skills DVD**, email <u>freedvd@mometrix.com</u> with "FREE STUDY SKILLS DVD" in the subject line and the following information in the body of the email:

    a.   The name of the product you purchased.

    b.   Your product rating on a scale of 1-5, with 5 being the highest rating.

    c.   Your feedback. It can be long, short, or anything in-between, just your impressions and experience so far with our product. Good feedback might include how our study material met your needs and will highlight features of the product that you found helpful.

    d.   Your full name and shipping address where you would like us to send your free DVD.

If you have any questions or concerns, please don't hesitate to contact me directly.

Thanks again!

Sincerely,

Jay Willis
Vice President
<u>jay.willis@mometrix.com</u>
1-800-673-8175

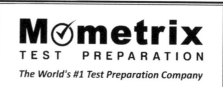

Sam J.

CEN Exam SECRETS

Study Guide
Your Key to Exam Success

CEN Test Review for the
Certification for Emergency
Nursing Examination

Published by
Mometrix Test Preparation
CEN Exam Secrets Test Prep Team

Written and edited by the CEN Exam Secrets Test Prep Staff

Printed in the United States of America

This paper meets the requirements of ANSI/NISO Z39.48-1992 (Permanence of Paper).

Mometrix offers volume discount pricing to institutions. For more information or a price quote, please contact our sales department at sales@mometrix.com or 888-248-1219.

CEN® is a registered trademark of the Board of Certification for Emergency Nursing (BCEN®), which was not involved in the production of, and does not endorse, this product.

ISBN 13: 978-1-60971-299-0
ISBN 10:1-60971-299-4

Dear Future Exam Success Story:

Congratulations on your purchase of our study guide. Our goal in writing our study guide was to cover the content on the test, as well as provide insight into typical test taking mistakes and how to overcome them.

Standardized tests are a key component of being successful, which only increases the importance of doing well in the high-pressure high-stakes environment of test day. How well you do on this test will have a significant impact on your future, and we have the research and practical advice to help you execute on test day.

The product you're reading now is designed to exploit weaknesses in the test itself, and help you avoid the most common errors test takers frequently make.

How to use this study guide

We don't want to waste your time. Our study guide is fast-paced and fluff-free. We suggest going through it a number of times, as repetition is an important part of learning new information and concepts.

First, read through the study guide completely to get a feel for the content and organization. Read the general success strategies first, and then proceed to the content sections. Each tip has been carefully selected for its effectiveness.

Second, read through the study guide again, and take notes in the margins and highlight those sections where you may have a particular weakness.

Finally, bring the manual with you on test day and study it before the exam begins.

Your success is our success

We would be delighted to hear about your success. Send us an email and tell us your story. Thanks for your business and we wish you continued success.

Sincerely,

Mometrix Test Preparation Team

Need more help? Check out our flashcards at: http://MometrixFlashcards.com/CEN

TABLE OF CONTENTS

Top 20 Test Taking Tips

1. Carefully follow all the test registration procedures
2. Know the test directions, duration, topics, question types, how many questions
3. Setup a flexible study schedule at least 3-4 weeks before test day
4. Study during the time of day you are most alert, relaxed, and stress free
5. Maximize your learning style; visual learner use visual study aids, auditory learner use auditory study aids
6. Focus on your weakest knowledge base
7. Find a study partner to review with and help clarify questions
8. Practice, practice, practice
9. Get a good night's sleep; don't try to cram the night before the test
10. Eat a well balanced meal
11. Know the exact physical location of the testing site; drive the route to the site prior to test day
12. Bring a set of ear plugs; the testing center could be noisy
13. Wear comfortable, loose fitting, layered clothing to the testing center; prepare for it to be either cold or hot during the test
14. Bring at least 2 current forms of ID to the testing center
15. Arrive to the test early; be prepared to wait and be patient
16. Eliminate the obviously wrong answer choices, then guess the first remaining choice
17. Pace yourself; don't rush, but keep working and move on if you get stuck
18. Maintain a positive attitude even if the test is going poorly
19. Keep your first answer unless you are positive it is wrong
20. Check your work, don't make a careless mistake

Cardiovascular Emergencies

Heart sounds

Auscultation of heart sounds can help to diagnose different cardiac disorders. Areas to auscultate include the aortic area, pulmonary area, Erb's point, tricuspid area, and the apical area. The normal heart sounds represent closing of the valves.
- The first heart sound (S1) "lub" is closure of the mitral and tricuspid valves (heard at apex/left ventricular area of the heart).
- The second heart sound (S2) "dub" is closure of the aortic and pulmonic valves (heard at the base of the heart). There may be a slight splitting of the S2.

The time between S1 and S2 is systole and the time between S2 and the next S1 is diastole. Systole and diastole should be silent although ventricular disease can cause gallops, snaps, or clicks and stenosis of the valves or failure of the valves to close can cause murmurs. Pericarditis may cause a friction rub.

Additional heart sounds:

Gallop rhythms	S3 occurs after S2 in children and young adults but may indicate heart failure or left ventricular failure in older adults (heard with patient lying on left side). S4 occurs before S1, during the contracting of the atria when there is ventricular hypertrophy, such as from coronary artery disease, hypertension, or aortic valve stenosis.
Opening snap	Unusual high-pitched sound occurring after S2 with stenosis of mitral valve from rheumatic heart disease.
Ejection click	Brief high-pitched sound occurring immediately after S1 with stenosis of the aortic valve.
Friction rub	Harsh, grating sound heard in systole and diastole with pericarditis.
Murmur	Sound caused by turbulent blood flow from stenotic or malfunctioning valves, congenital defects, or increased blood flow. Murmurs are characterized by location, timing in the cardiac cycle, intensity (rated from Grade I to Grade VI), pitch (low to high-pitched), quality (rumbling, whistling, blowing) and radiation (to the carotids, axilla, neck, shoulder, or back).

Administration of 12-lead ECG

The electrocardiogram provides a graphic representation of the electrical activity of the heart. It is indicated for chest pain, dyspnea, syncope, acute coronary syndrome, pulmonary embolism, and possible MI. The standard 12 lead ECG gives a picture of electrical activity from 12 perspectives through placement of 10 body leads:
- 4 limb leads are placed distally on the wrists and ankles (but may be placed more proximally if necessary)
- Precordial leads:
  - V1: right sternal border at 4th intercostal space
  - V2: left sternal border at 4th intercostal space
  - V3: Midway between V2 and V4

- V4: Left midclavicular line at 5th intercostal space.
- V5: Horizontal to V4 at left anterior axillary line.
- V6: Horizontal to V5 at left midaxillary line.

In some cases, additional leads may be used:
Right-sided leads are placed on the right in a mirror image of the left leads, usually to diagnose right ventricular infarction through ST elevation.

> **Review Video:** 12 Lead ECG
> *Visit **mometrix.com/academy** and enter **Code: 962539***

Intra-arterial BP monitoring

Intraarterial blood pressure monitoring is done for systolic, diastolic, and mean arterial pressure (MAP) for conditions that decrease cardiac output, tissue perfusion, or fluid volume. A catheter is inserted into an artery, such as the radial (most frequently used), dorsalis pedis, femoral, or axillary, percutaneously or through a cut-down. Before catheter insertion, collateral circulation must be assessed by Doppler or the Allen test (used for the hand). In the Allen test, both the radial and ulnar artery are compressed and the patient is asked to clench the hand repeatedly until it blanches, and then one artery is released, and the tissue on that side should flush. Then the test is repeated again, releasing the other artery. The MAP is most commonly used to evaluate perfusion as it shows pressure throughout the cardiac cycle. Systole is one-third and diastole two-thirds of the normal cardiac cycle. The MAP for a blood pressure of 120/60 (Normal range 70-100 mm Hg):

$$MAP = \frac{Diastole \times 2 + Systole}{3} = \frac{60 \times 2 + 120}{3} = \frac{240}{3} = 80$$

Jugular venous pressure

Jugular venous pressure (neck-vein) is used to assess the cardiac output and pressure in the right heart as the pulsations relate to changes in pressure in the right atrium. This procedure is usually not accurate if pulse rate is >100. This is a non-invasive estimation of central venous pressure and waveform. Measurement should be done with the internal jugular if possible; if not, the external jugular may be used.
- Elevate the patient's head to 45° (and to 90° if necessary) with patient's head turned to the right.
- Position light at an angle to illuminate veins and shadows.
- Measure the height of the jugular vein pulsation above the sternal joint, using a ruler.
  - Normal height is ≤ 4 cm above sternal angle

Increased pressure (> 4 cm) indicates increased pressure in right atrium, and right heart failure. It may also indicate pericarditis or tricuspid stenosis. Laughing or coughing may trigger the valsalva response and also cause an increase in pressure.

Perfusion pressure and pulse pressure

Perfusion pressure directly affects coronary blood flow, and coronary perfusion occurs during diastole. Coronary artery perfusion pressure is equal to the diastolic blood pressure minus the pulmonary artery occlusion pressure. Normal values are 60-80 mm Hg. During the cardiac cycle, aortic pressure causes the coronaries to be perfused, while ventricular pressure compresses the coronaries during systole, decreasing perfusion. The pulse pressure is the difference between systolic and diastolic pressures, and this can be an important indicator. For example, with a decrease in cardiac output, vasoconstriction takes place in the body's attempt to maintain the blood pressure. In this case, the MAP may remain unchanged, but the pulse pressure narrows. Necessary values for MAP include:

- >60 mm Hg to perfuse coronary arteries
- 70-90 mm Hg to perfuse the brain and other organs, such as the kidneys and to maintain cardiac patients and decrease the workload of the left ventricle.
- 90-110 to increase cerebral perfusion after neurosurgical procedures, such as carotid endarterectomy.

Patients should be assessed for changes in pulse pressure that may be precipitated by medications, such as diuretics that alter fluid volume.

Coronary artery syndromes

Stable angina
Impairment of blood flow through the coronary arteries leads to ischemia of the cardiac muscle and angina pectoris, and pain in the sternum, chest, neck, arms (especially the left), or back. The pain frequently occurs with crushing pain substernally, radiating down the left arm or both arms, although this type of pain is more common in males than females, whose symptoms may appear less acute and include nausea, dyspnea, and fatigue. Elderly or diabetic patients may also have pain in arms, no pain at all *(silent ischemia)*, or weakness and numbness in arms. Stable angina episodes usually last for fewer than 5 minutes and are caused by atherosclerotic lesions blocking more than 75% of the lumen of the affected coronary artery. Precipitating events include exercise, decrease in environmental temperature, heavy eating, strong emotions (such as fright or anger), or exertion, including coitus. Stable angina episodes usually resolve in fewer than 5 minutes by decreasing activity level and administering sublingual nitroglycerin. Angina decubitus occurs when the person lies supine because fluid redistribution increases cardiac workload.

Unstable and variant angina
Unstable angina (also known as preinfarction or crescendo angina) is a progression of coronary artery disease and occurs when there is a change in the pattern of stable angina. The pain may increase, may not respond to a single nitroglycerin, and may persist for more than 5 minutes. Usually pain is more frequent, lasts longer, and may occur at rest. Unstable angina may indicate rupture of an atherosclerotic plaque and the beginning of thrombus formation so it should always be treated as a medical emergency as it may indicate a myocardial infarction. Variant angina (also known as Prinzmetal's angina) results from spasms of the coronary arteries, in patients with or without atherosclerotic plaques, and is often related to smoking, alcohol, or illicit stimulants. Elevation of ST segments usually occurs with variant angina. Variant angina frequently occurs cyclically at the same time each day and often while the person is at rest. Nitroglycerin or calcium channel blockers are used for treatment.

Myocardial Infarction

Myocardial infarctions are classified according to their location and the extent of injury. Transmural myocardial infarction involves the full thickness of the heart (the endocardium, myocardium, and epicardium), often producing a series of Q waves on ECG. An MI most frequently damages the left ventricle and the septum, but the right ventricle may be damaged, depending upon the damaged area:

- Anterior wall infarction occurs with occlusion in the proximal left anterior descending artery, and may damage the left ventricle.
- Left lateral wall infarction occurs with occlusion of the circumflex coronary artery, often causing damage to anterior wall as well.
- Inferior wall infarction occurs with occlusion of the right coronary artery and causes conduction malfunctions.
- Right ventricular infarction occurs with occlusion of the proximal section of the right coronary artery and damages the right ventricle and the inferior wall.
- Posterior wall infarction occurs with occlusion in the right coronary artery or circumflex artery and may be difficult to diagnose.

Diagnosis of a myocardial infarction includes a complete physical examination and patient and family history with assessment of risk factors. Assessment may include:
- ECG obtained immediately to monitor heart changes over time. Typical changes include T-wave inversion, elevation of ST segment, and abnormal Q waves.
- Echocardiogram to evaluate ventricular function.
- Creatine kinase (CK) and isoenzyme (MB):
  o CK-MB (cardiac muscle) level increases within a few hours and peaks at about 24 hours (earlier with thrombolytic therapy or PTCA).
- Myoglobin (heme protein that transports oxygen) found in both skeletal and cardiac muscles. Levels increase in 1-3 hours after an MI and peak within 12 hours. While an increase is not specific to an MI, a failure to increase can be used to rule out an MI.
- Troponin (protein in the myocardium) and its isomers (C, I, and T) regulate contraction and levels increase as with CK-MB, but levels remains elevated for up to 3 weeks.

Clinical manifestations of myocardial infarction may vary considerably, with males having the more "classic" symptom of sudden onset of crushing chest pain and females and those under 55 often presenting with atypical symptoms. Diabetic patients may have reduced sensation of pain because of neuropathy and may complain primarily of weakness. Elderly patients may also have neuropathic changes that reduce sensation of pain. More than half of all patients present with acute MIs with no prior symptoms of cardiovascular disease. Symptoms may include:
- Angina with pain in chest that may radiate to neck or arms.
- Palpitations.
- Hypertension or hypotension
- ECG changes (ST segment and T-wave changes, tachycardia, bradycardia, and dysrhythmias).
- Dyspnea.
- Pulmonary edema, dependent edema
- Nausea and vomiting.
- Decreased urinary output.
- Pallor, skin cold and clammy, diaphoresis.
- Neurological/psychological disturbances: anxiety, light-headed, headache, visual abnormalities, slurred speech, and fear.

Myocardial infarctions (formerly classified as transmural or non-transmural) are currently classified as Q-wave or non-Q-wave:
- Q-wave
  o Characterized by series of abnormal Q waves (wider and deeper) on ECG, especially in the early AM (related to adrenergic activity).

[handwritten note in top margin: Coronary & blood vessels arteries & gets blood now branch the off aorta oxygen rich blood]

- o Infarction is usually prolonged and results in necrosis.
- o Coronary occlusion is complete in 80-90%.
- o Q-wave MI is often, but not always, transmural.
- o Peak CK levels occur in about 27 hours.
- o Mortality rates are about 10%.
- Non-Q-wave
    - o Characterized by changes in ST-T wave with ST depression (usually reversible within a few days).
    - o Usually reperfusion occurs spontaneously, so infarct size is smaller. Contraction necrosis related to reperfusion is common.
    - o Non-Q-wave MI is usually non-transmural.
    - o Coronary occlusion is complete in only 20-30%.
    - o Peak CK levels occur in 12-13 hours.
    - o Mortality rates are about 2-3%.
    - o Reinfarction is common, so 2-year survival rates are similar to Q-wave MI.

Aortic aneurysm

An aortic aneurysm occurs when a weakness in the wall of the aorta causes a ballooning dilation of the wall of the aorta. Aneurysms may result from infections or other trauma, although atherosclerosis is the most common cause for both thoracic and abdominal aortic aneurysms. There are a number of types: *False* is caused by a hematoma that may pulsate and erode the wall of the vessel. *True* is the bulging of 1 to 3 layers of the vessel wall. Fusiform is a symmetric bulging about the entire circumference of the vessel. Saccular is a ballooning on one side of the vessel wall. Dissecting splits the layers of the wall, usually caused by an expanding hematoma. About one-third of thoracic aneurysms (often dissecting) rupture, so surgical repair is indicated. Abdominal aneurysms may remain stable for years, so surgery may be delayed for those at risk until the aneurysm is 5 cm wide. Different classification systems are used to describe dissecting aneurysms: the DeBakey and the Daily (Stanford) systems.

- Type I begins in the ascending aorta but may spread to include the aortic arch and the descending aorta (60%). This is also considered a proximal lesion or Stanford type A.
- Type II is restricted to the ascending aorta (10% to 15%). This is also considered a proximal lesion or Stanford type A.
- Type III is restricted to the descending aorta (25% to 30%). This is considered a distal lesion or Stanford type B.

Types I and II are thoracic and type III is abdominal.

Dissecting aortic aneurysms

A dissecting aortic aneurysm occurs when the intima of the aorta is torn and blood flows between the layers of the wall, dilating and weakening it until it risks rupture (which has 90% mortality). Aortic aneurysms are more than twice as common in males as females, but females have a higher mortality rate, possibly because they are often older. The most common risk factor for a dissecting aortic aneurysm is hypertension, and other risk factors include inflammatory diseases, known aortic aneurysm (being followed/measured prior to dissection), collagen disorders (e.g. Marfan syndrome), and positive family history. Manifestations of a dissecting aortic aneurysm include a sharp/ripping posterior chest pain with a sudden onset, mediastinal widening on chest xray or other radiological studies, syncope, and impaired peripheral pulses or blood pressure differential.

If the dissection occurs in the ascending aorta there is often aortic valve regurgitation, cardiac tamponade, hemothorax, and MI.

Treatment

Once a dissecting aortic aneurysm is identified, and the type is determined, treatment may be medical management or surgical repair depending on type, location, and size:

- Antihypertensives to reduce systolic BP, such as beta-blockers (esmolol), or alpha-beta blocker combinations (labetalol) to reduce force of blood as it leaves the ventricle to reduce pressure against aortic wall. IV vasodilators (sodium nitroprusside) may also be needed.
- Intubation and ventilation may be required if the patient is hemodynamically unstable.
- Analgesia/Sedation to control anxiety and pain.
- Diagnostic tests, such as CT, MRI, transthoracic echocardiogram, and transesophageal echocardiograms may be needed.
- Types I and II are usually repaired surgically because of the danger of rupture and cardiac tamponade.
- Type III (abdominal) are often followed medically and surgery is delayed until aneurysm is greater than 5 cm, at which point either abdominal surgical repair or endoluminal stent may be done.

Cardiac dysrhythmias

Cardiac dysrhythmias, abnormal heart beats, in adults are frequently the result of damage to the conduction system during major cardiac surgery or as the result of a myocardial infarction. Bradydysrhythmias are pulse rates that are abnormally slow:

- Complete atrioventricular block (A-V block) may be congenital or a response to surgical trauma.
- Sinus bradycardia may be caused by the autonomic nervous system or a response to hypotension and decrease in oxygenation.
- Junctional/nodal rhythms often occur in post-surgical patients when absence of P wave is noted but heart rate and output usually remain stable, and unless there is compromise, usually no treatment is necessary.

Tachydysrhythmias are pulse rates that are abnormally fast:

- Sinus tachycardia is often caused by fever and infection.
- Supraventricular tachycardia (200-300 BPM) may have a sudden onset and result in congestive heart failure.

Conduction irregularities are irregular pulses that often occur post-operatively and are usually not significant. Premature contractions may arise from the atria or ventricles.

> ➤ **Review Video:** Pulse
> *Visit **mometrix.com/academy** and enter **Code: 342004***

Sinus node dysrhythmias

There are 3 primary types of sinus node dysrhythmias: sinus bradycardia, sinus tachycardia, and sinus arrhythmia.

SB

- 7 -

Sinus bradycardia (SB) is caused by a decreased rate of impulse from sinus node. The pulse and ECG usually appear normal except for a slower rate. SB is characterized by a regular pulse <50 to 60 with P waves in front of QRS, which are usually normal in shape and duration. PR interval is 0.12 to 0.20 seconds, QRS interval 0.04 to 0.11 seconds, and P:QRS ratio of 1:1.

SB may be caused by a number of factors:
- Conditions that lower the body's metabolic needs, such as hypothermia or sleep.
- Hypotension and decrease in oxygenation.
- Medications such as calcium channel blockers and β-blockers.
- Vagal stimulation that may result from vomiting, suctioning, or defecating.
- Increased intracranial pressure.
- Myocardial infarction.

Treatment involves eliminating cause if possible, such as changing medications. Atropine 0.5-1.0 mg may be given IV to block vagal stimulation.

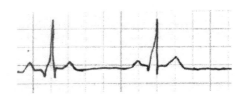

ST
Sinus tachycardia (ST) occurs when the sinus node impulse increases in frequency. ST is characterized by a regular pulse >100 with P waves before QRS but sometimes part of the preceding T wave. QRS is usually of normal shape and duration (0.04 to 0.11 seconds) but may have consistent irregularity. PR interval is 0.12-0.20 seconds and P: QRS ratio of 1:1. The rapid pulse decreases diastolic filling time and causes reduced cardiac output with resultant hypotension. Acute pulmonary edema may result from the decreased ventricular filling if untreated. ST may be caused by a number of factors:
- Acute blood loss, shock, hypovolemia, anemia.
- Sinus arrhythmia, hypovolemic heart failure.
- Hypermetabolic conditions, fever, infection.
- Exertion/exercise, anxiety.
- Medications, such as sympathomimetic drugs.

Treatment includes eliminating precipitating factors and calcium channel blockers and β-blockers to reduce heart rate.

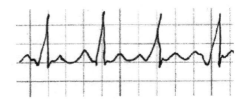

SA
Sinus arrhythmia (SA) results from irregular impulses from the sinus node, often paradoxical (increasing with inspiration and decreasing with expiration) because of stimulation of the vagal nerve during inspiration and rarely causes a negative hemodynamic effect. These cyclic changes in

the pulse during respiration are quite common in both children and young adults and often lesson with age but may persist in some adults. Sinus arrhythmia can, in some cases, relate to heart or valvular disease and may be increased with vagal stimulation for suctioning, vomiting, or defecating. Characteristics of SA include a regular pulse 50-100 BPM, P waves in front of QRS with duration (0.04 to 0.11 seconds) and shape of QRS usually normal, PR interval of 0.12 to 0.20 seconds, and P: QRS ratio of 1:1. Treatment is usually not necessary unless it is associated with bradycardia.

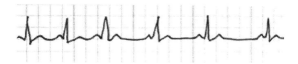

Atrial dysrhythmias

There are 3 primary types of atrial dysrhythmias, including premature atrial contractions, atrial flutter, and atrial fibrillation.

PAC
Premature atrial contraction (PAC) is essentially an extra beat precipitated by an electrical impulse to the atrium before the sinus node impulse. The extra beat may be caused by alcohol, caffeine, nicotine, hypervolemia, hypokalemia, hypermetabolic conditions, atrial ischemia or infarction. Characteristics include an irregular pulse because of extra P waves, shape and duration of QRS is usually normal (0.04 to 0.11 seconds) but may be abnormal, PR interval remains between 0.12 to 0.20, and P: QRS ratio is 1:1. Rhythm is irregular with varying P-P and R-R intervals. PACs can occur in an essentially healthy heart and are not usually cause for concern unless they are frequent (>6 hr) and cause severe palpitations. In that case, atrial fibrillation should be suspected.

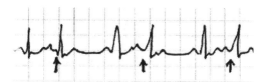

AFib
In atrial fibrillation (AFib), the ventricular rate increases with a decreased stroke volume, and cardiac output decreases with increased myocardial ischemia, resulting in palpitations and fatigue. AFib is characterized by very irregular pulse with atrial rate of 300-600 and ventricular rate of 120-200, shape and duration (0.04 to 0.11 seconds) of QRS is usually normal. The PR interval cannot be measured and the P: QRS ratio is highly variable. In the patient with new onset AFib, investigation into the precipitating and reversible causes of AFib should be investigated and corrected. Correcting rhythm, rate control, prevention of thromboembolism are the goals of AFib care. In the acute setting medications include: For pharmacologic cardioversion of AFib present <7 days: ibutilide, propafenone, dofetilide, flecainide. To control ventricular rate: β-blockers, diltiazem, and verapamil. (amiodarone and digoxin in patients with HF without accessory pathway) For maintenance of rhythm: amiodarone, disopyramide, dofetilide, flecainide, procainamide, propafenone, quinidine, sotalol.

For antithrombotic therapy:
- No risk factors: Aspirin
- Moderate Risk: Aspirin or Warfarin
- High Risk: Warfarin. (For patients on Warfarin, INR range is 2.0 to 3.0. High risk factors: MV stenosis, mechanical heart valve, history of CVA or embolism.)

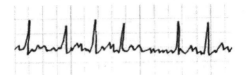

AFL

Atrial flutter (AFL) occurs when the atrial rate is faster, usually 250-400 beats per minute, than the AV node conduction rate so not all of the beats are conducted into the ventricles, effectively blocked at the AV node, preventing ventricular fibrillation although some extra ventricular impulses may pass though. AFL is caused by the same conditions that cause AFib: coronary artery disease, valvular disease, pulmonary disease, heavy alcohol ingestion, and cardiac surgery. AFL is characterized by atrial rates of 250-400 with ventricular rates of 75-150, with ventricular rate usually regular. P waves are saw-toothed (referred to as F waves), QRS shape and duration (0.04 to 0.11 seconds) are usually normal, PR interval may be hard to calculate because of F waves, and the P:QRS ratio is 2-4:1. Symptoms include chest pain, dyspnea, and hypotension. Treatment includes:
- Cardioversion if condition is unstable.
- Medications to slow ventricular rate and conduction through AV node: nondihydropyridine calcium channel blockers (Cardizem®, Calan®) and beta blockers.
- Medications to convert to sinus rhythm: Corvert® (this is the only med approved by FDA for converting AFL but the following are often used in practice: Cardioquin®, Norpace®, Cordarone®.)

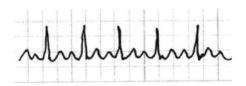

Junctional dysrhythmias

Premature junctional contractions

The area around the AV node is the junction, and dysrhythmias that arise from that are called junctional dysrhythmias. Premature junctional contractions (PJCs) occur when a premature impulse starts at the AV node before the next normal sinus impulse reaches the AV node. PJCs are similar to premature atrial contractions (PACs) and generally require no treatment although they may be an indication of digoxin toxicity. The ECG may appear basically normal with an early QRS complex that is normal in shape and duration (0.04 to 0.11 seconds). The P wave may be absent, precede, be part of, or follow the QRS with a PR interval of N0.12 seconds. The P: QRS ratio may vary from <1:1 to 1:1 (with inverted P wave). Rhythm is usually regular at a heart rate of 40 to 60. Significant symptoms related to premature junctional contractions are rare.

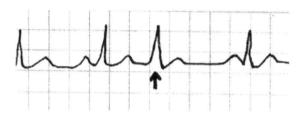

Junctional escape rhythm

Junctional escape rhythm occurs when the AV node becomes the pacemaker of the heart because the sinus node is depressed from increased vagal tone or a block at the AV node prevents sinus node impulses from being transmitted. While the sinus node normally sends impulses 60 to 100 beats per minute, the AV node junction sends impulses 40 to 60 beats per minute. Thus, junctional escape rhythm is characterized by:
- Regular atrial/ventricular rate of 40 to 60 beats per minute.
- QRS complex of usual shape and duration.
- P wave may be inverted and may be absent, hidden, or after the QRS.
- If the P wave precedes the QRS, the PR interval is less than 0.12 seconds.
- P to QRS ratio is 1:1 or 0:1.

The junctional escape rhythm is a protective mechanism preventing asystole with failure of the sinus node. While this rhythm is usually tolerated well, restoring a sinus rhythm is attempted and a pacemaker may be inserted in case AV failure occurs, leaving no backup system.

AV nodal reentry tachycardia

AV nodal reentry tachycardia occurs when an impulse conducts to area of the AV node, and the impulse is sent in a rapidly repeating cycle back to the same area and to the ventricles, resulting in a fast ventricular rate. The onset and cessation are usually rapid. AV nodal reentry tachycardia (also known as paroxysmal atrial tachycardia or supraventricular tachycardia if no P waves) is characterized by atrial rate of 150-250 with ventricular rate of 75-250, P wave that is difficult to see or absent, QRS complex that is usually normal and a PR interval of <0.12 if a P wave is present. The P: QRS ratio is 1-2:1. Precipitating factors include nicotine, caffeine, hypoxemia, and anxiety and underlying coronary artery disease and cardiomyopathy. Cardiac output may be decreased with a rapid heart rate, causing dyspnea, chest pain, and hypotension.

Treatment may include:
- Vagal maneuvers (carotid sinus massage, gag reflex, holding breath.)
- Medications (adenosine, verapamil, or diltiazem)
- Cardioversion if other methods unsuccessful.

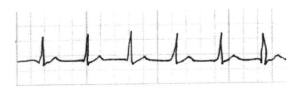

Ventricular dysrhythmias

PVCs
Premature ventricular contractions (PVCs) are those in which the impulse begins in the ventricles and conducts through them prior to the next sinus impulse. The ectopic QRS complexes may vary in shape, depending upon whether there is one site (unifocal) or more (multifocal) that is stimulating the ectopic beats. PVCs usually cause no morbidity unless there is underlying cardiac disease or an acute MI. PVCs are characterized by an irregular heart beat, QRS that is $\geq$0.12 seconds and oddly shaped, P wave that may be absent or may precede or follow the QRS, a PR interval of <0.12 seconds if P wave is present, and a P:QRS ratio of 0-1:1. Short-term therapy may include lidocaine, but PVCs are often not treated in otherwise healthy people. PVCs may be precipitated by caffeine, nicotine, or alcohol. Because PVCs may occur with any supraventricular dysrhythmia, the underlying rhythm (such as atrial fibrillation) must be noted as well as the PVCs.

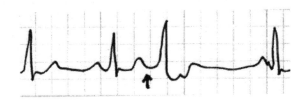

VF
Ventricular fibrillation (VF) is a rapid, very irregular ventricular rate >300 beats per minute with no atrial activity observable on the ECG, caused by disorganized electrical activity in the ventricles. The QRS complex is not recognizable as ECG shows irregular undulations. The causes are the same as for ventricular tachycardia (alcohol, caffeine, nicotine, underlying coronary disease), and VF may result if VT is not treated. VF may also result from an electrical shock or congenital disorder, such as Brugada syndrome. VF is accompanied by lack of palpable pulse, audible pulse, and respirations and is immediately life threatening without defibrillation. After emergency defibrillation, the cause should be identified and limited. Mortality is high if VF occurs as part of a myocardial infarction.

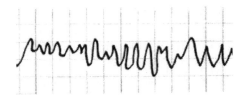

VT

Ventricular Tachycardia (VT) is at least 3 PVCs in a row with a ventricular rate of 100 to 200 beats per minute. Ventricular tachycardia may be triggered by the same things as PVCs and is often related to underlying coronary artery disease, but the rapid rate of contractions make VT dangerous as the ineffective beats may render the person unconscious with no palpable pulse. VT is characterized by:

- A detectable rate (100 to 200) is usually regular.
- QRS complex is at least 0.12 seconds and is usually abnormally shaped.
- P wave may be undetectable with an irregular PR interval if P wave is present.
- P to QRS ratio is often difficult to ascertain because of absence of P waves.

Treatment depends upon the degree of VT and the patient's tolerance and general condition. VT may convert spontaneously or may require cardioversion. Defibrillation is usually done as an emergency procedure if the patient is unconscious.

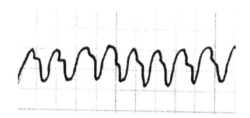

Ventricular asystole

Ventricular asystole is the absence of audible heartbeat, palpable pulse, and respirations, a condition often referred to as "flatlining" or "cardiac arrest." While the ECG may show some P waves initially, the QRS complex is absent although there may be an occasional QRS "escape beat." Cardiopulmonary resuscitation is required with intubation for ventilation and establishment of an intravenous line for fluids. Without immediate treatment, the patient will suffer from severe hypoxia and brain death within minutes. Identifying the cause is critical for the patient's survival and could include hypoxia, acidosis, electrolyte imbalance, hypothermia, or drug overdose. Even with immediate treatment, the prognosis is poor and ventricular asystole is often a sign of impending death.

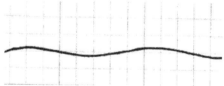

Additional treatment may include transcutaneous pacing and IV epinephrine, repeated at intervals of 3 to 5 minutes.

Idioventricular rhythm

Ventricular escape rhythm (idioventricular) occurs when the Purkinje fibers below the AV node create an impulse. This may occur if the sinus node fails to fire or if there is blockage at the AV node so that the impulse does not go through. Idioventricular rhythm is characterized by a regular ventricular rate of 20-40 BPM. Rates >40 BPM are called accelerated idioventricular rhythm. The P wave is missing and the QRS complex has a very bizarre and abnormal shape with duration of ≥0.12 seconds. The low ventricular rate may cause a decrease in cardiac output, often making the patient lose consciousness. In other patients, the idioventricular rhythm may not be associated with reduced cardiac output.

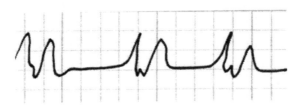

AV block

First-degree

First-degree AV block occurs when the atrial impulses are conducted through the AV node to the ventricles at a rate that is slower than normal. While the P and QRS are usually normal, the PR interval is greater than 0.2 seconds, and the P: QRS ratio is 1:1. A narrow QRS complex indicates a conduction abnormality only in the AV node, but a widened QRS indicates associated damage to the bundle branches as well. *Chronic* first-degree block may be caused by fibrosis/sclerosis of the conduction system related to coronary artery disease, valvular disease, and cardiac myopathies, and carries little morbidity. *Acute* first-degree block, on the other hand, is of much more concern and may be related to digoxin toxicity, beta-blockers, amiodarone, myocardial infarction, hyperkalemia, or edema related to valvular surgery. Incidence correlates with increasing age, and first-degree block is rare in young adults, although athletes have a higher rate (8.7%) than elderly persons (5%).

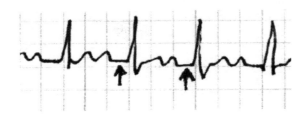

<u>Second-degree</u>

Second-degree AV block occurs when some of the atrial beats are blocked. Second-degree AV block is further subdivided according to the patterns of block:

- Mobitz type I block (Wenckebach): Each atrial impulse in a group of beats is conducted at a lengthened interval until one fails to conduct (the PR interval progressively increases), so there are more P waves than QRS, but the QRS complex is usual of normal shape and duration. The sinus node functions at a regular rate, so the P-P interval is regular, but the R-R interval usually shortens with each impulse. The P: QRS ratio varies, such as 3:2, 4:3, 5:4. This type of block by itself usually does not cause significant morbidity unless associated with inferior wall myocardial infarction, during which a temporary pacemaker may be utilized.

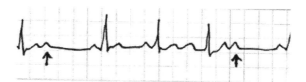

- Mobitz type II block: Only some of the atrial impulses are conducted unpredictably through the AV node to the ventricles, and the block always occurs below the AV node in the bundle of His, the bundle branches, or the Purkinje fibers. The PR intervals are the same if impulses are conducted, and QRS complex is usually widened. The P: QRS ratio varies 2:1, 3:1, and 4:1. Type II block is more dangerous than Type I because it may progress to complete AV block and may produce Stokes-Adams syncope. If the block is at the Purkinje fibers, there is no escape impulse. Usually a transcutaneous cardiac pacemaker and defibrillator should be at bedside. Symptoms may include chest pain if the heart block is precipitated by myocarditis or myocardial ischemia. At times there may be a 2:1 block: Every other atrial impulse (P:QRS ratio of 2.1) is conducted through the AV node, and a surface ECG cannot differentiate between Type I and Type II.

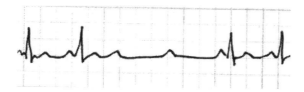

<u>Third-degree</u>

With third-degree AV block, there are more P waves than QRS with no clear relationship between them and an atrial rate 2 to 3 times the pulse rate, so the PR interval is irregular. If the SA node malfunctions, the AV node fires at a lower rate, and if the AV node malfunctions, the pacemaker site in the ventricles takes over at a bradycardic rate; thus, with complete AV block, the heart still contracts, but often ineffectually. With this type of block, the atrial P (sinus rhythm or atrial fibrillation) and the ventricular QRS (ventricular escape rhythm) are stimulated by different impulses, so there is AV dissociation. The heart may compensate at rest but cannot keep pace with exertion. The resultant bradycardia may cause congestive heart failure, fainting, or even sudden death, and usually conduction abnormalities slowly worsen. Symptoms include dyspnea, chest pain, and hypotension, which are treated with IV atropine. Transcutaneous pacing may be needed. Complete persistent AV block normally requires implanted pacemakers, usually dual chamber.

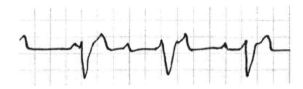

Endocarditis

Endocarditis is an infection of the lining of the heart that covers the heart valves and contains Purkinje fibers, known as the endocardium. Risk factors include being over 60 years of age, being male, IV drug use, and dental infections. Staphylococcal aureus is the most common cause of infective endocarditis. Etiology includes subacute bacterial endocarditis (often related to dental procedures), prosthetic valvular endocarditis (following valve replacement), and right sided endocarditis (often related to catheter infections and IV drug use). Organisms enter the bloodstream from portals of entry (surgery, catheterization, IV drug abuse) and migrate to the heart, growing on the endothelial tissue and forming vegetations (verrucae), collagen deposits, and platelet thrombi. With endocarditis, the valves frequently become deformed, but the pathogenic agents may also invade other tissues, such as the chordae tendineae. The lesions may invade adjacent tissue and break off, becoming emboli. The mitral valve is the most common valve affected, followed by aortic, tricuspid, and the pulmonary valve being the least often affected. Positive blood cultures, widened pulse pressures, ECG, murmurs, and vegetations seen on a transesophageal echocardiogram are used to make the diagnosis. After diagnosis is made, antibiotics are used for treatment, and when unsuccessful or heart failure is present valve repair may be warranted. Serious complications from endocarditis include emboli, sepsis, and heart failure. Untreated endocarditis is fatal.

Diagnosis of endocarditis is made on the basis of clinical presentation and diagnostic procedures that may include:
- Blood cultures should be done with 3 sets for both aerobic and anaerobic bacteria. Diagnosis is definitive if 2 cultures are positive, but a negative culture does not preclude bacterial endocarditis.
- Echocardiogram may identify vegetation on valves or increasing heart failure.
- ECG may demonstrate prolonged PR interval.
- Anemia (normochromic, normocytic).
- Elevated white blood cell count.
- Elevated erythrocyte sedimentation rate (ESR) and C-reactive protein (CRP).

Treatment includes general management of symptoms and the following:
- Antimicrobials specific to the pathogenic organism, usually administered IV for 4 to 6 weeks.
- Surgical replacement of aortic and/or mitral valves may be necessary (in 30% to 40% of cases) if there is no response to treatment and/or after infection is controlled if there are severe symptoms related to valve damage.

Clinical symptoms of endocarditis usually relate to the response to infection, the underlying heart disease, emboli, or immunological response. Typical symptoms include:
- Slow onset with unexplained low-grade and often intermittent fever.
- Anorexia and weight loss, difficulty feeding.
- General lassitude and malaise
- Splenomegaly present in 60% of patients; hepatomegaly may also be present.
- Anemia is present in almost all patients.
- Sudden aortic valve insufficiency or mitral valve insufficiency.
- Cyanosis with clubbing of fingers.
- Embolism of other body organs (brain, liver, bones).
- Congestive heart failure.
- Dysrhythmias.
- New or change in heart murmur.
- Immunological responses
- Janeway lesions: painless areas of hemorrhage on palms of hands and soles of feet.
- Splinter hemorrhages: thin, brown-black lines on nails of fingers and toes.
- Petechiae: pinpoint-sized hemorrhages on oral mucous membranes, as well as hands and trunk.
- Roth spots: retinal hemorrhagic lesions caused by emboli on nerve fibers. Glomerulonephritis: microscopic hematuria.

Myocarditis

Myocarditis is inflammation of the cardiac myocardium (muscle tissue), usually triggered by a viral infection, such as the influenza virus, Coxsackie virus, and HIV. Myocarditis can also be caused by bacteria, fungi, or parasites, or an allergic response to medications. In some cases, it is also a complication of endocarditis. It may also be triggered by chemotherapy drugs and some antibiotics. Myocarditis can result in dilation of the heart, development of thrombi on the heart walls (known as mural thrombi), and infiltration of blood cells around the coronary vessels and between muscle fibers, causing further degeneration of the muscle tissue. The heart may become enlarged and weak, as the ability to pump blood is impaired, leading to congestive heart failure. Symptoms depend upon the extent of damage but may include fatigue, dyspnea, pressure and discomfort in chest or epigastric area, and palpitations.

Diagnosis of myocarditis depends upon the clinical picture, as there is no test specific for myocarditis, although a number of tests may be done to verify the clinical diagnosis:
- Chest radiograph may indicate cardiomegaly or pulmonary edema.
- ECG may show nonspecific changes.
- Echocardiogram may indicate cardiomegaly and demonstrate defects in functioning.
- Cardiac catheterization and cardiac biopsy will yield confirmation in 65% of cases, but not all of the heart muscle may be affected, so a negative finding does not rule out myocarditis.

- Viral cultures of nasopharynx and rectal may help to identify organism.
- Viral titers may increase as disease progresses.
- Polymerase chain reaction (PCR) of biopsy specimen may be most effective for diagnosis.

Treatment:
- As indicated for underlying cause (such as antibiotics).
- Restriction of activities.
- Careful monitoring for heart failure and medical treatment as indicated (e.g., diuretics, digoxin).
- Oxygen as needed to maintain normal oxygen saturation.
- IV gamma globulin for acute stage.

Pericarditis

Pericarditis is inflammation of the pericardial membrane that surrounds the heart. The outer fibrous pericardium is connective tissue that is continuous with the outer layers of the great vessels and serves to protect and anchor the heart. The inner serous pericardium has 2 layers separated with serous pericardial fluid to lubricate the heart and prevent friction. With pericarditis, the layers may become attached to each other (dry), or the serous fluid may be replaced by purulent material, calcifications, fibrinous material, or blood. Pericarditis is frequently associated with surgical repair of cardiac structural abnormalities, but it may also result from other systemic viral, bacterial, fungal, or parasitic infections, or may be caused by direct trauma. Some chronic connective tissue disorders, such as lupus erythematosus, may also cause pericarditis. When pericarditis is related to a viral etiology, patients usually present with flu-like symptoms. The most common sign of pericarditis is a sharp chest pain that is worse with inspiration and is improved when the patient is leaning forward while sitting up. Pericardial effusion may be seen on imaging, a friction rub may be heard on auscultation, and new ST elevations or PR depression may be seen on ECG.

Pericarditis is treated according to the cause and the type and extent of inflammation. Diagnostic procedures are similar to those for endocarditis and myocarditis. Treatment includes:
- Analgesics as indicated to control pain.
- NSAIDS (usually ibuprofen, aspirin, or indomethacin) are recommended for patients with pericarditis unless contraindicated to reduce inflammation and pain.
- Colchicine 0.5 mg every twice a day for six months is often prescribed in adjunct to NSAID therapy, as it decreases the incidence of recurrent pericarditis.
- Corticosteroids are used in some cases if there is no response to anti-inflammatory drugs.
- Extreme physical activity can trigger pain and should be avoided until conclusion of medication treatment and symptoms have subsided (generally 6 months).

Patients that have idiopathic pericarditis or viral pericarditis have a good prognosis with medication alone, however high risk patients may require surgical intervention like a pericardiocentesis, which is removing fluid from the pericardial sac in order to relieve increasing pressure and to diagnose the causative agent. In some cases, a small opening may be made into the pericardium to allow continuous drainage of exudate into the chest cavity. In severe cases, the outer layer of the pericardium may need to be removed if it is preventing functioning of the ventricles.

HF

Heart failure (formerly congestive heart failure) is a cardiac disease that includes disorders of contractions (systolic dysfunction) or filling (diastolic dysfunction) or both and may include pulmonary, peripheral, or systemic edema. The most common causes are coronary artery disease, systemic or pulmonary hypertension, cardiomyopathy, and valvular disorders. The incidence of chronic heart failure correlates with age. The 2 main types of HF are systolic and diastolic. HF is classified according to symptoms and prognosis:

- Class I: The patient is essentially asymptomatic during normal activities with no pulmonary congestion or peripheral hypotension. There is no restriction on activities, and prognosis is good.
- Class II: Symptoms appear with physical exertion but are usually absent at rest, resulting in some limitations of activities of daily living (ADLs). Slight pulmonary edema may be evident by basilar rales. Prognosis is good.
- Class III: Obvious limitations of ADLs and discomfort on any exertion. Prognosis is fair.
- Class IV: Symptoms at rest. Prognosis is poor.

Treatment may include:

- Careful monitoring of fluid balance and weight to determine changes in fluid retention
- Low sodium diet
- Restriction of activity
- Medications may include diuretics, vasodilators, or ACE inhibitors to decrease the heart's workload, digoxin may be given to increase contractibility
- Anticoagulant therapy if distended atria, enlarged ventricles, or atrial fibrillation to decrease the danger of thromboembolia.

> ➤ **Review Video:** Congestive Heart Failure
> *Visit mometrix.com/academy and enter Code: 924118*

Systolic heart failure

Systolic heart failure is the typical "left-sided" failure and reduces the amount of blood ejected from the ventricles during contraction (decreased ejection fraction), stimulating the sympathetic nervous system to produce epinephrine and norepinephrine to support the myocardium. However, this eventually causes down regulation in which beta and adrenergic receptor sites are destroyed, causing further myocardial damage. Because of reduced perfusion, the kidneys produce renin, which promotes angiotensin I, which is converted into angiotensin II, a vasoconstrictor, by the blood vessels. This in turns stimulates production of aldosterone, causing sodium and fluid retention. The end result of these processes is an increase in preload and afterload, increasing the workload on the heart, especially the ventricles. The heart muscle begins to lose contractibility and blood begins to pool in the ventricles during, stretching the myocardium and enlarging the ventricles (ventricular remodeling). The heart compensates by thickening the muscle (hypertrophy) without an adequate increase in capillary blood supply because of the vasoconstriction of the coronary arteries, leading to ischemia. Symptoms include: Activity intolerance, dyspnea, edema, heart sounds S3 and S4, hepatomegaly, JVD, LOC changes, rales, and tachycardia.

Diastolic heart failure

Diastolic heart failure may be difficult to differentiate from systolic heart failure based on clinical symptoms, which are similar. With diastolic heart failure, the myocardium is unable to sufficiently <u>relax</u> to facilitate filling of the ventricles. This may be the end result of systolic heart failure as myocardial hypertrophy stiffens the muscles, and the causes are similar. Diastolic heart failure is more common in females >75. Typically, intracardiac pressures at rest are within normal range but increase markedly on exertion. Because the relaxation of the heart is delayed, the ventricles do not expand enough for the fill-volume, and the heart cannot increase stroke volume during exercise, so symptoms (dyspnea, fatigue, pulmonary edema) are often pronounced on exertion. Ejection fractions are usually >40-50% with increase in left ventricular end-diastolic pressure (LVEDP) and decrease in left ventricular end-diastolic volume (LVEDV). The major goal with all types of heart failure is to prevent further damage and remodeling, prevent exacerbations, and improve the patient's long term prognosis.

Hypertensive crises

Hypertensive crises are marked elevations in blood pressure than can cause severe organ damage if left untreated. Hypertensive crises may be related to primary or secondary hypertension, which may result from kidney or endocrine disorders. Other diseases that may precipitate hypertensive crises include dissection of an aortic aneurysm, pulmonary edema, CNS disorders (subarachnoid hemorrhage, stroke), eclampsia, and failure to take medications properly. There are 2 classifications:
- Hypertensive emergency occurs when acute hyper-tension (1.5 x the 95th percentile), usually >120 mm Hg diastolic, must be treated immediately to lower blood pressure in order to prevent damage to vital organs, such as the heart, brain, or kidneys.
- Hypertensive urgency occurs when acute hypertension must be treated within a few hours but the vital organs are not in immediate danger. Blood pressure is lowered more slowly to avoid hypotension, ischemia of vital organs, or failure of autoregulation.
  - 1/3 reduction in 6 hours
  - 1/3 reduction in next 24 hours
  - 1/3 reduction over days 2-4

Diagnostics include ECG, Chest x-ray, CBC, BMP, Urinalysis (looking for blood and casts). Hypertensive crisis may be managed by a variety of different medications, depending upon the cause and whether the hypertension is an emergency or urgency. In some cases, medications may be combined. Patients with hypertensive emergency receive IV medications and oxygen.

Medications include:
- Initial: Sodium nitroprusside (Nipride®) for fast-acting vasodilation.
- Short acting β-blockers (labetalol, esmolol) for dissecting aortic aneurysm.
- ACE inhibitors (enalaprilat) for heart failure.
- Nitroglycerin for chest pain.
- Dopamine-receptor antagonist (fenoldopam) for renal disease to increase circulation to kidneys.
- Hydralazine for eclampsia.
- Calcium channel blocker (nicardipine) CNS disorders.

- Enalaprilat and labetalol for CNS disorders.
- Alpha-blocker (phentolamine) for pheochromocytoma.
- Diuretics, such as Lasix® and bumetanide to reduce edema.

Continuous monitoring of BP must be done and patient observed for hypotension cause by treatment. If the patient had a stroke, thrombolytic therapy (t-PA) should not be given if the systolic BP is >185 mm Hg and/or the diastolic BP is >110 mm Hg.

Cardiac tamponade

Cardiac tamponade occurs with pericardial effusion in which fluid accumulates in the pericardial sac, causing pressure against the heart. It may be a complication of trauma, pericarditis, cardiac surgery, or heart failure. About 50 mL of fluid normally circulates in the pericardial area to reduce friction, and a sudden increase in this volume can compress the heart and cause a number of cardiac responses:
- Increased end-diastolic pressure in both ventricles.
- Decrease in venous return.
- Decrease in ventricular filling.

Symptoms may include a feeling of pressure or pain in the chest as well as dyspnea, and pulsus paradoxus greater than 10 mm Hg (systolic BP heard during exhalation but not during inhalation). Beck's triad (increased central venous pressure with distended neck veins, muffled heart sounds, and hypotension) is commonly found. Treatment includes pericardiocentesis with large bore needle or surgical repair to control bleeding and relieve cardiac compression.

> **Review Video:** Cardiac Tamponade
> *Visit **mometrix.com/academy** and enter **Code:** 920182*

Peripheral vascular insufficiency

Peripheral vascular insufficiency involves both arterial and venous disease; however, venous disease is a chronic condition that rarely causes critical care crises. Peripheral arterial disease involves the aorta, its branches, arteries, and arterioles. Peripheral arterial disease often involves occlusion of the arteries of the lower extremities, resulting in severe pain and ischemia. The arteries most often affected by peripheral arterial disease are the femoral, the popliteal, the distal aorta, and the iliac arteries. The most common cause of arterial occlusion is atherosclerosis. Symptoms of peripheral arterial disease include:
- Intermittent claudication, a cramping pain while walking.
- Rest pain, a progression of intermittent claudication that includes pain even at rest. This requires catheter or surgical treatment to repair blockage.
- Tissue changes include thickening of nails, hair loss, and dry skin. Ulcerations may occur.
- Acute occlusion, with pain, lack of pulses, decreased skin temperature, pallor, and loss of sensation and function. This requires immediate surgical intervention.

Assessment of lower extremities

Pulse and bruit

Evaluation of the pulses of the lower extremities is an important part of assessment for peripheral arterial disease/trauma. Pulses should be first evaluated with the patient in supine position and then again with the legs dependent, checking bilaterally and proximal to distal to determine if intensity of pulse decreases distally. Pedal pulses should be examined at both the posterior tibialis and the dorsalis pedis. The pulse should be evaluated as to the rate, rhythm, and intensity, which is usually graded on a 0 to 4 scale:

- 0: pulse absent
- 1: weak, difficult to palpate
- 2: normal as expected
- 3: full
- 4: strong and bounding

Pulses may be palpable or absent with peripheral arterial disease. Absence of pulse on both palpation and Doppler probe does indicate peripheral arterial disease. Bruits may be noted by auscultating over major arteries, such as femoral, popliteal, peroneal, and dorsalis pedis, indicating peripheral arterial disease.

Perfusion of lower extremities

Assessment of perfusion can indicate venous or arterial abnormalities:

- Venous refill time: Begin with the patient lying supine for a few moments and then have the patient sit with the feet dependent. Observe the veins on the dorsum of the foot and count the seconds before normal filling. Venous occlusion is indicated with times greater than 20 seconds.
- Capillary refill: Grasp the toenail bed between the thumb and index finger and apply pressure for several seconds to cause blanching. Release the nail and count the seconds until the nail regains normal color. Arterial occlusion is indicated with times of more than 2 to 3 seconds. Check both feet and more than one nail bed.
- Skin temperature: Using the palm of the hand and fingers, gently palpate the skin, moving distally to proximally and comparing both legs. Arterial disease is indicated by decreased temperature (coolness) or a marked change from proximal to distal. Venous disease is indicated by increased temperature about the ankle.

ABI

The ankle-brachial index (ABI) examination is done to evaluate peripheral arterial disease of the lower extremities. Apply BP cuff to one arm, palpate brachial pulse, and place conductivity gel over the artery. Place the tip of a Doppler device at a 45-degree angle into the gel at the brachial artery and listen for the pulse sound. Inflate the cuff until the pulse sound ceases and then inflate 20 mm Hg above that point. Release air and listen for the return of the pulse sound. This reading is the brachial systolic pressure. Repeat the procedure on the other arm, and use the higher reading for calculations. Repeat the same procedure on each ankle with the cuff applied above the malleoli and the gel over they posterior tibial pulse to obtain the ankle systolic pressure. Divide the ankle systolic pressure by the brachial systolic pressure to obtain the ABI. Sometimes, readings are taken both before and after 5 minutes of walking on a treadmill.

Once the ABI examination is completed, the ankle systolic pressure must be divided by the brachial systolic pressure. Ideally, the BP at the ankle should be equal to that of the arm or slightly higher.

With peripheral arterial disease, the ankle pressure falls, affecting the ABI. Additionally, some conditions that cause calcification of arteries, such as diabetes, can cause a false elevation. Calculation is simple; if the ankle systolic pressure is 90 and the brachial systolic pressure is 120: $90 \div 120 = 0.75$

The degree of disease relates to the score:
- >1.3: Abnormally high, may indicate calcification of vessel wall
- 1 to 1.3: Normal reading, asymptomatic
- < 0.95: Indicates narrowing of one or more leg blood vessels
- < 0.8: Moderate, often associated with intermittent claudication during exercise
- < than or equal to 0.6 to 0.8: Borderline perfusion
- <0.5 to 0.75: Severe disease, ischemia
- < 0.5: Pain even at rest, limb threatened
- < 0.25: Critical, limb-threatening condition

Arterial and venous insufficiency

Characteristics that distinguish arterial from venous insufficiency

Characteristic	Arterial	Venous
Type of pain	Ranges from intermittent claudication to severe constant.	Aching and cramping.
Pulses	Weak or absent.	Present.
Skin of extremity	Rubor on dependency but pallor of foot on elevation. Skin pale, shiny, and cool with loss of hair on toes and foot. Nails thick and ridged.	Brownish discoloration around ankles and anterior tibial area.
Ulcers	Pain, deep, circular, often necrotic ulcers on toe tips, toe webs, heels, or other pressure areas.	Varying degrees of pain in superficial, irregular ulcers on me-dial or lateral malleolus and sometimes the anterior tibial area.
Extremity edema	Minimal.	Moderate to severe.

VTE

Acute venous thromboembolism (VTE) is a condition that includes both deep vein thrombosis (DVT) and pulmonary emboli (PE). VTE may be precipitated by invasive procedures, lack of mobility, and inflammation, so it is a common complication in critical care units. Virchow's triad comprises common risk factors: blood stasis, injury to endothelium, and hypercoagulability. Some patients may be initially asymptomatic, but symptoms may include:
- Aching or throbbing pain.
- Positive Homan's sign (pain in calf when foot is dorsiflexed).
- Erythema and edema.
- Dilation of vessels.
- Cyanosis.

Diagnosis may be made by ultrasound and/or D-dimer test, which test the serum for cross-linked fibrin derivatives. CT scan, pulmonary angiogram, and ventilation-perfusion lung scan may be used to diagnose pulmonary emboli. Prophylaxis is very important, but once diagnosed; treatment involves bed rest, elevation of affected limb, anticoagulation therapy, and analgesics. Elastic stockings are worn when patient begins ambulating.

Pharmacologic measures to maximize perfusion

The primary focus of pharmacologic measures to maximize perfusion is to reduce the risk of thromboses:
- Antiplatelet agents, such as aspirin, Ticlid®, and Plavix®, which interfere with the function of the plasma membrane, interfering with clotting. These agents are ineffective to treat clots but prevent clot formation.
- Vasodilators may divert blood from ischemic areas, but some may be indicated, such as Pletal®, which dilates arteries and decreases clotting, and is used for control of intermittent claudication.
- Antilipemic, such as Zocor® and Questran®, slow progression of atherosclerosis.
- Hemorheologics, such as Trental®, reduce fibrinogen, reducing blood viscosity and rigidity of erythrocytes; however, clinical studies show limited benefit. It may be used for intermittent claudication.
- Analgesics may be necessary to improve quality of life. Opioids may be needed in some cases.
- Thrombolytics may be injected into a blocked artery under angiography to dissolve clots.
- Anticoagulants, such as Coumadin® and Lovenox®, prevent blood clots from forming.

Fibrinolytic (thrombolytic) infusions

Fibrinolytic infusion is indicated for acute myocardial infarction under these conditions:
- Symptoms of MI, <6-12 hours since onset of symptoms.
- $\geq$1 mm elevation of ST in $\geq$2 contiguous leads.
- No contraindications and no cardiogenic shock.

Fibrinolytic agents should be administered as soon as possible, within 30 minutes is best. All agents convert plasminogen to plasmin, which breaks down fibrin, dissolving clots:
- Streptokinase & anistreplase (1st generation).
- Alteplase or tissue plasminogen activator (tPA) (second generation).
- Reteplase & tenecteplase (3rd generation).

Contraindications	Relative contraindications
Present or recent bleeding or history of severe bleeding. History of intracranial hemorrhage. History of stroke (<3 months unless within 3 hours). Aortic dissection or pericarditis. Itracranial/intraspinal surgery or trauma within 3 months or neoplasm, aneurysm, or AVM.	Active peptic ulcer. >10 minutes of CPR. Advanced renal or hepatic disease. Pregnancy. Anticoagulation therapy. Acute uncontrolled hypertension or chronic poorly controlled hypertension. Recent (2-4 weeks) internal bleeding. Noncompressible vascular punctures.

PTCA and stent insertion

Percutaneous transluminal coronary angioplasty (PTCA) is a reperfusion option for patients. The decision to use PTCA versus CABG is based on multiple factors, including symptoms, severity of CAD, EF, comorbidities, number of blocked arteries, and degree of narrowing of arteries. This procedure is done to increase circulation to the myocardium by breaking through an atheroma if there is collateral circulation. Cardiac catheterization is done with a hollow catheter (sheath), usually inserted into the femoral vein or artery and fed through the vessels to the coronary arteries. When the atheroma is verified by fluoroscopy, a balloon-tipped catheter is fed over the sheath and the balloon is inflated with a contrast agent, to a specified pressure to compress the atheroma. The balloon may be inflated a number of times to ensure that residual stenosis is <20%. Laser angioplasty using the excimer laser is also used to vaporize plaque. Stents may be inserted during the angioplasty to maintain patency. Stents may be flexible plastic or wire mesh and are typically placed over the catheter, which is inflated to expand the stent against the arterial wall.

Papillary muscle rupture

The atrioventricular valves separate the atria from the ventricles with the tricuspid valve on the right and the bicuspid (mitral) valve on the left. The papillary muscles are located on the sides of ventricular walls and connect to the valves with fibrous bands called chordae tendineae. During systole, the papillary muscles contract, tightening the chordae tendineae and closing the valves. One complication of an MI is papillary muscle rupture, usually on the left affecting the mitral valve, with the posteromedial papillary muscle more often affected than the anterolateral. Dysfunction of the papillary muscles occurs in about 40% of those with a posterior septal infarction, but rupture can occur with infarction of the inferior wall or an anterolateral MI. Rupture on the right side results in tricuspid regurgitation and right ventricular failure, while rupture on the left side leads to mitral regurgitation with resultant pulmonary edema and cardiogenic shock. Early identification and surgical repair is critical.

Blunt cardiac trauma

Blunt cardiac trauma, including myocardial contusions, concussions and ruptures, most often occurs as the result of motor vehicle accidents, falls, or other blows to the chest, which can result in respiratory distress as well as hypovolemia from rupture of the great vessels or the heart and/or cardiac failure from cardiac tamponade or increasing intrathoracic pressure. The heart is particularly vulnerable to chest trauma, with the right atrium and right ventricle the most commonly injured because they are anterior to the rest of the heart. Cardiac trauma may be difficult to diagnose because of other injuries, but if suspected, the patient should be evaluated and an ECG should be done and if any abnormalities (dysrhythmias, ST changes, sinus tachycardia, or heart block) are present, continuous monitoring with should be done for 24-48 hours. Although the most effective test to evaluate for blunt cardiac trauma isn't agreed upon, echocardiogram in conjunction with CPK MB levels is useful in predicting complications. Decreased cardiac output and cerebral oxygenation may result in severe agitation with combative behavior, so changes in mentation should be monitored. Medications may be needed to control arrhythmias and pain.

Penetrating cardiac injuries

The incidence of penetrating cardiac injuries has been on the rise, primarily associated with gun shot injuries and stabbings. The extent of damage caused by a stab wound is often easier to assess than gunshot wounds, which may be multiple and often result in unpredictable and widespread damage not only to the heart but other structures. The primary complications:

- Exsanguination is frequently related to gunshot wounds, and prognosis is very poor. This may lead to hemothorax and hemorrhagic shock.
- Cardiac tamponade (compression of the heart from bleeding into the pericardial sac) is more common with knife wounds, but prognosis is fairly good with surgical repair. Cardiac tamponade often presents with three classic symptoms, known as Beck's triad that should be quickly recognized: muffled heart sounds, low arterial blood pressure, and jugular vein distention.
- Pneumothorax is an irregular amount of air coming between the lungs and chest wall that forces the lung to collapse. Small injuries will heal in time, and more complicated injuries require a tube or syringe for removal of excess air.

Mortality rates are very high in the first hour after a penetrating cardiac injury, so it is imperative the injured be taken immediately to a trauma center rather than attempts made to stabilize the person at the site. Management includes controlling bleeding, giving fluids and pressors for bp, preparing patient for surgery, and monitoring for the above mentioned complications.

Traumatic injury to the great vessels

Traumatic injuries to the great vessels most commonly result from severe decelerating blunt force or penetrating injuries, with aortic trauma the most common. If the aorta is torn, it will result in almost instant death, but in some cases, there is an incomplete laceration to the intimal lining (innermost membrane) of the aorta, causing an aortic hematoma or bulging. This lining, the adventitia, is quite strong and often will contain the rupture long enough to allow surgical repair. Other vessels may be injured as well, so careful examination must be done. Diagnosis is made initially with chest x-ray or CT, which may show widening of the mediastinum and a misshapen aorta. If there are indications of injury, an aortogram or a combination of CT and transesophageal echocardiogram may be used to verify the injury. Treatment requires surgical repair to avoid eventual rupture, during which other vessels are examined for clotting or internal injuries.

Emergency department thoracotomy

Survival rates for emergency thoracotomy are low but sometimes there is no time to transfer the patient to surgery. Prehospital intubation with CPR increases survival rates. Contraindications include asystole with blunt trauma without vital signs prehospital. Indications may include blunt and penetrating cardiac injuries, air embolism, major vascular injuries, blunt and penetrating abdominal injury, and failure to resuscitate nontraumatic cardiac arrest with external CPR. The thoracotomy tray should be available in the emergency department. The procedure includes:

- Establishment of airway with orotracheal tube and mechanical ventilation.
- Anesthesia, including analgesics and muscle relaxing agents (ketamine 2 mg/kg IV and midazolam 0.1 to 0.2 mg/kg IV).
- Universal precautions.
- Suctioning for blood.
- Closed chest compressions to continue until the incision is made.

- Incision is usually anterolateral over 5th rib and into the 4th intercostal space.
- Ventilation stopped briefly before pleura opened so lung is not contacting chest wall.
- Rib retractors to provide exposure.
- Clots from hemothorax removed manually, with suctioning of blood and towels used to absorb drainage.

Pericardiocentesis

Pericardiocentesis is done with ultrasound guidance to diagnose pericardial effusion or with ECG or ultrasound guidance to relieve cardiac tamponade. In the emergency setting, pericardiocentesis is indicated in the patient with cardiac tamponade accompanied by hemodynamic collapse, often with cardiac arrest or presentation of pulseless electrical activity (PEA) with increased jugular venous pressure. For patients with clinical deterioration related to cardiac tamponade, if ultrasound is not available immediately, blind pericardiocentesis can be performed, although it may not be as effective and carries higher risk. Nonhemorrhagic tamponade may be relieved in 60% to 90% of cases, but hemorrhagic tamponade requires thoracotomy as blood will continue to accumulate until cause of hemorrhage is corrected. Resuscitation equipment must be available, including a defibrillator, an IV line in place, and cardiac monitoring. Of note, following pericardiocentesis for cardiac tamponade, there is a sudden drop in preload that can cause hemodynamic instability and even cardiac arrest.

Procedure for pericardiocentesis:
- Elevate chest to 45 degrees to bring heart closer to chest wall.
- Premedication with atropine may prevent vasovagal reactions.
- If abdominal distention is present, a NG tube should be inserted.
- The lower xiphoid and epigastric areas should be prepped with 10% povidone-iodine and draped if possible.
- Local anesthetic should be applied if the patient is conscious.
- Three approaches include the parasternal approach (left 5th intercostal space), subxiphoid approach (between xiphoid process and left costal margin), or apical approach.
- After insertion of the needle, the obturator is removed and a syringe attached for aspiration.
- A sterile alligator clamp is attached from the needle to any precordial lead of the ECG for monitoring to ensure that the ventricle is not punctured.
- The needle is slowly advanced while aspirating gently. The conscious patient may experience pain when the pericardium is breached.
- If fluoroscopy is available, a small amount of contrast may be injected to ensure correct placement if blood is aspirated.
- A catheter may be threaded into the space or the needle is used directly for aspiration of fluid.
- A chest x-ray should be done after removal of the needle to check for pneumothorax.

Cardiopulmonary arrest and SCD

More than 60% of sudden cardiac deaths (SCDs) from cardiovascular disease result from cardiopulmonary arrest, usually involving those with underlying cardiac disease, such as coronary atherosclerosis and/or enlarged heart. There are a number of causative events:

- Ventricular tachyarrhythmias, such as tachycardia or fibrillation, which may result from left ventricular hypertrophy.
  - Treatment: Prompt CPR and defibrillation.
- Brady asystole (cardiac rate less than 60 with periods of asystole) with failure of the electrical system of the heart, resulting from ischemia of the right coronary artery, ischemia of the AV node, systemic disease, hypoxia and hypercarbia, vagal stimulation, or sick sinus syndrome, which is a range of pacemaker disorders.
  - Treatment: Atropine, dopamine, or epinephrine for sick sinus syndrome. Permanent ventricular or AV pacing is usually necessary.
- Pulseless electrical activity (PEA) is the present of organized rhythm without detectable pulse caused by marked decrease in cardiac output resulting from hypovolemia, shock, acidosis, hypothermia, electrolyte imbalances, cardiac dysfunction, or cardiotoxins (beta-blockers, calcium channel blockers, and tricyclic antidepressants).
  - Treatment: Identify and treat underlying cause.

ALTE and SIDS

Apparent life-threatening event (ALTE) occurs when an infant is limp, cyanotic, and not breathing, but is resuscitated. Sudden infant death syndrome (SIDS) is a terminal event. Studies indicate that ALTE and SIDS are usually related to respiratory failure with ventilation disturbances and hypoxemia rather than initial cardiac dysrhythmias. Risk factors for ALTE include:

- Hypoventilation with resultant chronic hypoxemia.
- Inadequate ventilatory response to carbon dioxide.
- More than 15 seconds of sleep apnea, accompanied by pallor or cyanosis.
- Increased episodes of periodic breathing with 3-second periods of pauses and apnea for more than 20 seconds, accompanied by bradycardia.
- Prolonged expiratory apnea.
- Respiratory infection resulting in apnea.

Risk factors for SIDS include:

- Full-term infants with ALTE.
- Premature infants with low-birth weight.
- Siblings of an infant who died of SIDS.
- Infants whose mothers are substance abusing.
- About 10% of SIDS is related to child abuse.
- Prone sleeping may cause airway obstruction or rebreathing of CO_2, leading to respiratory and cardiac arrest.

Emergency defibrillation/automated external defibrillation

Emergency defibrillation is non-synchronized shock which is given to treat acute ventricular fibrillation, pulseless ventricular tachycardia, or polymorphic ventricular tachycardia with a rapid rate and decompensating hemodynamics. Defibrillation can be given at any point in the cardiac cycle. Defibrillation causes depolarization of myocardial cells, which can then repolarize to regain a normal sinus rhythm. Defibrillation delivers an electrical discharge through pads/paddles. In an acute care setting, the preferred position to place the pads is the anteroposterior position. In this position one pad is placed to the right of the sternum, about the second to third intercostal space and the other pad is placed between the left scapula and the spinal column. This decreases the chances of damaging implanted devices, such as pacemakers, and this positioning has also been shown to be more effective for external cardioversion (if indicated at some point during resuscitation). There are two main types of defibrillator shock waveforms, monophasic and biphasic. Biphasic defibrillators deliver a shock one direction for half of the shock, and then in the return direction for the other half, making them more effective, and able to be used at lower energy levels. Monophasic defibrillation is given at 200-360 J and biphasic defibrillation is given at 100-200 J.

Endotracheal administration of medications

Endotracheal administration of medications should be reserved for emergency situations in which rapid administration is necessary and other means, such as IV, are not readily available. There are a number of issues to consider:
- Dosages usually should be 2 to 2.5 times higher than those used for IV administration.
- Diluent may be needed to increase effectiveness but must be limited to avoid complications. The American Heart Association (AHA) recommends a total volume of 10 mL for adults, 5 mL for pediatrics, and 1 mL for neonates.
- Choice of diluent affects absorption and complications. Distilled water increases delivery of the drug, but normal saline produces less pulmonary dysfunction.
- Various delivery methods, including direct instillation or catheter inserted into the tube, are used and studies regarding effectiveness are contradictory. Drugs that are effective endotracheally include atropine, diazepam, epinephrine, flumazenil, lidocaine, and naloxone.

Length-based resuscitation tape

Length-based resuscitation tape is used to estimate weight according to length in infants and small children. The measurement is taken from head to heel with the child in supine position. The results are used to determine dosages of drugs and sizes of equipment. Dosages of common emergency drugs are printed on the tape for different lengths, although some calculations for volume and concentration may be required. The Broselow tape is commonly used by emergency departments and first responders. The marked tape is usually extended alongside the child while the child is in the supine position with the top end (Red in color if the Broselow tape) placed at the top of the child's head and held in place and the bottom end at the patient's heel (not the toes). A straight edge should be used when possible and the tape should be smoothed straight to increase accuracy. Lengths are divided by colors into different "zones" related to length/estimated weight. In some emergency departments, pediatric carts are color-coded to correspond to the zones on the tape. It is important to use the tape properly, and those using it should have training to make sure they understand how to use it accurately.

Pacemakers

Pacemakers are used to stimulate the heart when the normal conduction system of the heart is defective. Pacemakers may be used temporarily or permanently implanted. Temporary pacemakers for external cardiac pacing are commonly used in the emergency setting. Temporary pacemakers may be used prophylactically or therapeutically to treat a cardiac abnormality. Clinical uses include:
- To treat persistent dysrhythmias not responsive to medications.
- To increase cardiac output with bradydysrhythmia by increasing rate.
- To decrease ventricular or supraventricular tachycardia by "overdrive" stimulation of contractions.
- To treat secondary heart block caused by myocardial infarction, ischemia, and drug toxicity.
- To improve cardiac output after cardiac surgery.
- To provide diagnostic information through electrophysiology studies, which induce dysrhythmias for purposes of evaluation.
- To provide pacing when a permanent pacemaker malfunctions.

> ➢ **Review Video:** Pacemaker Care
> *Visit* **mometrix.com/academy** *and enter* **Code: 979075**

AICD

The automatic implantable cardioverter defibrillator (AICD) is similar to the pacemaker and is implanted in the same way with one or more leads to the ventricular myocardium or the epicardium, but it is used to control tachycardia and/or fibrillation. Most AICDs consist of a pacing/sensing electrode, a pulse generator, and defibrillation electrodes. Severe tachycardia may be related to electrical disturbances, cardiomyopathy, or postoperative response to repair of congenital disease. In some cases, it is not responsive to medications. When the pulse reaches a certain preset rate, then the device automatically provides a small electrical impulse to the atrial or ventricular myocardium to slow the heart. If fibrillation occurs, a higher energy shock is delivered. It takes 5 to 15 seconds for the device to detect abnormalities in the pulse rate, and more than one shock may be required so fainting can occur. Contemporary devices can function as both a pacemaker and an ICD, especially important for those who have both episodes of bradycardia and tachycardia. The use of adjunctive antiarrhythmics or ablation is important to prevent AICD shocks.

Cardioversion

Cardioversion is a timed electrical stimulation to the heart to convert a tachydysrhythmia (such as atrial fibrillation) to a normal sinus rhythm. Usually anticoagulation therapy is done for at least 3 weeks prior to elective cardioversion to reduce the risk of emboli and digoxin is discontinued for at least 48 hours prior to cardioversion. Usually anticoagulation therapy should be continued for 3 weeks after procedure as well. If the arrhythmia is causing hypotension, altered mental status, shock, angina or HF, emergent synchronized cardioversion is done (unless it is a regular narrow complex and then vagal maneuvers and adenosine can be considered). During the procedure, the patient is usually sedated and/or anesthetized, if conditions allow. Electrodes in the form of gel-covered paddles or pads are placed in the anteroposterior position, with one pad placed to the right of the sternum, about the 2nd to 3rd intercostal space and the other pad is placed between the left scapula and the spinal column, connected by leads to a computerized ECG and cardiac monitor with a defibrillator. The defibrillator is synchronized with the ECG so that the electrical current is delivered during ventricular depolarization (QRS). The timing must be precise in order to prevent

- 30 -

ventricular tachycardia or ventricular fibrillation. Sometimes, drug therapy is used in conjunction with cardioversion; for example, antiarrhythmics (Cardizem®, Cordarone®) may be given before the procedure to slow the heart rate. Cardiology consult usually follows cardioversion. Risk for embolic stroke for patients with afib who undergo cardioversion must be considered and is lowest when the onset of dysrhythmia is less than 48 hours. Guidelines for cardioversion:

Arrhythmia	Beginning Biphasic Shock
Narrow Regular	50-100 J
Narrow Irregular	120-200 J (200 J if monophasic)
Wide Regular (monomorphic asymptomatic)	100 J

Shock

There are a number of different types of shock, but there are general characteristics that they have in common. In all types of shock, there is a marked decrease in tissue perfusion related to hypotension, so that there is insufficient oxygen delivered to the tissues and, in turn, inadequate removal of cellular waste products, causing injury to tissue:

- Hypotension (systolic below 90 mm Hg). This may be somewhat higher (110 mm Hg) in those who are initially hypertensive.
- Decreased urinary output (<0.5 mL/kg/hr), especially marked in hypovolemic shock
- Metabolic acidosis.
- Hypoxemia <90 mm Hg for children and adults birth-50; < 80mm Hg for those 51 to 70 and <70 for those over 70.
- Peripheral/cutaneous vasoconstriction/vasodilation resulting in cool, clammy skin.
- Alterations in level of consciousness.

	Distributive	Cardiogenic	Hypovolemic
Preload	decrease(sometimes stays same)	increase	decrease
Cardiac Output	increase	decrease	decrease
SVR	decrease	increase	increase

Cardiogenic shock

Cardiogenic shock in adults most often is secondary to myocardial infarction damage that reduces the contractibility of the ventricles, interfering with the pumping mechanism of the heart, decreasing oxygen perfusion. Cardiogenic shock has 3 characteristics: Increased preload, increased afterload, and decreased contractibility. Together these result in a decreased cardiac output and an increase in systemic vascular resistance (SVR) to compensate and protect vital organs. This results in an increase of afterload in the left ventricle with increased need for oxygen. As the cardiac output continues to decrease, tissue perfusion decreases, coronary artery perfusion decreases, fluid backs up and the left ventricle fails to adequately pump the blood, resulting in pulmonary edema and right ventricular failure. Decreasing oxygen consumption is a major initial goal of cardiogenic shock. Symptoms include:

- Hypotension with systolic BP <90 mm Hg.
- Tachycardia > 100 beats/min with weak thready pulse and dysrhythmias.
- Decreased heart sounds.

- Chest pain.
- Tachypnea and basilar rales.
- Cool, moist skin, pallor.

Cardiogenic shock usually results from MI damaging more than 40% of the left ventricle. Diagnosis includes ruling out other causes for symptom:
- ECG: MI-related shock shows initial ST elevation and eventual Q waves. Clinical examination. ABGs
- B-type natriuretic peptide (BNP) correlates with left ventricular end-diastolic pressure and pulmonary artery occlusion.
- Echocardiogram shows impaired contractility of left ventricle.
- Hemodynamic monitoring.

Treatment includes stabilizing patient but may vary according to presenting symptoms and underlying cause:
- Supplemental oxygen and mechanical ventilation if in respiratory failure.
- IV access, arterial line, and urinary catheter.
- Antidysrhythmics if needed.
- Nitroglycerin for chest pain.
- ASA and FD-heparin for MI.
- Inotropes for stabilization: dopamine, dobutamine.
- Diuretics as indicated.
- Thrombolytic therapy followed by intra-aortic balloon counterpulsation and revascularization surgery by percutaneous coronary intervention or coronary bypass.
- Rapid transfer if necessary to facility equipped to do invasive cardiac revascularization.

Respiratory Emergencies

Aspiration pneumonitis/pneumonia

There are a number of risk factors that can lead to aspiration pneumonitis/pneumonia:
- Altered level of consciousness related to illness or sedation.
- Depression of gag, swallowing reflex.
- Intubation or feeding tubes.
- Ileus or gastric distention.
- Gastrointestinal disorders, such as gastroesophageal reflux disorders (GERD).

Diagnosis is based on clinical findings, ABGs showing hypoxemia, infiltrates observed on x-ray, and increased WBC if infection present. Symptoms are similar to other pneumonias, depending upon the site of inflammation:
- Cough often with copious sputum
- Respiratory distress, dyspnea.
- Cyanosis.
- Tachycardia.
- Hypotension.

Treatment includes:
- Suctioning as needed to clear upper airway.
- Supplemental oxygen.
- Antibiotic therapy as indicated after 48 hours if symptoms not resolving.
- Symptomatic respiratory support.

Foreign body aspiration

Foreign body aspiration can cause obstruction of the pharynx, larynx or trachea, leading to acute dyspnea or asphyxiation and the object may be drawn distally into the bronchial tree. With adults, most foreign bodies migrate more readily down the right bronchus. Food is the most frequently aspirated, but other small objects, such as coins or needles, may also be aspirated. Sometimes the object causes swelling, ulceration, and general inflammation that hamper removal. Symptoms are as follows:
- Initial: Severe coughing, gagging, sternal retraction, wheezing. Objects in the larynx may cause inability to breathe or speak and lead to respiratory arrest. Objects in the bronchus cause cough, dyspnea, and wheezing.
- Delayed: Hours, days, or weeks later, an undetected aspirant may cause an infection distal to the aspirated material. Symptoms depend on the area and extent of the infection.

Treatment includes:
- Removal with laryngoscopy or bronchoscopy (rigid is often better than flexible).
- Antibiotic therapy for secondary infection.
- Surgical bronchotomy (rarely required).
- Symptomatic support.

> ➢ **Review Video:** Aspiration of a Foreign Body
> Visit **mometrix.com/academy** and enter **Code: 539288**

- 33 -

Status asthmaticus

Status asthmaticus is a severe acute attack of asthma that does not respond to conventional therapy, such as inhaled bronchodilators, and progresses to respiratory failure. The 3 primary symptoms of asthma are cough, wheezing, and dyspnea. An acute attack of asthma is precipitated by some stimulus, such as an antigen that triggers an allergic response, resulting in an inflammatory cascade that causes edema of the mucous membranes (swollen airway), contraction of smooth muscles (bronchospasm), increased mucus production (cough and obstruction), and hyperinflation of airways. Symptoms include:

- Airway obstruction.
- Sternal and intercostal retractions with forced expirations.
- Tachypnea and dyspnea with increasing cyanosis.
- Cardiac decompensation with increased LV afterload and increased pulmonary edema resulting from alveolar-capillary permeability. Hypoxia may trigger and increase in PVR with increased RV afterload.
- Pulsus paradoxus (decreased pulse on inspiration and increased on expiration) with extra beats on inspiration detected through auscultation but not detected radially. BP normally decreases slightly during inspiration, but this response is exaggerated. Pulsus paradoxus indicates increasing severity of asthma.
- Hypoxemia (with impending respiratory failure).
- Hypocapnia followed by hypercapnia (w impending resp failure).
- Metabolic acidosis.

> ➤ **Review Video:** Asthma and Allergens
> *Visit* ***mometrix.com/academy*** *and enter* ***Code: 799141***

Mechanical ventilation (MV) for status asthmaticus should be avoided if possible because of the danger of increased bronchospasm as well as barotrauma and decreased circulation. However, there are some absolute indications for the use of intubation and ventilation and a number of other indications that are evaluated on an individual basis. Absolute indications for MV are:

- Cardiac and/or pulmonary arrest.
- Markedly depressed mental status (obtundation).
- Severe hypoxia and/or apnea.
- Bradycardia

Relative indications for MV are:

- Exhaustion/muscle fatigue from exertion of breathing.
- Sharply diminished breath sounds and no audible wheezing.
- Pulse paradoxus >20-40 mm Hg.
- If pulse paradoxus is absent, this is an indication of imminent respiratory arrest.
- PaO_2 <70 mm Hg on 100% oxygen.
- Dysphonia.
- Central cyanosis.
- Increased hypercapnia.
- Metabolic/respiratory acidosis: pH <7.20.

In this patient population, ventilator goal is to minimize airway pressures while oxygenating the patient. Vent settings include: low tidal volume (6-8 ml/kg), low respiratory rate (10-14 respirations/minute), and high inspiratory flow rate (80-100 L/min).

Pharmacological agents used for asthma

Numerous pharmacological agents are used for control of asthma, some long acting to prevent attacks and others that are short-acting to provide relief for acute episodes. Listed with each are the standard med and dosage used for urgent care:
- β-Adrenergic agonists include both long-acting and short-acting preparations used for relaxation of smooth muscles and bronchodilation, reducing edema and aiding clearance of mucus. Medications include salmeterol (Serevent), sustained release albuterol (Volmax ER®) and short-acting albuterol (Proventil®) and levalbuterol (Xopenex®). Albuterol 2.5 to 5 mg q 20 minutes x 3 doses by nebulizer.
- Anticholinergics aid in preventing bronchial constriction and potentiate the bronchodilating action of β-Adrenergic agonists. The most-commonly used medication is ipratropium bromide (Atrovent®) 500 mcg q 20 minutes x 3 doses by nebulizer.
- Corticosteroids provide anti-inflammatory action by inhibiting immune responses, decreasing edema, mucus, and hyper-responsiveness. Because of numerous side effects, glucocorticosteroids are usually administered orally or parentally for >5 days (prednisone, prednisolone, methylprednisolone) and then switched to inhaled steroids. If a person receives glucocorticoids for more than 5 days, then dosages are tapered. Methylprednisone 60 to 125 mg IV is the standard dose for respiratory failure.
- Methylxanthines are used to improve pulmonary function and decrease need for mechanical ventilation. Medications include aminophylline and theophylline.
- Magnesium sulfate is used to relax smooth muscles and decrease inflammation. If administered intravenously, it must be given slowly to prevent hypotension and bradycardia. Inhaled, it potentiates the action of albuterol. Standard dosage: 2 g (8 mmol) IV x 1 dose over 20 minutes.
- Heliox (helium-oxygen) is administered to decrease airway resistance with airway obstruction, thereby decreasing respiratory effort. Heliox improves oxygenation of those on mechanical ventilation.
- Leukotriene inhibitors are used to inhibit inflammation and bronchospasm for long-term management. Medications include montelukast (Singulair®).

COPD

Chronic obstructive pulmonary disease (COPD) is a disease that causes limitations in airflow and may include both emphysema and chronic bronchitis, or more often a combination. The primary components to COPD include:
- Progressive airflow limitation.
- Inflammatory response that causes a narrowing of the peripheral airways and thickening of the vessel walls of the pulmonary vasculature.
- Exertional dyspnea and chronic cough.

Acute exacerbation can result in decompensation with increased hypoxemia (arterial oxygen saturation [SaO_2] less than 90% with tachycardia, tachypnea, cyanosis, change in mental status), and hypercapnia (mental status change and hypopnea). Dyspnea and orthopnea are common symptoms. Diagnosis for severity includes pulmonary function tests, ABGs, chest x-ray (to rule out pneumonia or other complications), and echocardiogram.

Treatments include: Oxygen with nasal cannula, face mask, venturi mask, or non-rebreathing mask to elevate PaO_2 greater than 60 mm HG or SaO_2 greater than 90%. Beta-2 adrenergic agonists per nebulizer for bronchodilation. Anticholinergics: ipratropium bromide per metered inhaler. Corticosteroids: 60 to 180 mg/day for 7 to 14 days in decreasing doses. Antibiotics for signs of infection. Assisted ventilation for muscle fatigue and respiratory acidosis.

Bronchiolitis

Bronchiolitis is inflammation of the bronchiolar level and is usually caused by RSV, although adenoviruses, parainfluenza, and Mycoplasma pneumoniae have also been implicated. It is most common in very small children between the ages of 2 months and 2 years and rarely occurs after that age. Most children who require hospitalization are infants younger than 6 months of age. The infection is usually seasonal and is usually mild, although it can result in severe respiratory complications so children should be observed carefully. Symptoms include dyspnea, a paroxysmal cough that is nonproductive, tachypnea, and wheezing. The infection is usually self-limiting and runs its course in 8 to 15 days, but is highly contagious.

Treatment is usually symptomatic and includes:
- Antipyretics, such as acetaminophen.
- Oxygen therapy with intubation and mechanical ventilation may be required in the presence of severe disease and respiratory compromise.
- Ribavirin aerosol is used for severe disease.

Bronchiolitis in adults is different from that in infants. Adult bronchiolitis results in inflammation of the small airways, which are 1-2 mm in diameter, sometimes affecting adjacent alveoli and causing fibrotic changes. The cause of adult bronchiolitis is unclear but may be precipitated by infection or chronic rejection response after transplantation.

Croup syndromes

Acute epiglottitis
Acute epiglottitis (supraglottitis) requires immediate medical attention as it can rapidly become obstructive. The onset is usually very sudden and often occurs suddenly during the night with a fever but not usually a cough. Symptoms include:
- Tripod position: Person sits upright, leaning forward with chin out, mouth open, and tongue protruding.
- Agitation: Person appears restless, tense, and agitated.
- Drooling: Excess secretions combined with pain or dysphagia and mouth in open position, which causes drooling.
- Voice: Voice sounds thick and "froglike."
- Cyanosis: Color is usually pale and sallow initially progressing to frank cyanosis.
- Throat: Epiglottis bright red and swollen.

Diagnosis is by direct examination with nasopharyngoscopy.

Historically, most cases were viral, caused by *H. influenza* type B, but infections can also be bacterial, with infections caused by *Streptococci* becoming more common. Acute epiglottitis has declined in children since the Hib vaccine was introduced, and is now more common in adults.

Treatment: Because this condition can lead to acute respiratory failure and carries a risk of death, immediate treatment is necessary. Treatments include:
- Antibiotics for suspected bacterial infections or as indicated by epiglottal cultures.
- Respiratory support, which may require intubation or tracheostomy and mechanical ventilation (especially for viral infection). Intubation may be very difficult because of the excessive swelling, so immediate tracheostomy may be required.
- Corticosteroids are usually administered during intubation.

Swelling induced by bacteria usually recedes within 24 hours and returns to normal within 3 days.

Acute tracheitis

Acute tracheitis occurs in children from 1 month to 6 years and is usually caused by *Staphylococcus aureus*, with an increase in community-acquired MRSA (CA-MRSA), although group A beta-hemolytic *Streptococci* and *H. influenzae* and other organisms are implicated. This disorder may present with symptoms similar to acute laryngotracheobronchitis, but often fails to respond to the same treatment and can result in airway obstruction and respiratory arrest, so diagnosis and treatment are critical. This condition is usually preceded by an upper respiratory tract infection with croupy cough and strider, as well as a high fever. One difference between this and other forms of croup is the production of copious amounts of thick purulent tracheal exudate, which are implicated in dyspnea and obstruction. Treatment includes:
- Intubation and mechanical ventilation to ensure patency of airway. Tracheostomy may be necessary in some cases.
- Antibiotic therapy should include vancomycin if there are signs of multiorgan failure or increased incidence of CA-MRSA.

Acute laryngotracheobronchitis

Acute laryngotracheobronchitis occurs in children from 3 months to 8 years (usually younger than 5). It is a viral infection, usually caused by the human parainfluenza viruses types 1, 2, and 3, and accounts for about 75% of the total cases. It usually follows an upper respiratory tract infection that slowly encompasses the larynx, resulting in swelling of the mucosa and a progressive onset of low-grade fever with characteristic "croupy" cough. Swelling can cause respiratory obstruction, resulting in acute respiratory acidosis and respiratory failure. Treatment includes:
- Cool humidified air is usually best, but some respond to a warm steamy atmosphere or cool outside air.
- Nebulized racemic epinephrine may be used in the hospital setting, but it is very short acting and can have a rebound effect, so children should not be treated in the emergency department and released until at least the two hour window of its effects have worn off so that they will be able to be treated if airway obstruction remains.
- Glucocorticoids are the new cornerstone of treatment, and a single IM dose of dexamethasone is adequate for most.
- Intubation and ventilation as needed.

Acute respiratory tract infections

Acute bronchitis

Acute bronchitis is an inflammation of the bronchial tree in which swelling and exudate cause a partial obstruction that prevents the lung from fully inflating. Causes include viruses (most common), bacteria, yeasts, and fungi, and noninfectious things, such as smoke or air pollutants. In adults, the most common viral triggers are influenza virus, adenovirus, and respiratory syncytial virus (RSV). Symptoms vary but may include:

- Dyspnea and tachypnea.
- Cyanosis.
- Heavy productive moist or raspy cough.
- Sputum clear, white, yellow, green, or bloody.
- Localized crackling rales and expiratory high-pitched sibilant wheezes.
- Fever may or may not be present, but prolonged or high fever may indicate a bacterial infection.

Since most cases of acute bronchitis are caused by viruses and are self-limiting in 2 to 3 weeks, antibiotics are not helpful, but treatment may include:

- Bronchial dilators (albuterol) to improve air exchange.
- Cough suppressant and/or expectorants to relieve cough.
- Antihistamines for those with allergic triggers.
- Antibiotics for bacterial infections.

Pneumonia

Pneumonia is inflammation of the lung parenchyma, filling the alveoli with exudate. It is common throughout childhood and adulthood. Pneumonia may be a primary disease or may occur secondary to another infection or disease, such as lung cancer. Pneumonia may be caused by bacteria, viruses, parasites, or fungi.

Common causes for community-acquired pneumonia (CAP) include:

- Streptococcus pneumoniae.
- Legionella species.
- Haemophilus influenzae.
- Staphylococcus aureus.
- Mycoplasma pneumoniae.
- Viruses.

Pneumonia may also be caused by chemical damage. Pneumonia is characterized by location:

- Lobar involves one or more lobes of the lungs. If lobes in both lungs are affected, it is referred to as "bilateral" or "double" pneumonia.
- Bronchial/lobular involves the terminal bronchioles and exudate can involve the adjacent lobules. Usually the pneumonia occurs in scattered patches throughout the lungs.
- Interstitial involves primarily the interstitium and alveoli where white blood cells and plasma fill the alveoli, generating inflammation and creating fibrotic tissue as the alveoli are destroyed.

Viral pneumonia

Viral pneumonia is more common in adults than children. However, the respiratory syncytial virus (RSV), which causes upper respiratory tract infections and bronchiolitis, can progress to pneumonia and is most commonly found in children younger than 5. A number of other viruses, such as adenoviruses, parainfluenza, cytomegalovirus, and coronavirus, may be implicated. The viruses invade the cells that line the airways and alveoli, causing death of the cells. Symptoms related to viral pneumonia are similar to those of bacterial pneumonia, although the onset is often slow with pneumonia preceded by a respiratory infection that progressively worsens, with increasing cough, fever, dyspnea, cyanosis, and respiratory distress. There are few effective treatments for viral pneumonia, and one danger is that a viral pneumonia increases susceptibility to bacterial infection of the lungs.

Treatment may include:
- Rest and adequate fluids and nutrition.
- Antipyretics, such as acetaminophen.
- Oxygen therapy with intubation and mechanical ventilation may be required in the presence of severe disease and respiratory compromise.
- Ribavirin aerosol is used for severe RSV disease and pneumonia.

Community-acquired pneumonia

Streptococcus pneumoniae (pneumococcus)
S. pneumoniae (a gram-positive coccus) is part of the normal flora of the upper respiratory tract and is the most frequent cause of bacterial pneumonia, often secondary to an upper respiratory tract infection. The overall incidence has dropped since the heptavalent pneumococcal conjugate vaccine (PCV-7) was introduced in 2000, with the most significant effect on those younger than 2 years of age (78% drop in cases). However, a vaccinated infant that is febrile with toxic symptoms and a leukocyte count of at least 15,000 cells/mL is at risk for pneumonia. The bacteria induce an acute inflammatory response causing the alveoli and interstitium to fill with protein-rich fluid. The infection spreads quickly, often to multiple lobes, causing consolidation, pleural effusions, super infections, and bacteremia (15% to 25%). Pericarditis may occur. Symptoms include an abrupt onset with high fever (at least 105°F), chills, diaphoresis, cyanosis, chest pain, tachypnea, tachycardia, altered consciousness, and cough productive of rusty or green-tinged mucus. Although testing positive for sputum cultures and consolidations on chest x-ray indicate pneumonia, diagnosis is differentiated by blood culture or urinary antigen. Treatment may include:
- Antipyretics and analgesics.
- Respiratory support.
- Antibiotics: penicillins or others.

Mycoplasma pneumoniae (atypical)
Mycoplasma pneumoniae is caused by pleomorphic (variously shaped) microorganisms that interfere with the function of the cilia and produce hydrogen peroxide, which disrupts cell functions. They also activate an inflammatory response. Only about 3% of those infected develop pneumonia, affecting primarily children and young adults between the ages of 4 and 20. Mycoplasma pneumoniae occurs seasonally in the fall in a regular 4- to 8-year cycle of epidemics. The onset is usually gradual, and children tend to be less obviously ill than with other types of pneumonia. Symptoms may include a paroxysmal cough, low-grade fever, myalgia, diarrhea, erythematous rash, and pharyngitis. The pneumonia presents as interstitial infiltrates on x-ray.

While complications, such as myocarditis, endocarditis, and aseptic meningitis and encephalitis, may occur, most infections clear without sequelae.

Treatment includes:
- Antibiotic therapy: erythromycin, tetracycline, macrolide, or fluoroquinolone.
- Symptomatic support: antidiarrheals, antipyretics, and analgesics.

MRSA

Community-acquired methicillin-resistant *Staphylococcus aureus (MRSA)* has emerged as a documented cause of pneumonia since 1997, although, pneumococcus remains the most predominant pathogen for community acquired pneumonia. CA-MRSA tends to be more susceptible to antibiotics than hospital acquired, but it is often more destructive with higher mortality, often causing a necrotizing pneumonia. CA-MRSA is suspected when a patient who is already known to be colonized with CA-MRSA (often those living in crowded places, prisoners, those who play contact sports) develops pneumonia. CA-MRSA pneumonia also often follows influenza in patients that are elderly or very young, and should be suspected, especially if pulmonary necrosis is present on imaging. Symptoms are the same for other types of pneumonia. Diagnosis: Blood cultures, Chest x-ray, assessment, history, and sputum cultures (will show gram-positive cocci in clusters).

Treatment includes:
- Linezolid (treatment of choice) 600 mg IV every 12 hours for 7-21 days.
- Vancomycin 45-60 mg/kg/day divided every 8 hours for 7-21 days, and keeping target trough levels between 15-20 mcg/mL.

Inhalation injuries

Inhalation injuries most often result from exposure to smoke in closed spaces, and are often associated with conditions that affect mentation, such as intoxication or head injury. People also often suffer thermal burn injuries. Thermal injuries occur to the upper airway, but inhalation causes injury below the vocal cords. Toxic inhalants can include tissue asphyxiants, pulmonary irritants, and systemic toxins. Patients may suffer from carbon monoxide and hydrogen cyanide poisoning. Symptoms of inhalation injuries include:
- Dyspnea with bronchospasm.
- Coma from brain hypoxia (carbon monoxide poisoning).
- Rapid upper airway edema and delayed (24 hours or less) lower airway edema.

Diagnosis includes clinical examination, ABGs and carboxyhemoglobin levels, and chest radiograph. Treatments include:
- Humidified oxygen, 100%.
- Evaluation or hyperbaric oxygen therapy (carbon monoxide poisoning).
- Endotracheal intubation if indicated by severity of burns or respiratory status.
- Anti-toxin therapy according to inhalant.

> **Review Video:** Inhalants
*Visit **mometrix.com/academy** and enter **Code: 926725***

Pleural effusion

Pleural effusion is the collection of fluid in the area between the visceral and parietal pleurae. The fluid may be high protein exudates from pleural irritation (such as from neoplasms, infections, pulmonary embolism, empyema, uremia, pancreatitis, or drugs such as amiodarone) or low protein transudates from congestive heart failure (CHF), cirrhotic ascites, peritoneal dialysis, or nephrotic syndrome. Symptoms may be lacking or present as dyspnea and chest pain. Diagnosis is by clinical findings of decreased breath sounds and dullness on percussion, upright chest radiograph, ultrasound (especially useful for small pockets of fluid), CT scan, and thoracentesis if necessary to diagnose condition or infections.

Treatment includes:
- Therapy directed at underlying cause, such as diuretics for CHF.
- Needle/catheter thoracentesis to drain excessive fluid for large pleural effusions.
- Insertion of chest tube indicated for large amounts of fluid.
- Antibiotics as indicated for infection.

Acute pulmonary embolism

Acute pulmonary embolism occurs when a pulmonary artery or arteriole is blocked by a blood clot originating in the venous system or the right heart. While most pulmonary emboli are from thrombus formation, other causes may be air, fat, or septic embolus (from bacterial invasion of a thrombus). Common originating sites for thrombus formation are the deep veins in the legs, the pelvic veins, and the right atrium. Causes include stasis related to damage to endothelial wall and changes in blood coagulation factors. Atrial fibrillation poses a serious risk because blood pools in the right atrium, forming clots that travel directly through the right ventricle to the lungs. The obstruction of the artery/arteriole causes an increase in alveolar dead space in which there is ventilation but impairment of gas exchange because of the ventilation/perfusion mismatching or intrapulmonary shunting. This results in hypoxia, hypercapnia, and the release of mediators that cause bronchoconstriction. If more than 50% of the vascular bed becomes excluded, pulmonary hypertension occurs. Clinical manifestations of acute pulmonary embolism (PE) vary according to the size of the embolus and the area of occlusion.

Symptoms include:
- Dyspnea with tachypnea.
- Tachycardia.
- Anxiety and restlessness.
- Chest pain.
- Fever.
- Rales.
- Cough (sometimes with hemoptysis).
- Hemodynamic instability.

Diagnostic tests include:
- ABG analysis may show hypoxemia (Decreased PaO_2), hypocarbia (Decreased $PaCO_2$) and respiratory alkalosis (Increased pH).
- D-dimer (will show elevation with PE).
- ECG may show sinus tachycardia or other abnormalities.

- Echocardiogram can show emboli in the central arteries and can assess the hemodynamic status of the right side of the heart.
- Chest x-ray is of minimal value.
- Spiral CT may provide definitive diagnosis.
- V/Q scintigraphy can confirm diagnosis.
- Pulmonary angiograms also can confirm diagnosis.

Medical management of pulmonary embolism starts with preventive measures for those at risk, including leg exercises, elastic compression stockings, and anticoagulation therapy (Coumadin®). Most pulmonary emboli present as medical emergencies, so the immediate task is to stabilize the patient. Medical management may include:
- Oxygen to relieve hypoxemia.
- Intravenous infusions: Dobutamine (Dobutrex®) or dopamine (Intropin®) to relieve hypotension.
- Cardiac monitoring for dysrhythmias and issues due to right sided heart failure.
- Medications as indicated: digitalis glycosides, diuretic, and antiarrhythmics.
- Intubation and mechanical ventilation may be required.
- Analgesia (such as morphine sulfate) or sedation to relieve anxiety.
- Anticoagulants to prevent recurrence (although it will not dissolve clots already present), including heparin and warfarin (Coumadin®).
- Placement of percutaneous venous filter (Greenfield) in the inferior vena cava to prevent further emboli from entering the lungs may be done if anticoagulation therapy is contraindicated.
- Thrombolytic therapy, recombinant tissue-type plasminogen activator (rt-PA) or streptokinase, for those severely compromised, but these treatments have limited success and pose the danger of bleeding.

ARDS

Patients presenting with acute respiratory distress syndrome (ARDS) may initially present with only mild tachypnea, but more serious symptoms develop as respiratory function becomes more compromised:
- Crackling rales or wheezing may be heard throughout lungs.
- Decrease in pulmonary compliance (lung volume), referred to as "baby lung," results in increasing tachypnea with expiratory grunting.
- Cyanosis may develop with characteristic blue discoloration of lips and skin mottling.
- Hypotension and tachycardia may occur.
- Symptoms associated with volume overload are missing (third heart sound or jugular venous distention).
- Respiratory alkalosis is often an early sign but is replaced as the disease progresses with hypercarbia and respiratory acidosis.
- X-ray studies may be normal at first but then show diffuse infiltrates in both lungs, but the heart and vessels appear normal.

Acute lung injury (ALI) comprises a syndrome of respiratory distress culminating in acute respiratory distress syndrome (ARDS). ARDS is damage to the vascular endothelium and an increase in the permeability of the alveolar-capillary membrane when damage to the lung results in toxic substances (gastric fluids, bacteria, chemicals, or toxins emitted by neutrophils as part of the inflammatory-mediated response) reducing surfactant and causing pulmonary edema as the alveoli fill with blood and protein-rich fluid and collapse. Atelectasis with hyperinflation and areas of normal tissue occur as the lungs "stiffen." The fluid in the alveoli becomes a medium for infection. Inadequate ventilation and perfusion, leads to increasing hypoxemia and tachypnea as the body tries to compensate to maintain a normal $PaCO_2$. Symptoms are characterized by respiratory distress within 72 hours of surgery or a serious injury to a person with otherwise normal lungs and no cardiac disorder. Untreated, the condition results in respiratory failure, MODS, and a mortality rate of 5-30%.

The management of acute respiratory distress syndrome (ARDS) involves providing adequate gas exchange and preventing further damage to the lung from forced ventilation. Treatment includes:

- No drug has proved effective in the clinical management or prevention of ARDS. The following are therapies that are commonly used but per ARDS network there is insufficient evidence that they decrease mortality rates: corticosteroids (may increase mortality rates in some patient populations, though this is the most common given), nitrous oxide, inhaled surfactant, and anti-inflammatory medications.
- Treatment of the underlying condition is the only proven treatment, especially identifying and treating with appropriate antibiotics any infection, as sepsis is most common etiology for ARDS, but prophylactic antibiotics are not indicated.
- Conservative fluid management is indicated to reduce days on the ventilator, but does not reduce overall mortality.
- Pharmacologic preventive care: enoxaparin 40 mg subcutaneously QD, sucralfate 1 g NGT four times daily or omeprazole 40 mg IV QD, and enteral nutrition support within 24 hours of ICU admission or intubation.

ABGs

Arterial blood gases (ABGs) are monitored to assess effectiveness of oxygenation, ventilation, and acid-base status, and to determine oxygen flow rates. Partial pressure of a gas is that exerted by each gas in a mixture of gases, proportional to its concentration, based on total atmospheric pressure of 760 mm Hg at sea level. Normal values include:

- Acidity/alkalinity (pH): 7.35-7.45.
- Partial pressure of carbon dioxide ($PaCO_2$): 35-45 mm Hg.
- Partial pressure of oxygen (PaO_2): $\geq$80 mg Hg.
- Bicarbonate concentration (HCO_3-): 22-26 mEq/L.
- Oxygen saturation (SaO_2): $\geq$95%.

The relationship between these elements, particularly the $PaCO_2$ and the PaO_2 indicates respiratory status. For example, $PaCO_2$ >55 and the PaO_2 <60 in a patient previously in good health indicates respiratory failure. There are many issues to consider. Ventilator management may require a higher $PaCO_2$ to prevent barotrauma and a lower PaO_2 to reduce oxygen toxicity.

Respiratory acidosis

Respiratory acidosis is precipitated by inadequate ventilation of alveoli, interfering with gaseous exchange so that carbon dioxide increases and oxygen decreases, causing excess carbonic acid (H_2CO_3) levels. The body maintains a normal pH by balancing bicarbonate (renal) with $PaCO_2$ (pulmonary) in a 20:1 ratio. If the pH alters, the system (renal or pulmonary) that is not causing the problem compensates. Respiratory acidosis is most common in acute respiratory disorders, such as pulmonary edema, pneumothorax, sleep apnea syndrome, atelectasis, aspiration of foreign objects,

- 43 -

severe pneumonia, ARDS, administration of oxygen to treat chronic hypercapnia, or mechanical ventilation. Diseases with respiratory muscle impairment may also cause respiratory acidosis, such as muscular dystrophy, severe Guillain-Barre, and myasthenia gravis. Respiratory acidosis may be acute or chronic:

- Acute: Increased $PaCO_2$ with decreased pH caused by sudden decrease in ventilation.
- Chronic: Increased $PaCO_2$ with normal pH and serum bicarbonate (HCO_3-) >30 mm Hg with renal compensation.

ABG values in respiratory acidosis:
- pH <7.35.
- $PaCO_2$ >42 mm Hg.
- Increased H_2CO_3.

Symptoms include:
- Acute respiratory acidosis:
    o Increased heart rate.
    o Tachypnea.
    o Hypertension.
    o Confusion and pressure in head related to cerebrovascular vasodilation, especially if $PaCO_2$ > 60 mm Hg.
    o Increased intracranial pressure with papilledema.
    o Ventricular fibrillation.
    o Hyperkalemia.
- Chronic respiratory acidosis:
    o Symptoms may be subtler with chronic respiratory acidosis because of the compensatory mechanisms. If the $PaCO_2$ remains >50 mm Hg for long periods, the respiratory center becomes increasingly insensitive to CO_2 as a respiratory stimulus, replaced by hypoxemia, so supplemental oxygen administration should be monitored carefully to ensure that respirations are not depressed.

Treatment includes:
- Improving ventilation.
- Mechanical ventilation may be used with care.
- Medications as indicated (depending on cause): bronchodilators, anticoagulation therapy, diuretics, and antibiotics.
- Pulmonary hygiene.

Respiratory alkalosis

Respiratory alkalosis results from hyperventilation, during which extra CO_2 is excreted, causing a decrease in carbonic acid (H_2CO_3) concentration in the plasma. Respiratory alkalosis may be acute or chronic. Acute respiratory alkalosis is precipitated by anxiety attacks, hypoxemia, salicylate intoxication, bacteremia (Gram-negative), and incorrect ventilator settings. Chronic respiratory alkalosis may result from chronic hepatic insufficiency, cerebral tumors, and chronic hypocapnia. Characteristics include:

- Decreased $PaCO_2$.
- Normal or decreased serum bicarbonate (HCO_3^-) as kidneys conserve hydrogen and excrete HCO_3^-.
- Increased pH.

Symptoms include:
- Vasoconstriction with decreased cerebral blood flow resulting in lightheadedness, alterations in mentation, and/or unconsciousness.
- Numbness and tingling.
- Tinnitus.
- Tachycardia and dysrhythmias.

Treatment includes:
- Identifying and treating underlying cause. If respiratory alkalosis is related to anxiety, breathing in a paper bag may increase CO_2 level.
- Some people may require sedation.
- ABG values in respiratory alkalosis:
  - pH >7.45.
  - $PaCO_2$ < 38 mm Hg.
  - Decreased H_2CO_3.

Management of thoracic trauma

Pulmonary contusion
Pulmonary contusion is the result of direct force to the lung, resulting in parenchymal injury and bleeding and edema that impact the capillary-alveoli juncture, resulting in intrapulmonary shunting as the alveoli and interstitium fill with fluid. Parenchymal injury reduces compliance and impairs ventilation. Diagnosis may be more difficult if other injuries, such as fractured ribs or pneumothorax are also present because they may all contribute to respiratory distress. CT scans provide the best diagnostic tool. Symptoms vary widely depending upon the degree of injury but may include:
- Mild dyspnea/
- Severe progressive dyspnea.
- Hemoptysis.
- Acute respiratory failure.

Treatment varies according to the injury but can include:
- Close monitoring of arterial blood gases and respiratory status.
- Supplemental oxygen.
- Intubation and mechanical ventilation with positive-end expiratory pressure (PEEP) for more severe respiratory distress.
- Fluid management and diuretics to control pulmonary edema.
- Respiratory physiotherapy to clear secretions.

Hemothorax
Hemothorax occurs with bleeding into the pleural space, usually from major vascular injury such as tears in intercostal vessels, lacerations of great vessels, or trauma to lung parenchyma. A small bleed may be self-limiting and seal, but a tear in a large vessel can result in massive bleeding, followed quickly by hypovolemic shock. The pressure from the blood may result in inability of the lung to ventilate and a mediastinal shift. Often a hemothorax occurs with a pneumothorax, especially in severe chest trauma. Further symptoms include severe respiratory distress, decreased breath sounds, and dullness on auscultation. Treatment includes placement of a chest tube to drain the hemothorax, but with large volumes, the pressure may be preventing exsanguination, which can

occur abruptly as the blood drains and pressure is reduced, so a large bore intravenous line should be in place and typed and cross-matched blood immediately available. Autotransfusion may be used, contraindicated if wound is older than three hours, possibility of bowel/stomach contamination, liver failure, and malignancy. Thoracotomy may be indicated after chest tube insertion if there is still hemodynamic instability, tension hemothorax, more than 1500 mL blood initially on insertion, or bleeding continues at a rate of >300 ml/hr.

Flail chest
Flail chest is a more common injury in adults and older teens than children. It occurs when at least 3 adjacent ribs are fractured, both anteriorly and posteriorly, so that they float free of the rib cage. There may be variations, such as the sternum floating with ribs fractured on both sides. Flail chest results in a failure of the chest wall to support changes in intrathoracic pressure so that there paradoxical respirations occur with the flail area contracting on inspiration and expanding on expiration. The lungs are not able to expand properly, decreasing ventilation, but the degree of respiratory distress may relate to injury to underlying structures more than the flail chest alone.

Treatment:
- Initial stabilization with tape, one side only, don't wrap chest.
- Analgesia for pain relief.
- Respiratory physiotherapy to prevent atelectasis.
- Mechanical ventilation is usually not indicated unless needed for underlying injuries.
- Surgical fixation is usually done only in those requiring thoracotomy for underlying injuries.

Fractured ribs
Fractured ribs are usually the result of severe trauma, such as blunt force from a motor vehicle accident or physical abuse. Underlying injuries should be expected according to the area of fractures:
- Upper 2 ribs: Injuries to trachea, bronchi, or great vessels.
- Right-sided $\geq$rib 8: Trauma to liver.
- Left-sided $\geq$ rib 8: Trauma to spleen.

Pain, often localized or experienced on respirations or compression of chest way may be the primary symptom of rib fractures, resulting in shallow breathing that can lead to atelectasis or pneumonia. Diagnostics: Chest x-ray or CT scan.

Treatment is primarily supportive as rib fractures usually heal in about 6 weeks: however, preventing pulmonary complications (pneumothorax, hemothorax) often necessitates adequate pain control. Underlying injuries are treated according to the type and degree of injury:
- Supplemental oxygen.
- Analgesia may include NSAIDs, intercostal nerve blocks, and narcotics.
- Pulmonary physiotherapy.
- Rib Belts
- Surgical fixation (ORIF) is usually done only in those requiring thoracotomy for underlying injuries.
- Splinting

Tracheal perforation/injury

Tracheal perforation/injury may result from external injury, such as from trauma from a vehicle accident or from an assault, such as a gunshot or knife wound or in some cases a laceration as a complication of percutaneous dilation tracheostomy (PDT) or other endotracheal tubes. In some cases, an inhaled foreign object may become lodged in the trachea and eventually erode the tissue. If the injury is severe, respiratory failure may cause death in a very short period of time, so rapid diagnosis and treatment is critical. Symptoms include:

- Severe respiratory distress.
- Hemoptysis.
- Strider with progressive dysphonia.
- Pneumothorax, pneumomediastinum.
- Subcutaneous emphysema from air leaking from the pleural space into the tissues of the chest wall, neck, face, and even into the upper extremities.

Treatment includes:

- Intubation and non-surgical healing for small lacerations.
- Surgical repair for larger wounds or severe respiratory distress.

Ruptured diaphragm

The diaphragm separates the chest from the abdominal cavity, and ruptured diaphragm is usually caused by blunt trauma, often associated with rib fractures and/or ruptured spleen. Injuries to the left diaphragm are more common because the liver provides some underlying protection on the right. Because of the extent of injuries and/or the use of mechanical ventilation, symptoms may be overlooked initially, so careful abdominal examination should be done every 30 minutes for 4 hours, hourly for 4 to 6 hours, and then every 2 to 4 hours for the first 24 hours after injury.

Symptoms include:

- Respiratory and circulatory impairment.
- Herniation of abdominal organs into the chest cavity often associated with nausea and vomiting and abdominal pain, sometimes radiating to the left shoulder from pressure on the phrenic nerve.

Diagnosis may be by radiograph after insertion of radiopaque NG tube, CT, MRI, and/or diagnostic peritoneal lavage. Treatment requires surgical consultation and immediate surgical repair, usually with laparotomy, as there are often other abdominal injuries. Delayed repair may require thoracotomy.

Pneumothorax

Pneumothorax is a complete or partial collapse of a lung that occurs as a result of a leak between the lung tissue and the chest wall so that extraneous air is in the pleural space. Types include:

- Spontaneous/Simple pneumothorax is a breach of the parietal or visceral pleura, such as when an air-filled bleb on the lung surface ruptures or with a bronchopleural fistula without connection to outside air, often related to smoking and COPD.
- Traumatic pneumothorax is a lacerating wound of the chest wall, such as a gunshot or knife wound. It can also result from invasive procedures, such as thoracentesis or lung biopsies or from barotrauma related to ventilation or chest surgery. Open pneumothorax occurs when air passes in and out, causing the lung to collapse, a sucking sound, and paradoxical movement of the chest wall with respirations.

- Tension pneumothorax is similar to traumatic open pneumothorax; however, the air can enter the pleural sac but cannot be expelled, causing a pronounced mediastinal shift to the unaffected side with severe compromise of cardiac and respiratory function.

Symptoms vary widely depending on the cause and degree of the pneumothorax and whether or not there is underlying disease:
- Acute pleuritic pain (95%), usually on the affected side.
- Decreased breath sounds.
- Tension pneumothorax: tracheal deviation and hemodynamic compromise.

Diagnosis:
- Clinical findings.
- Radiograph: 6-foot upright posterior-anterior.
- Ultrasound may detect traumatic pneumothorax.

Treatment includes:
- Chest-tube thoracostomy with underwater seal drainage is the most common treatment for all types of pneumothorax.
- Tension pneumothorax: Immediate needle decompression and chest tube thoracostomy.
- Small pneumothorax, patient stable: Oxygen administration and observation for 3-6 hours. If no increase shown on repeat x-ray, patient may be discharged with another x-ray in 24 hours.
- Primary spontaneous pneumothorax: catheter aspiration or chest tube thoracostomy.

ETC

The esophageal tracheal Combitube® (ETC) is an intermediate airway that contains two lumens and can be inserted into either the trachea or the esophagus (≤91%). The twin-lumen tube has a proximal cuff providing a seal of the oropharynx and a distal cuff providing a seal about the distal tube. Prior to insertion, the Combitube® cuffs should be checked for leaks (15 ml of air into distal and 85 ml of air into proximal). The patient should be non-responsive and with absent gag reflex with head in neutral position. The tube is passed along the tongue and into the pharynx, utilizing markings on the tube (black guidelines) to determine depth by aligning the ETC with the upper incisors or alveolar ridge. Once in place the distal cuff is inflated (10-15 ml) and then placement in the trachea or esophagus should be determined, so the proper lumen for ventilation can be used. The proximal cuff is inflated (usually to 50-75 ml) and ventilation begun. Capnogram should be used to confirm ventilation.

LMA

The laryngeal-mask airway (LMA) is an intermediate airway allowing ventilation but not complete respiratory control. The LMA consists of an inflatable cuff (the mask) with a connecting tube. It may be used temporarily before tracheal intubation or when tracheal intubation can't be done. It can also be a conduit for later blind insertion of an endotracheal tube. The head and neck must be in neutral position for insertion of the LMA. If the patient has a gag reflex, conscious sedation or topical anesthesia (deep oropharyngeal) is required. The LMA is inserted by sliding along the hard palate, using the finger as a guide, into the pharynx, and the ring is inflated to create a seal about the opening to the larynx, allowing ventilation with mild positive-pressure. The ProSeal® LMA has a modified cuff that extends onto the back of the mask to improve seal. LMA is contraindicated in morbid obesity, obstructions or abnormalities of oropharynx, and non-fasting patients, as some aspiration is possible even with the cuff seal inflated.

RSI

RSI is the simultaneous giving of a sedative and a paralytic in order to facilitate emergency intubation, and is considered to be the standard of care for emergency airway management (except in patients with anticipated difficult intubation or in those with contraindications to sedatives/paralytics). Initial preparation includes inserting 2 IV lines, and establishing cardiac monitoring, oximetry, and capnography. The patient should be preoxygenated (100%) for at least 3 minutes, but without pressure ventilation that may cause aspiration of stomach contents. Procedure includes:

- Induction agent: thiopental, ketamine, etomide, propofol.
- Paralysis: succinylocholine, rocuronium, other NMBAs.
- Sellick's maneuver (pressure applied externally with thumb and index finger to cricoid) to close off the esophagus and prevent aspiration.
- Suction to clear mouth if necessary.
- Laryngoscopy to visual vocal cords.
- EET inserted, cuff inflated, and ETT secured.

Proper placement verified by capnometer or capnograph. Breath sounds should be auscultated. Post intubation chest x-ray to assess depth of tube and check for any trauma or issue. Induction agents and use of additional sedation may vary from one institution to another, but the primary goal is to safely anesthetize and intubate while preventing regurgitation of stomach contents.

Tracheal intubation

Tracheal intubation is often necessary with respiratory failure for control of hypoxemia, hypercapnia, hypoventilation, and/or obstructed airway. Equipment should be assembled and tubes and connections checked for air leaks with a 10 ml syringe. The mouth and/or nose should be cleaned of secretions and suctioned if necessary. The patient should be supine with the patient's head level with the lower sternum of the clinician. With orotracheal/endotracheal intubation, the clinician holds the laryngoscope (in left hand) and inserts it into right corner of mouth, the epiglottis is lifted and the larynx exposed. A thin flexible intubation stylet may be used and the endotracheal tube (ETT) (in right hand) is inserted through the vocal cords and into the trachea, cuff inflated to minimal air leak (10 ml initially until patient stabilizes), and placement confirmed through capnometry or esophageal detection devices. The correct depth of insertion is verified: 21 cm (female), 23 cm (male). After insertion, the tube is secured.

There are a number of methods to confirm correct placement of endotracheal tubes. Clinical assessment alone is not adequate.

- Capnometry utilizes an end-tidal CO_2 (ETCO$_2$) detector that measures the concentration of CO_2 in expired air, usually through pH sensitive paper that changes color (commonly purple to yellow). The capnometer is attached to the ETT and a bag-valve-mask (BVM) ventilator attached. The patient is provided 6 ventilations and the CO_2 concentration checked.
- Capnography is attached to the ETT and provides a waveform graph, showing the varying concentrations of CO_2 in real time throughout each ventilation (with increased CO_2 on expiration) and can indicate changes in respiratory status.

- Esophageal detection devices fit over the end of the ETT so that a large syringe can be used to attempt to aspirate. If the ETT is in the esophagus, the walls collapse on aspiration and resistance occurs whereas the syringe fills with air if the ETT is in the trachea. A self-inflating bulb (Ellick® device) may also be used.

Ventilators

Non-invasive positive pressure ventilators provide air through a tight-fitting nasal or facemask, usually pressure cycled, avoiding the need for intubation and reducing the danger of hospital-acquired infection and mortality rates. It can be used for acute respiratory failure and pulmonary edema. There are 2 types of non-invasive positive pressure ventilators:
- CPAP (Continuous positive airway pressure) provides a steady stream of pressurized air throughout both inspiration and expiration. CPAP improves breathing by decreasing preload for patients with congestive heart failure. It reduces the effort required for breathing by increasing residual volume and improving gas exchange.
- Bi-PAP (Bi-level positive airway pressure) provides a steady stream of pressurized air as CPAP but it senses inspiratory effort and increases pressure during inspiration. Bi-PAP pressures for inspiration and expiration can be set independently. Machines can be programmed with a backup rate to ensure a set number of respirations per minute.

A mask size guide should be used to ensure proper fit. The patient should breathe with mouth closed with nasal mask.

> **Review Video:** Ventilators: Best and Worst Times to Use Them
> *Visit **mometrix.com/academy** and enter **Code: 679637***

Tracheostomy

Tracheostomy, surgical tracheal opening, may be utilized for mechanical ventilation. Tracheostomy tubes are inserted into the opening to provide a conduit and maintain the opening. Tracheostomy tubes are usually silastic or plastic, most lacking an inner cannula because they are non-adherent. The tube is secured with ties around the neck. Because the air entering the lungs through the tracheostomy bypasses the warming and moistening effects of the upper airway, air is humidified through a room humidifier or through delivery of humidified air through a special mask or mechanical ventilation. The patient with a tracheostomy must have continuous monitoring of vital signs and respiratory status to ensure patency of tracheostomy. Regular suctioning is needed, especially initially, to remove secretions:
- Suction catheter should be 50% the size of the tracheostomy tube to allow ventilation during suctioning.
- Vacuum pressure: 80-100 mm Hg.
- Catheter should only be inserted ≤ 0.5 cm beyond tube to avoid damage to tissues or perforation.
- Catheter should be inserted without suction and intermittent suction on withdrawal.

Neurological Emergencies

Dementia/Alzheimer disease

Dementia may be related to medications, drug abuse, metabolic disorders, depression, or Alzheimer disease, and differentiating requires a careful history and examination. Cognitive impairment related to sudden onset with changes typical of depression (loss of appetite, sleep disturbances, suicidal thoughts) may be dementia of depression. Patients with Alzheimer disease may have a slower progression of symptoms and exhibit mild to pronounced cognitive impairment. They may be brought to the ED when they are found confused and wandering. History from family or caregiver may be helpful in determining the cause of dementia and recent changes. Patients should be kept in an environment with limited distractions. Questions and explanations should be simple and direct, tone of questioner's voice low and pleasant, and the patient should not be left alone. Nonverbal cues, such as facial expression and body language, may help to determine if the patient has pain or injury. The patient should be oriented frequently as to place and purpose and reassured.

Multiple sclerosis

Multiple sclerosis is an autoimmune disorder of the CNS in which the myelin sheath around the nerves is damaged and replaced by scar tissue that prevents conduction of nerve impulses. Symptoms vary widely and can include problems with balance and coordination, tremors, slurring of speech, cognitive impairment, vision impairment and nystagmus, pain, and bladder and bowel dysfunction. Symptoms may be relapsing-remitting or progressive or a combination. Onset is usually at 20 to 30 years of age, with incidence higher in females. Patient may initially present with problems walking or falling or optic neuritis (30%) causing loss of central vision. Males may complain of sexual dysfunction as an early symptom. Others have dysuria with urinary retention. Diagnosis is based on clinical and neurological examination and MRI. Treatment is symptomatic and includes treatment to shorten duration of episodes and slow progress.
- Glucocorticoids: methylprednisolone.
- Immunomodulator: interferon beta, glatiramer acetate, natalizumab.
- Immunosuppressant: mitoxantrone.
- Hormone: estriol (for females).

ALS

ALS is a progressive degenerative disease of the upper and lower motor neurons, resulting in progressively severe symptoms, such as spasticity; hyperreflexia, muscle weakness, and paralysis that can cause dysphagia; cramping; muscular atrophy; and respiratory dysfunction. ALS may be sporadic or familial (rare). Speech may become monotone; however, cognitive functioning usually remains intact. Eventually, patients become immobile and cannot breathe independently. Diagnosis is based on history, electromyography, nerve conduction studies, and MRI. Treatment includes riluzole to delay progression of the disease. Patients in the ED usually have been diagnosed and have developed an acute complication, such as acute respiratory failure, aspiration pneumonia, or other trauma. Treatment includes:
- Nebulizer treatments with bronchodilators and steroids.
- Antibiotics for infection.
- Mechanical ventilation.

If ventilatory assistance is needed, it is important to determine if the patient has a living will expressing the wish to be ventilated or not or has assigned power of attorney for health matters to someone to make this decision.

Parkinson's disease

Parkinson's disease (PD) is an extrapyramidal movement motor system disorder caused by loss of brain cells that produce dopamine. Typical symptoms include tremor of face and extremities, rigidity, bradykinesia, akinesia, poor posture, and lack of balance and coordination, causing increasing problems with mobility, talking, and swallowing. Some may suffer depression and mood changes. Tremors usually present unilaterally in an upper extremity. Diagnosis includes:
- Cogwheel rigidity test: extremity put through passive range of motion, which causes increased muscle tone and ratchet-like movements.
- Physical and neurological exam.
- Complete history to rule out drug-induced Parkinson akinesia.

Treatment includes:
- Symptomatic support.
- Dopaminergic therapy: levodopa, amantadine, and carbidopa.
- Anticholinergics: trihexyphenidyl, benztropine.
- Drug-induced Parkinson disease: terminate drugs.

Drug therapy tends to decrease in efficiency over time, and patients may present with marked increase in symptoms. Discontinuing the drugs for 1 week may exacerbate symptoms initially, but functioning may improve when drugs are reintroduced.

> ➤ **Review Video:** Parkinson's Disease
> *Visit **mometrix.com/academy** and enter **Code:** 110876*

Myasthenia gravis

Myasthenia gravis is an autoimmune disorder of the neuromuscular system in which acetylcholine receptors are damaged at neural synapses, preventing transmission of impulses to contract muscles. The thymus gland develops abnormalities and sometimes thymoma. Symptoms of myasthenia gravis are muscle weakness, which decreases with rest. Eye muscles are often affected first, resulting in ptosis and visual disturbances such as diplopia. General weakness in extremities, neck, and face, as well as dysphagia and slurred speech occur. Acute respiratory failure can occur as part of myasthenic crisis before diagnosis or related to fever, infection, or drug therapy. Diagnosis of myasthenia gravis is from history, neurological exam, antibody testing, edrophonium chloride testing to differentiate exacerbation of disease from cholinergic crisis, electromyogram, and pulmonary function tests. Treatments include:
- Crisis: mechanical ventilation and treatment of underlying cause.
- Thymectomy: relieves symptoms in 70%.
- Immunosuppressants: azathioprine, cyclosporine, and prednisone.
- Acetylcholinesterase inhibitors: pyridostigmine.

Many drugs can trigger respiratory failure, so drug lists should be checked and ventilatory equipment available when treating MG patients.

> ➤ **Review Video:** Myasthenia Gravis
> *Visit **mometrix.com/academy** and enter Code:* **162510**

Guillain-Barré syndrome

Guillain-Barré syndrome (GBS) is an autoimmune disorder of the myelinated motor peripheral nervous system, often triggered by a viral gastroenteritis or *Campylobacter jejuni* infection. Symptoms include numbness and tingling with increasing weakness of lower extremities that may become generalized, sometimes resulting in complete paralysis and inability to breathe without ventilatory support. Deep tendon reflexes are typically absent and some people experience facial weakness and ophthalmoplegia (paralysis of muscles controlling movement of eyes). Diagnosis is by history, clinical symptoms, and lumbar puncture, which often shows increased protein with normal glucose and cell count, although protein may not increase for a week or more. Treatment is supportive. Patients should be hospitalized for observation and placed on ventilator support if forced vital capacity is less than 2 L. In patients with GBS, avoid succinylcholine during anesthesia and intubation. While there is no definitive treatment, plasma exchange or IV immunoglobulin shorten the duration of symptoms and decrease mechanical ventilator need.

Headaches

Headaches may be primary or secondary. Primary headaches include migraines, and cluster and tension headaches, usually with low rates of morbidity; however, secondary headaches, such as those caused by brain tumors, meningitis, sinusitis, severe hypertension, dental abscesses, and other disorders, may result in severe morbidity and death. Symptoms of secondary headache include sudden onset and severe pain, and may be associated with fever, nausea and vomiting, and altered mental status. It may occur after head trauma. Diagnosis includes complete history and physical, including neurological examination. A complete description of the headache should be included: location, quality, frequency, precipitating factors, aggravating factors, time of day, and associated symptoms. Allergy and family history may provide clues to the cause as well. If there are abnormalities on the neurological exam or severe onset of symptoms, CT, angiography, or MRI may be indicated as well as CBC, ESR, and chemical panels. Treatments:
- NSAIDs.
- Triptans and ergotamines for migraines).
- Corticosteroids (cerebral arteritis).
- Neurological consult as needed.

Head trauma

A variety of different injuries can occur as a result of head trauma:
- Concussions are the most common injury and are usually relatively transient, causing no permanent neurological damage. They may result in confusion, disorientation, and mild amnesia, but last only minutes or hours.
- Contusions/Lacerations are bruising and tears of cerebral tissue. There may be petechial areas at the impact site (coup) or larger bruising. Contrecoup injuries are less common in children than in adults. Areas most impacted by contusions and lacerations are the occipital, frontal, and temporal lobes. The degree of injury relates to the amount of vascular damage, but initial symptoms are similar to concussion; however, symptoms may persist and progress, depending upon the degree of injury. Lacerations are often caused by fractures.

Complications
Head injuries that occur at the time of trauma include fractures, contusions, hematomas, and diffuse cerebral and vascular injury. These injuries may result in hypoxia, increased intracranial pressure, and cerebral edema. Open injuries may result in infection. Patients often suffer initial hypertension, which increases intracranial pressure, decreasing perfusion. Often the primary problem with head trauma is a significant increase in swelling, which also interferes with perfusion, causing hypoxia and hypercapnia, which trigger increased blood flow. This increased volume at a time when injury impairs autoregulation increases cerebral edema, which, in turn, increases intracranial pressure and results in a further decrease in perfusion with resultant ischemia. If pressure continues to rise, the brain may herniate. Concomitant hypotension may result in hypoventilation, further complicating treatment. Diffuse axonal injuries involve widespread brain damage, caused by traumatic shearing of neural axons. CT may be normal, but patient may be unconscious. Diffuse axonal injuries can result in chronic vegetative states.

Fractures are a common cause of penetrating wounds causing cerebral lacerations. Open fractures are those in which the dura is torn, and closed is when the dura remain intact. While fractures by themselves do not cause neurological damage, force is needed to fracture the skull, often causing damage to underlying structures. Meningeal arteries lie in groves on the underside of the skull, and a fracture can cause an arterial tear and hemorrhage. Skull fractures include:
- Basilar: Occurs in bones at the base of the brain and can cause severe brainstem damage.
- Comminuted: Skull fractures into small pieces.
- Compound: Surface laceration extends to a skull fracture.
- Depressed: Pieces of the skull are depressed inward on the brain tissue, often producing dural tears.
- Linear/Hairline: Skull fracture forms a thin line without any splintering.

> **Review Video:** Behaviors Associated with Brain Damage
> *Visit **mometrix.com/academy** and enter **Code: 891782***

GCS

The Glasgow coma scale (GCS) measures the depth and duration of coma or impaired level of consciousness and is used for post-operative assessment. The GCS measures three parameters: Best eye response, best verbal response, and best motor response, with a total possible score that ranges from 3 to 15:

Eye opening	4: Spontaneous. 3: To verbal stimuli. 2: To pain (not of face). 1: No response.
Verbal	5: Oriented. 4: Conversation confused, but can answer questions. 3: Uses inappropriate words. 2: Speech incomprehensible. 1: No response.
Motor	6: Moves on command. 5: Moves purposefully respond pain. 4: Withdraws in response to pain. 3: Decorticate posturing (flexion) in response to pain. 2: Decerebrate posturing (extension) in response to pain. 1: No response.

Injuries/conditions are classified according to the total score: 3-8 Coma; ≤ 8 Severe head injury; 9-12 Moderate head injury; 13-15 Mild head injury.

Neurological motor testing and testing for nuchal rigidity

Neurological motor testing requires careful observation for involuntary or spastic movements and examination of muscles for lack of symmetry or atrophy with observation of gait. Muscle tone is examined by flexing and extending the upper and lower extremities, observing for flaccid or spastic changes. Muscle strength is examined by having the patient press fingers, wrists, elbows, hips, knees, ankles, and plantar area against resistance, graded 0 (no movement) to 5 (normal). Pronator drift is an indication of disease of the upper motor neurons. The patient stands with eyes closed and both arms extended horizontally in front with the palms facing upwards (supination). The patient should be told to hold the arms still and not move them while the examiner taps downward on the arm. If motor neuron disease is present, the patient's arms will drift downward and hands will drift toward pronation. Nuchal rigidity is tested by placing the hands behind the patient's head and flexing the neck gently to determine if there is increased resistance.

ICP monitoring

Increasing intracranial pressure (ICP) is a frequent complication of brain injuries, tumors, or other disorders affecting the brain, so monitoring the ICP is very important. Increased ICP can indicate cerebral edema, hemorrhage, and/or obstruction of cerebrospinal fluid. The Monroe-Kellie hypothesis states that in order to maintain a normal ICP, a change in volume in one compartment must be compensated by a reciprocal change in volume in another compartment. There are 3 compartments in the brain: the brain tissue, cerebrospinal fluid (CSF), and blood.The CSF and blood can change more easily to accommodate changes in pressure than tissue, so medical intervention focuses on cerebral blood flow and drainage. Normal ICP is 0-15 mm Hg on transducer or 80-180 mm H_2O on manometer. As intracranial pressure increases, symptoms include:

- Headache.
- Alterations in level of consciousness.
- Restlessness.
- Slowly reacting or nonreacting dilated or pinpoint pupils.
- Seizures.
- Motor weakness.
- Cushing's triad (late sign):
  o Increased systolic pressure with widened pulse pressure.
  o Bradycardia in response to increased pressure.
  o Decreased respirations.

Increased intracranial pressure must be treated quickly to prevent irreversible brain damage and death. Identifying and treating the cause, such as repair of a ruptured aneurysm or removal of a tumor is of primary importance. Measures to decrease intracranial pressure include:

- Elevating the head of the bed 30 degrees to promote drainage, keeping head midline.
- Oral intubation instead of nasotracheal if ventilation required.
- Analgesia to control pain and reduce agitation.
- Sedation: propofol (adults only), benzodiazepines.
- Respiratory support, including ventilation with oxygen administration to increase perfusion. Hyperventilation is used only if herniation of the brain is imminent.
- Drainage of cerebrospinal fluid as indicated.
- Diuretics, such as mannitol or furosemide.
- Induction of coma with pentobarbital (10 mg/kg in 30 minutes and then 5 mg/kg over 60 minutes x 3 doses, then a maintenance dose of 1 to 3 mg/kg every hour).
- Volume replacement.
- Careful monitoring and replacement of electrolytes.

Epidural hematoma

Epidural hematoma occurs with bleeding between the skull and the dura mater. Epidural hematomas usually result from blunt trauma and usually are associated with skull fractures. Symptoms can include loss of consciousness after trauma with a lucent period and then a relapse into unconsciousness, although some never lose consciousness and others never regain consciousness. Diagnosis is by CT scan. Epidural hematomas are usually arterial but may be venous (20%) and are always medical emergencies and require craniotomy with evacuation before compression damage to the brain occurs. Prognosis is good if corrected early because underlying brain damage is rarely severe. Treatment: Evacuation of hematomas can be done in a number of different ways, including burr holes, needle aspiration, direct surgical craniotomy, or endoscope. If

- 56 -

no neurosurgical care is available, bilateral burr holes may need to be done in the ED to prevent herniation from arterial bleeding.

Ventricular-peritoneal shunt dysfunction

Ventricular-peritoneal shunt is commonly used to treat hydrocephalus. This procedure consists of placement of a ventricular catheter directly into the ventricles (usually lateral) at one end, with the other end in the peritoneal area to drain away excess CSF. There is a one-way valve near the proximal end that prevents backflow but opens when pressure rises to drain fluid. In some cases, the distal end drains into the right atrium. An implantable flush pump may be in place. Ventricular-peritoneal shunts may become occluded or disconnected, the catheter may be positioned incorrectly, and the valve pressure may not be adequate. If the shunt does not function properly, signs of hydrocephalus and increased intracranial pressure can occur. If there is a flush valve, this may relieve the obstruction, but obstruction may be difficult to assess with radiography, so a neurosurgical consult may be indicated for revision of the shunt.

Spinal cord injuries

Spinal cord injuries may result from blunt trauma (such as automobile accidents), falls from a height, sports injuries, and penetrating trauma (such as gunshot or knife wounds). Damage results from mechanical injury and secondary responses resulting from hemorrhage, edema, and ischemia. The type of symptoms relate to the area and degree of injury:
- Anterior cord: The posterior column functions remains so there is sensation of touch, vibration, and position remaining below injury but with complete paralysis and loss of sensations of pain and temperature. Prognosis is poor.
- Brown-Séguard: The cord is hemisected, resulting in spastic paresis, loss of sense of position and vibration on the injured side, and loss of pain and temperature on the other side. Prognosis is good.
- Cauda equina: Damage is below L1 with variable loss of motor ability and sensation, and bowel and bladder dysfunction. Injury is to peripheral nerves that can regenerate, so prognosis is better than for other lesions of the spinal cord.
- Central cord: Results from hyperextension and ischemia or stenosis of cervical spine, causing quadriparesis (more severe in upper extremities) with some loss of sensations of pain and temperature). Prognosis is good but fine motor skills are often impaired in upper extremities.
- Conus medullaris: Injury to lower spine (lower lumbar and sacral nerves).
- Posterior cord: Motor function is preserved but without sensation.
- Spinal shock: Injury at T6 or above results in flaccid paralysis below lesion with loss of sensations and rectal tone, bradycardia, and hypotension.

Patients with spinal cord injuries should immediately be evaluated for airway control, and the spine kept immobilized. Treatment includes:
- Intubation and ventilation (usually with sedation) to prevent respiratory failure for injuries at C5 or above.
- IV fluids to prevent and treat hypotension.
- Examination, blood cell count, chest x-ray and abdominal ultrasound and/or lavage to evaluate blood loss.
- Complete neurological exam after patient is stabilized.
- X-ray or CT scans.

- MRI to examine nerve or ligamentous injury.
- Corticosteroids for neurological deficits from blunt trauma:
- Begin within 8 hours of injury.
- Methylprednisolone 30 mg/kg bolus IV over 15 minutes.
- 45-minute break.
- Methylprednisolone 5.4 mg/kg per hour for 23 hours.
- Surgical decompression as needed for penetrating wounds.
- Antibiotics as indicated for penetrating stab wounds.
- Nonoperative spinal stabilization as indicated.

Spinal stabilization/immobilization

Spinal stabilization/immobilization is frequently done in some form by first responders but devices may need to be applied or modified in the emergency department:
- Cervical spine: The head should be immobilized midline, secured with a cervical extrication collar and supporting backboard, with rolls, tape, or bolsters to prevent lateral movement for injuries to head and neck. Cervical collars include hard collar, Philadelphia collar, and Miami J collar. Subluxations are reduced with Gardner-Wells tongs and weights. Cervicothoracic braces or the halo cervical immobilizer may be necessary for unstable fractures.
- Upper thoracic spine: Thoracic corsets may be used for minor disorders, Jewett and Taylor braces for more moderate injuries, and Risser jacket and body cast for severe injuries requiring more immobilization.
- Thoracolumbar, sacral spine: Initially the patient is secured to a full-length backboard, and a thoracolumbosacral orthosis may be applied, primarily to provide support and restrict movement, when external immobilization is difficult.

Autonomic dysreflexia

Autonomic dysreflexia is a complication of central cord lesions at or above T6. This may be precipitated by urinary infection, bladder distention, or kidney stones or fecal impaction, but numerous other stresses, such as ingrown toenail, pressure ulcers, sunburns, sexual intercourse, or tight clothing, can cause the disorder. Symptoms include hypertension with increase of 20 to 40 mm Hg systolic BP, vasoconstriction, pallor, piloerection below lesion, severe pounding headache, nasal congestion, restlessness, and apprehension. Diagnosis is based on clinical findings and hypertension. Treatment:
- Antihypertensives: nitroprusside, nitrates.
- Placement of urinary catheter if necessary (using lidocaine jelly to decrease stimulation) or checking catheter for obstruction.
- Check for fecal impaction after BP is stabilized, placing lidocaine jelly into the rectum 5 minutes before disimpaction.
- If there are no bladder or bowel problems, a complete examination needs to be done to identify other causes.
- Patient should be monitored for 2 hours after hypertension and symptoms subside.

Strokes

Strokes (brain attacks, cerebrovascular accidents) result when there is interruption of the blood flow to an area of the brain. The two basic types are ischemic and hemorrhagic.

Ischemic
About 80% are ischemic, resulting from blockage of an artery supplying the brain:
- Thrombosis in large artery, usually resulting from atherosclerosis, may block circulation to a large area of the brain. It is most common in the elderly and may occur suddenly or after episodes of transient ischemic attacks.
- Lacunar infarct (penetrating thrombosis in small artery) is most common in those with diabetes mellitus and/or hypertension.
- Embolism travels through the arterial system and lodges in the brain, most commonly in the left middle cerebral artery. An embolism may be cardiogenic, resulting from cardiac arrhythmia or surgery. An embolism usually occurs rapidly with no warning signs.
- Cryptogenic has no identifiable cause.

Hemorrhagic
Hemorrhagic strokes account for about 20% and result from a ruptured cerebral artery, causing not only lack of oxygen and nutrients but also edema that causes widespread pressure and damage:
- Intracerebral is bleeding into the substance of the brain from an artery in the central lobes, basal ganglia, pons, or cerebellum. Intracerebral hemorrhage usually results from atherosclerotic degenerative changes, hypertension, brain tumors, anticoagulation therapy, or some illicit drugs, such as crack and cocaine. Onset is often sudden and may cause death.
- Intracranial aneurysm occurs with ballooning cerebral artery ruptures, most commonly at the Circle of Willis.
- Arteriovenous malformation (AVM) is a tangle of dilated arteries and veins without a capillary bed. This is a congenital abnormality. Rupture of AVMs is a cause of brain attack in young adults.
- Subarachnoid hemorrhage is bleeding in the space between the meninges and brain, resulting from aneurysm, AVM, or trauma. This type of hemorrhage compresses brain tissue.

Symptoms
Brain attacks most commonly occur in the right or left hemisphere, but the exact location and the extent of brain damage affects the type of presenting symptoms. If the frontal area of either side is involved, there tends to be memory and learning deficits. Some symptoms are common to specific areas and help to identify the area involved:
- Right hemisphere: This results in left paralysis or paresis and a left visual field deficit that may cause spatial and perceptual disturbances, so people may have difficulty judging distance. Fine motor skills may be impacted, resulting in trouble dressing or handling tools. People may become impulsive and exhibit poor judgment, often denying impairment. Left-sided neglect (lack of perception of things on the left side) may occur. Depression is common as well as short-term memory loss and difficulty following directions. Language skills usually remain intact.
- Left hemisphere: Results in right paralysis or paresis and a right visual field defect. Depression is common and people often exhibit slow, cautious behavior, requiring repeated instruction and reinforcement for simple tasks. Short-term memory loss and difficulty learning new material or understanding generalizations is common. Difficulty with

- 59 -

mathematics, reading, writing, and reasoning may occur. Aphasia (expressive, receptive, or global) is common.

- Brain stem: Because the brain stem controls respiration and cardiac function, a brain attack frequently causes death, but those who survive may have a number of problems, including respiratory and cardiac abnormalities. Strokes may involve motor or sensory impairment or both.
- Cerebellum: This area controls balance and coordination. Brain attacks in the cerebellum are rare but may result in ataxia, nausea and vomiting, and headaches and dizziness or vertigo.

Classification system for extent of stroke injury
The American Stroke Association developed a brain attack outcome classification system to standardize descriptions of stroke injuries:

- Number of impaired domains (motor, sensory, vision, language, cognition, and affect): Level 0: none; Level 1: one impaired; Level 2: two impaired; Level 3: greater than 2 impaired;
- Degree of impairment: A (minimal); B (moderate), 1 or more domains involved; or C (severe), 1 or more domains involved.

Assessment of function determines the ability to live independently:

Level III requires much assistance and Levels IV and V cannot live independently.

I. Independent in basic activities of daily living (BADL), such as bathing, eating, toileting, and walking; and instrumental activities of daily living (IADL), such as telephoning, shopping, maintaining a household, socializing, and using transportation.
II. Independent in BADL but partially dependent in IADL.
III. Partially dependent in BADL (less than 3 areas) and IADL
IV. Partially dependent in BADL (3 or more areas).
V. Completely dependent in BADL (5 or more areas) and IADL.

Medical management
Medical management of ischemic brain attacks with tissue plasminogen activator (tPA) (alteplase), the primary treatment, should be initiated within 3 hours:

- Thrombolytic medication (tPA) is produced by recombinant DNA and is used to dissolve fibrin clots. It is given IV (0.9 mg/kg up to 90 mg) with 10% injected as an initial bolus and the rest over the next hour. Antihypertensives if MAP greater than 130 mm HG or systolic BP greater than 220. Cooling to reduce hyperthermia.
- Osmotic diuretics (mannitol), hypertonic saline, loop diuretics (furosemide), and/or corticosteroids (dexamethasone) to decrease cerebral edema and intracranial pressure.
- Aspirin/Anticoagulation may be used with embolism.
- Stool softeners to prevent constipation.
- Monitor and treat hyperglycemia.

Contraindications to thrombolytic therapy include:
- Evidence of cerebral or subarachnoid hemorrhage or other internal bleeding. Recent stroke, head trauma, or surgery.
- History of intracranial hemorrhage. Uncontrolled hypertension.
- Seizures. Intracranial AVM, neoplasm, or aneurysm.
- Current anticoagulation therapy.
- Low platelet count (less than 100,000 mm³).

NIHSS

The National Institutes of Health Stroke Scale (NIHSS) is administered with careful attention to directions. The examiner should record the answers and avoid coaching or repeating requests, although demonstration may be used with aphasic patients. The scale comprises 11 sections, with scores for each section ranging from 0 (normal) to 2 to 4:
- Level of consciousness: response to noxious stimulation (0 to 3), request for month and his/her age (0 to 2), request to open and close eyes, grip and release unaffected hand (0 to 2).
- Best gaze: Horizontal eye movement (0 to 2).
- Visual: Visual fields (0 to 3).
- Facial palsy: Symmetry when patient shows teeth, raises eyebrows, and closes eyes (0 to 3).
- Motor, arm: Drift while arm extended with palms down (0 to 4).
- Motor, leg: Leg drift at 30 degrees while patient supine (0 to 4).
- Limb ataxia: Finger-nose and heel-shin (0 to 2).
- Sensory: Grimace or withdrawal from pinprick (0 to 2).
- Best language: Describes action of pictures (0 to 3).
- Dysarthria: Reads or describes words on list (0 to 2).
- Distinction and inattention: Visual spatial neglect (0 to 2).

AVM

Arteriovenous malformation (AVM) is a congenital abnormality within the brain consisting of a tangle of dilated arteries and veins without a capillary bed. AVMs can occur anywhere in the brain and may cause no significant problems. Usually the AVM is "fed" by one or more cerebral arteries, which enlarge over time, shunting more blood through the AVM. The veins also enlarge in response to increased arterial blood flow because of the lack of a capillary bridge between the two. Because vein walls are thinner and lack the muscle layer of an artery, the veins tend to rupture as the AVM becomes larger, causing a subarachnoid hemorrhage. Chronic ischemia that may be related to the AVM can result in cerebral atrophy. Sometimes small leaks, usually accompanied by headache and nausea and vomiting, may occur before rupture. AVMs may cause a wide range of neurological symptoms, including changes in mentation, dizziness, sensory abnormalities, confusion, and, increasing ICP, and dementia.

Treatment includes:
- Supportive management of symptoms.
- Surgical repair or focused irradiation (definitive treatments).

Ruptured cerebral aneurysms

Cerebral aneurysms, weakening and dilation of a cerebral artery, are usually congenital (90%) while the remaining (10%) result from direct trauma or infection. Aneurysms usually range from 2-7 mm and occur in the Circle of Willis at the base of the brain. A rupturing aneurysm may decrease perfusion as well as increasing pressure on surrounding brain tissue. Cerebral aneurysm is classified as follows:

- Berry/saccular: The most common congenital type occurs at a bifurcation and grows from the base on a stem, usually at the Circle of Willis.
- Fusiform: Large and irregular (>2.5 cm) and rarely ruptures but causes increased intracranial pressure. Usually involves the internal carotid or vertebrobasilar artery.
- Mycotic: Rare type that occurs secondary to bacterial infection and aseptic emboli.
- Dissecting: Wall is torn apart and blood enters layers. This may occur during angiography or secondary to trauma or disease.
- Traumatic Charcot-Bouchard (pseudoaneurysm): small lesion resulting from chronic hypertension.

Bacterial meningitis

Bacterial meningitis may be caused by a wide range of pathogenic organisms, with the predominant agents varying with age:

- 1 month or younger: E.coli, group B streptococci, Listeria monocytogenes, and Neisseria meningitidis.
- 1 to 2 months: group B streptococci.
- Older than 2 months: Streptococcus pneumoniae, N. meningitidis.
- Unvaccinated (Hib vaccine) children are at risk for *Haemophilus influenzae*. These are most common in adults.

Bacterial infections usually arise from spread distant infections, although they can enter the CNS from surgical wounds, invasive devices, nasal colonization, or penetrating trauma. The infective process includes inflammation, exudates, white blood cell accumulation, and tissue damage with the brain showing evidence of hyperemia and edema. Purulent exudate covers the brain and invades and blocks the ventricles, obstructing CSF and leading to increased intracranial pressure. Since antibodies specific to bacteria do not cross the blood/brain barrier, the body's ability to fight the infection is very poor. Diagnosis is usually based on lumbar puncture examination of cerebrospinal fluid and symptoms.

Bacterial meningitis may manifest differently, depending upon age.

- Neonates: Signs may be very nonspecific, such as weight loss, hypo- or hyperthermia, jaundice, irritability, lethargy, irregular respirations with periods of apnea. More specific signs may include increasing signs of illness, difficulty feeding with loss of suck reflex, hypotonia, weak cry, seizures, and bulging fontanels (may be a late sign). Nuchal rigidity does not usually occur with neonates.
- Infants and young children: Classic symptoms usually do not appear until at least 2 years. Signs may include fever, poor feeding, vomiting, irritability, and bulging fontanel. Nuchal rigidity in some children.

- Older children and adolescents/adults: Abrupt onset, including fever, chills, headache, and alterations of consciousness with seizures, agitation, and irritability. May have photophobia, hallucinations, aggressive or stuporous behavior, and lapsing into coma. Nuchal rigidity progressing to opisthotonos. Reflexes are variable but positive Kernig and Brudzinski signs. Signs may relate to particular bacteria, such as rashes, sore joints, or draining ear.

Seizures

Seizures are sudden involuntary abnormal electrical disturbances in the brain that can manifest as alterations of consciousness, spastic tonic and clonic movements, convulsions, and loss of consciousness. Seizures may be partial, affecting part of the brain, or generalized, affecting the whole brain. Seizures are a symptom of underlying pathology. Many seizures are transient. Some seizures may result from pathology, such as meningitis, cerebral edema, brain trauma, or brain tumors. Others are idiopathic, predisposing the person to recurrent seizures, usually of the same type. Seizures are characterized as focal (localized), focal with rapid generalization (spreading), and generalized (widespread). Seizure disorders with onset in childhood younger than 4 years usually cause more neurological damage than those that have a later onset.

Diagnosis may include:
- Serum glucose, pregnancy test, serum electrolytes, BUN, toxicology screening.
- CT or MRI to rule out lesions.
- EEG.

Treatment includes protecting patient from injury during active seizures:
- Anticonvulsives: phenytoin, carbamazepine, phenobarbital, primidone, valproic acid.
- Referral to neurologist for new onset.

> ➤ **Review Video:** Seizures
> *Visit **mometrix.com/academy** and enter **Code: 977061***

Partial seizures
Partial seizures are caused by an electrical discharged to a localized area of the cerebral cortex, such as the frontals, temporal, or parietal lobes with seizure characteristics related to area of involvement. They may begin in a focal area and become generalized, often preceded by an aura.
- Simple partial: Unilateral motor symptoms including somatosensory, psychic, and autonomic.
  - Aversive: Eyes and head turned away from focal side
  - Sylvan (usually during sleep): Tonic-clonic movements of the face, salivation, and arrested speech.
- Special sensory: Various sensations (numbness, tingling, prickling, or pain) spreading from one area. May include visual sensations, posturing or hypertonia.

Complex (Psychomotor): No loss of consciousness, but altered consciousness and non-responsive with amnesia. May involve complex sensorium with bad tastes, auditory or visual hallucinations, feeing of déjà vu, strong fear. May carry out repetitive activities, such as walking, running, smacking lips, chewing, or drawling. Rarely aggressive. Seizure usually followed by prolonged drowsiness and confusion. Most common ages 3 through adolescence.

<u>SE</u>
Status epilepticus (SE) is usually generalized tonic-clonic seizures that are characterized by a series of seizures with intervening time too short for regaining of consciousness. The constant assault and periods of apnea can lead to exhaustion, respiratory failure with hypoxemia and hypercapnia, cardiac failure, and death. Causes include:

- Uncontrolled epilepsy or non-compliance with anticonvulsants.
- Infections, such as encephalitis.
- Encephalopathy or stroke.
- Drug toxicity (isoniazid).
- Brain trauma.
- Neoplasms.
- Metabolic disorders.

Treatment includes:

- Anticonvulsants usually beginning with fast-acting benzodiazepine (Ativan®), often in steps, with administration of medication every 5 minutes until seizures subside.
- If cause is undetermined, acyclovir and ceftriaxone may be given.
- If there is no response to the first 2 doses of anticonvulsants (refractory SE), rapid sequence intubation (RSI), which involves sedation and paralytic anesthesia, may be done while therapy continues. Combining phenobarbitol and benzodiazepine can cause apnea, so intubation may be necessary.
- Phenytoin and phenobarbitol are added.

<u>Generalized seizures</u>
Generalized seizures lack a focal onset and appear to involve both hemispheres, usually presenting with loss of consciousness and no preceding aura.

- Tonic-clonic (Grand Mal): Occurs without warning.
  - Tonic period (10-30 seconds): Eyes roll upward with loss of consciousness, arms flexed; stiffen in symmetric tonic contraction of body, apneic with cyanosis and salivating.
  - Clonic period (10 seconds to 30 minutes, but usually 30 seconds). Violent rhythmic jerking with contraction and relaxation. May be incontinent of urine and feces. Contractions slow and then stop.
  - Following seizures, there may be confusion, disorientation, and impairment of motor activity, speech and vision for several hours. Headache, nausea, and vomiting may occur. Person often falls asleep and awakens conscious.
- Absence (Petit Mal): Onset between 4-12 and usually ends in puberty. Onset is abrupt with brief loss of consciousness for 5-10 seconds and slight loss of muscle tone but often appears to be daydreaming. Lip smacking or eye twitching may occur.

Neurogenic shock

Neurogenic shock is a type of distributive shock that occurs when injury to the CNS (from trauma resulting in acute spinal cord injury (from both blunt and penetrating injuries), neurological diseases, drugs, or anesthesia, impairs the autonomic nervous system that controls the cardiovascular system. The degree of symptoms relates to the level of injury with injuries above T1 capable of causing disruption of the entire sympathetic nervous system and lower injuries causing various degrees of disruption. Even incomplete spinal cord injury can cause neurogenic shock.

Symptoms include:
- Hypotension and warm dry skin related to lack of vascular tone that results in hypothermia from loss of cutaneous heat.
- Bradycardia is a common but not universal symptom.

Treatment includes:
- ABCDE (airway, breathing, circulation, disability evaluation, exposure)
- Rapid fluid administration with crystalloid to keep mean arterial pressure at 85-90 mm Hg.
- Placement of pulmonary artery catheter to monitor fluid overload.
- Inotropic agents (dopamine, dobutamine) if fluids don't correct hypotension.
- Atropine for persistent bradycardia.

Gastrointestinal, Genitourinary, Gynecology, and Obstetrical Emergencies

Appendicitis

Appendicitis is inflammation of the appendix often caused by luminal obstruction and pressure within the lumen; secretions build up and can eventually perforate the appendix. Diagnosis can be made difficult by the fact that there is some variation in the exact location of the appendix in some patients. Appendicitis can occur in all ages, but children younger than 2 years usually present with peritonitis or sepsis because of difficulty in early diagnosis. Symptoms include:
- Acute abdominal pain, which may be epigastric, periumbilical, right lower quadrant, or right flank with rebound tenderness.
- Anorexia.
- Nausea and vomiting.
- Positive psoas and obturator signs.
- Fever may develop after 24 hours.
- Malaise.
- Bowel irregularity and flatulence.

Diagnosis is based on clinical presentation, CBC (although leukocytosis may not be present), urinalysis, and imaging studies (usually an abdominal CT with contrast).

Peritonitis

Peritonitis (inflammation of the peritoneum) may be primary (from infection of blood or lymph) or, more commonly, secondary, related to perforation or trauma of the gastrointestinal tract, Common causes include perforated bowel, ruptured appendix, abdominal trauma, abdominal surgery, peritoneal dialysis or chemotherapy, or leakage of sterile fluids, such as blood, into the peritoneum. Diagnosis is made according to clinical presentation, abdominal x-rays, which may show distention of the intestines or air in the peritoneum, and laboratory findings, such as leukocytosis. Blood cultures may indicate sepsis. Symptoms of peritonitis are those of an acute abdomen. Symptoms include:
- Diffuse abdominal pain with rebound tenderness (Blumberg's sign).
- Abdominal rigidity.
- Paralytic ileus.
- Fever (with infection).
- Nausea and vomiting.
- Sinus tachycardia.

Treatment includes:
- Intravenous fluids and electrolytes.
- Broad-spectrum antibiotics.
- Laparoscopy as indicated to determine cause of peritonitis and effect repair.

Cholecystitis

Cholecystitis can result in obstruction of the bile duct related to calculi as well as pancreatitis from obstruction of the pancreatic duct. In acute cholecystitis, there is fever, leukocytosis, right upper quadrant abdominal pain, and inflammation of the gallbladder. The disease is most common in overweight women 20 to 40 years of age, but can occur in pregnant women and people of all ages, especially those who are diabetic or elderly. Cholecystitis may develop secondary to cystic fibrosis, obesity, or total parenteral nutrition. Many times, cholecystitis may resolve in about 7-10 days on its own, but acute cholecystitis may need surgical intervention to prevent complications such as gangrene in the gallbladder or perforation. Diagnosis is confirmed by ultrasound of gallbladder showing thickening of gallbladder walls or positive Murphy's sign, or a HIDA scan showing failure to fill. Symptoms include:

- Severe right upper quadrant or epigastric pain (ranging from 2-6 hours per episode).
- N/V
- Jaundice
- Altered mental status
- Positive Murphy's sign

Treatment includes:

- Antibiotics for sepsis/ ascending cholangitis.
- Antispasmodic agents (glycopyrrolate) for biliary colic and vomiting.
- Analgesics (note that opioids result in increased sphincter of Oddi pressure). Antiemetics
- Surgical consultation for possible laparoscopic or open cholecystectomy.

Acute pancreatitis

Acute pancreatitis is related to chronic alcoholism or cholelithiasis in 90% of patients. Pancreatitis may be triggered by a variety of drugs (tetracycline,thiazides, acetaminophen, oral contraceptives). Pain is usually acute and may be in mid-epigastric, left upper abdominal, or more generalized. Nausea and vomiting as well as abdominal distention may be present. Complications may include shock, acute respiratory distress syndrome, and multi-organ failure. Diagnostic tests include:

- Serum lipase >2 X normal value.
- Serum amylase (less accurate than lipase).
- CT with contrast to determine if there is pancreatic necrosis.
- Ultrasound to check bile duct for obstruction.
- MR cholangiopancreatography may be used in place of CT and ultrasound where available.

Treatment is usually supportive with oral intake NPO or restricted to clear liquids to help manage vomiting, ileus, and aspiration. Rehydration with intravenous fluids may be needed or TPN. Hemodynamic support as needed. Biliary obstruction needs to be removed with cholecystectomy. Antibiotics are given if necrosis is related to infection. Analgesia may be indicated, but avoid morphine and as it may cause spasms in the sphincter of Oddi.

Diverticulitis

Diverticular disease is a condition in which diverticula (saclike pouchings of the bowel lining that extend through a defect in the muscle layer) occur anywhere within the GI tract. About 20% of patients with diverticular disease will develop acute diverticulitis, which occurs as diverticula become inflamed when food or bacteria are retained within diverticula. This may result in abscess, obstruction, perforation, bleeding, or fistula.

Diagnosis is best confirmed by abdominal CT with contrast (showing a localized thickening of the bowel wall, increased density of soft tissue, and diverticula in the colon). Many patients have normal lab studies, but some present with leukocytosis, elevated serum amylase, and pyuria on urinalysis. Symptoms are similar to appendicitis:
- Steady pain in left lower quadrant.
- Change in bowel habits.
- Tenesmus.
- Dysuria from irritation.
- Recurrent urinary infections from fistula.
- Paralytic ileus from peritonitis or intraabdominal irritation.
- Toxic reactions: fever, severe pain, leukocytosis.

Treatment includes:
- Rehydration and electrolytes per IV fluids
- Nothing by mouth initially.
- Antibiotics, broad spectrum (IV if toxic reactions).
- NG suction if necessary for obstruction.
- Careful observation for signs of perforation or obstruction.

Hepatic cirrhosis

Cirrhosis may be either compensated or decompensated. Compensated cirrhosis usually involves non-specific symptoms, such as intermittent fever, epistaxis, ankle edema, indigestion, abdominal pain, and palmar erythema. Hepatomegaly and splenomegaly may also be present.

Compensated
Cirrhosis is a chronic hepatic disease in which normal liver tissue is replaced the fibrotic tissue that impairs liver function. There are 3 types:
- Alcoholic (from chronic alcoholism) is the most common type and results in fibrosis about the portal areas. The liver cells become necrotic, replaced by fibrotic tissue, with areas of normal tissue projecting in between, giving the liver a hobnail appearance.
- Postnecrotic with broad bands of fibrotic tissue is the result of acute viral hepatitis.
- Biliary, the least common type is caused by chronic biliary obstruction and cholangitis, with resulting fibrotic tissue about the bile ducts.

Decompensated
Decompensated cirrhosis occurs when the liver can no longer adequately synthesize proteins, clotting factors, and other substances so that portal hypertension occurs.

Symptoms include:
- Hepatomegaly. Chronic elevated temperature. Clubbing of fingers.
- Purpura resulting from thrombocytopenia, with bruising and epistaxis.
- Portal obstruction resulting in jaundice and ascites. Bacterial peritonitis with ascites. Esophageal varices.

- Edema of extremities and presacral area resulting from reduced albumin in the plasma. Vitamin deficiency from interference with formation, use, and storage of vitamins, such as A, C, and K.
- Anemia from chronic gastritis and decreased dietary intake.
- Hepatic encephalopathy with alterations in mentation.
- Hypotension.
- Atrophy of gonads.

Treatment varies according to the symptoms and is supportive rather than curative as the fibrotic changes in the liver cannot be reversed:
- Dietary supplements and vitamins.
- Diuretics (potassium sparing), such as Aldactone® and Dyrenium®, to decrease ascites.
- Colchicine to reduce fibrotic changes.
- Liver transplant (the definitive treatment).

Fulminant hepatitis

Fulminant hepatitis is a severe acute infection of the liver that can result in hepatic necrosis, encephalopathy, and death within 1 to 2 weeks. Most hepatitis is caused by infection with hepatitis viruses A, B, C, D, or E, but it can also be caused by numerous viruses, toxic chemicals (carbon tetrachloride), metabolic diseases (Wilson disease), and drugs, such as acetaminophen. Fulminant hepatitis can result from any of these factors. Fulminant hepatitis can be divided into 3 stages according to the duration from jaundice to encephalopathy:
- Hyperacute liver failure: 0 to 7 days.
- Acute liver failure: 8 to 28 days.
- Subacute liver failure: 28 to 72 days.

Symptoms include:
- Poor feeding/anorexia.
- Increased intracranial pressure with cerebral edema and encephalopathy.
- Coagulopathies.
- Renal failure.
- Electrolyte imbalances.

Treatment:
- Identify and treat underlying cause.
- Intracranial pressure monitoring and treatment.
- Diuresis.
- Liver transplantation may be necessary.

Survival rates vary from 50% to 85%.

GERD

Gastroesophageal reflux disease (GERD) is involuntary regurgitation of stomach contents into the esophagus, usually caused by decreased tone in the gastroesophageal valve and hiatal hernia, causing damage to the mucosal lining of the esophagus. Chronic esophagitis, strictures, Barrett esophagus (abnormal changes in cells of distal esophagus), and esophageal cancer may develop.

Symptoms include:
- Epigastric pain
- Heartburn
- Dysphagia
- Chronic cough, especially at night
- Hoarseness
- Earache
- Sinusitis

Treatment includes:
- Avoiding large meals or after-dinner snacking and eating at least 3 hours before going to bed or lying down.
- Modifying food intake to avoid coffee, alcohol, fatty food, spicy foods, and cruciferous vegetables.
- Sleeping with head of the bed elevated and on left side.
- Medications include histamine-2 receptor blockers (famotidine and ranitidine), proton pump inhibitors, alginic acid, and antacids (without aluminum).
- Surgical repair (fundoplication) may be needed if medical treatment is not adequate.

Peptic ulcer disease

Peptic ulcer disease (PUD)/gastritis includes both ulcerations of the duodenum and stomach. They may be primary (usually duodenal) or secondary (usually gastric). Gastric ulcers are commonly associated with *H. pylori* infections (80%) but may be caused by aspirin and NSAIDs. *H. pylori* are spread in the fecal-oral route from person to person or contaminated water, and cause a chronic inflammation and ulcerations of the gastric mucosa. PUD is 2 to 3 times more common in males and is associated with poor economic status that results in a crowded, unhygienic environment, although it can occur in others. Usually other family members have a history of ulcers as well. Symptoms include abdominal pain, nausea, vomiting, and GI bleeding in children younger than 6 years with epigastric and postprandial pain and indigestion in older children and adults.

Treatment includes:
- Antibiotics for H. pylori: amoxicillin, clarithromycin, metronidazole.
- Proton pump inhibitors: lansoprazole or omeprazole.
- Bismuth.
- Histamine-receptor antagonists: cimetidine, ranitidine, famotidine.

> **Review Video:** Peptic Ulcers and GERD
*Visit **mometrix.com/academy** and enter **Code: 184332***

Acute GI hemorrhage

SRES
Stress-related erosive syndrome (SRES) (stress ulcers) occurs most frequently in those who are critically ill, such as those with severe or multi-organ trauma, mechanical ventilation, sepsis, severe burns, and head injury with increased intracranial pressure. Stress induces changes in the gastric mucosal lining and decreased perfusion of the mucosa, causing ischemia. SRES involves

hemorrhage in ≥30% with mortality rates of 30-80% so prompt identification and treatment is critical. The lesions tend to be diffuse, so they are more difficult to treat than peptic ulcers.

Symptoms include:
- Coffee ground emesis.
- Hematemesis.
- Abdominal discomfort.

Treatment includes:
- Prophylaxis in those at risk:
  - Sucralfate (Carafate®) protects mucosa against pepsin.
  - Famotidine (Pepcid®), nizatidine (Axid®), ranitidine (Zantac®) or cimetidine (Tagamet®) reduces gastric secretions.
- Treatment for active bleeding includes:
  - Intraarterial infusion of vasopressin.
  - Intraarterial embolization.
  - Oversewing of ulcers or total gastrectomy if bleeding persists.

Peptic ulcers
Gastrointestinal (GI) hemorrhage may occur in the upper or lower gastrointestinal track. The primary cause (50-70%) of GI hemorrhage is peptic ulcer disease (gastric and duodenal ulcers), which results in deterioration of the gastromucosal lining, compromising the glycoprotein mucous barrier and the gastroduodenal epithelial cells that provide protection from gastric secretions. The secretions literally digest the mucosal and submucosal layers, damaging blood vessels and causing hemorrhage. The primary causes are NSAIDs and infection with *Helicobacter pylori*. Symptoms include:
- Abdominal pain and distention.
- Hematemesis.
- Bloody or tarry stools.
- Hypotension with tachycardia.

Treatment includes:
- Fluid replacement with transfusions if necessary.
- Antibiotic therapy for *Helicobacter pylori*.
- Endoscopic thermal therapy to cauterize or injection therapy (hypertonic saline, epinephrine, ethanol) to cause vasoconstriction.
- Arteriography with intraarterial infusion of vasopressin and/or embolizing agents, such as stainless stell coils, platinum microcoils, or Gelfoam pledgets.
- Vagotomy and pyloroplasty if bleeding persists.

Esophageal varices
Esophageal varices are torturous dilated veins in the submucosa of the esophagus (usually the distal portion), a complication of cirrhosis of the liver in which obstruction of the portal vein causes an increase in collateral vessels, a decrease in circulation to the liver, and an increase in pressure in the collateral vessels in the submucosa of the esophagus and stomach. This causes the vessels to dilate. Because they tend to be fragile and inelastic, they tear easily, causing sudden massive esophageal hemorrhage. Bleeding from varices occurs in 19-50% with associated mortality rates of 40-70%.

Treatment may include:
- Fluid and blood replacement.
- Intravenous vasopressin, somatostatin, and octreotide to decreased portal venous pressure and provide vasoconstriction.
- Endoscopic injection with sclerosing agents.
- Endoscopic variceal band ligation.
- Esophagogastric balloon tamponade to apply direct pressure.

Transjugular intrahepatic portosystemic shunting (TIPS) creates a channel between systemic and portal venous systems to reduce portal hypertension. A variety of other shunts may be done surgically if bleeding persists.

Inflammatory bowel disease

Ulcerative colitis
Ulcerative colitis is superficial inflammation of the mucosa of the colon and rectum, causing ulcerations in the areas where inflammation has destroyed cells. These ulcerations, ranging from pinpoint to extensive, may bleed and produce purulent material. The mucosa of the bowel becomes swollen, erythematous, and granular. Patients may present emergently with severe ulcerative colitis (having >6 blood stools a day, fever, tachycardia, anemia) or with fulminant colitis (>10 blood stools per day, sever bleeding, and toxic symptoms) These patients are at high risk for megacolon and perforation. For patients with severe and fulminant ulcerative colitis symptoms include:
- Abdominal pain.
- Anemia.
- F&E depletion.
- Bloody diarrhea/rectal bleeding.
- Diarrhea.
- Fecal urgency.
- Tenesmus.
- Anorexia.
- Weight loss.
- Fatigue.
- Systemic disorders: Eye inflammation, arthritis, liver disease, and osteoporosis as immune system triggers generalized inflammation.

Treatment includes:
- Glucocorticoids.
- Aminosalicylates.
- Antibiotics if s/s of toxicity.
- D/C anticholinergics, NSAIDS, and antidiarrheals.
- If fulminant: Admitted & monitored for deterioration. Kept NPO, and given IV F&E replacement. NGT for decompression if intestinal dilation is present. Knee-elbow position to reposition gas in bowel. Colectomy for those with megacolon or unresponsive to therapy.

Crohn's disease
Crohn's disease manifests with inflammation of the GI system. Inflammation is transmural (often leading to intestinal stenosis and fistulas), focal, and discontinuous with aphthous ulcerations progressing to linear and irregular-shaped ulcerations. Granulomas may be present. Common sites

of inflammation are the terminal ileum and cecum. The condition is chronic, but patients with severe or fulminant disease (fevers, persistent vomiting, abscess, obstruction) often present emergently for treatment.

Symptoms include:
- Perirectal abscess/fistula in advanced disease.
- Diarrhea.
- Watery stools.
- Rectal hemorrhage.
- Anemia.
- Abdominal pain (commonly RLQ).
- Cramping.
- Weight Loss.
- N/V.
- Fever.
- Night Sweats.

Treatment includes:
- Triamcinolone for oral lesions, aminosalicylates, glucocorticoids, antidiarrheals, probiotics, avoiding lactose and identify and eliminate food triggers.
- For patients who present with toxic symptoms: hospitalization for careful monitoring, IV glucocorticoids, aminosalicylates, antibiotics, bowel rest. Parenteral nutrition for malnourished.
- For repeated relapses (refractory): Immunomodulatory agents (azathioprine, mercaptopurine, methotrexate). Or Biologic therapies (infliximab). Bowel resection if unresponsive to all treatment or with ischemic bowel.

Hernias

Hernias are protrusions into or through the abdominal wall and may occur in children and adults. Hernias may contain fat, tissue, or bowel. There are a number of types:
- Direct inguinal hernias occur primarily in adults and rarely incarcerate.
- Indirect inguinal hernias related to congenital defect is most common on the right in males and can incarcerate, especially during the first year and in females.
- Femoral hernias occur primarily in women and may incarcerate.
- Umbilical hernias occur in children, especially those of African-American descent, and rarely incarcerate. They may also occur in adults, primarily women, and may incarcerate.
- Incisional hernias are usually related to obesity or wound infections, and may incarcerate.

Hernias are evident on clinical examination. Symptoms of incarceration include:
- Severe pain.
- Nausea and vomiting.
- Soft mass at hernia site.
- Tachycardia.
- Temperature.

Treatment for hernias includes:
- Reduction if incarceration very recent with patient in Trendelenburg position and gentle compression
- Surgical excision and fixation.
- Broad-spectrum antibiotics.

Intussusception

Intussusception is a telescoping of one portion of the intestine into another, usually at the ileocecal valve, causing an obstruction. As the walls of the intestine come in contact, inflammation and edema cause decreased perfusion, which can result in infarction with peritonitis and death. Fecal material cannot move past the obstruction. It is most common between 3 and 12 months but can occur until 6 years and may relate to viral infections.

Symptoms include:
- "Current jelly stool" composed of blood/mucous (occurs in 60%).
- Sudden, acute episodes of severe abdominal pain during which child pulls knees to chest.
- Vomiting.
- Lethargy and weakness.
- Distended abdomen, painful to palpation.
- Sausage-shaped mass in right upper quadrant of abdomen.
- Progressive fever and prostration if peritonitis occurs.

Treatment includes:
- Barium or air enema to diagnose and apply pressure that may resolve the intussusception.
- Surgical repair if there is shock, peritonitis, intestinal perforation, or failure to resolve with barium/air enema.

Constipation

Constipation is a condition with bowel movements less frequent than normal for a person, or hard, small stool that is evacuated fewer than 3 times weekly. Food moves through the GI from the small intestine to the colon in semi-liquid form. Constipation results from the colon, where fluid is absorbed. If too much fluid is absorbed, the stool can become too dry. People may have abdominal distention and cramps and need to strain for defecation.

Fecal impaction occurs when the hard stool moves into the rectum and becomes a large, dense, immovable mass that cannot be evacuated even with straining, usually as a result of chronic constipation. In addition to abdominal cramps and distention, the person may feel intense rectal pressure and pain accompanied by a sense of urgency to defecate. Nausea and vomiting may also occur. Hemorrhoids will often become engorged. Fecal incontinence, with liquid stool leaking about the impaction, is common. Medical procedures to evaluate causes of constipation should be preceded by a careful history as this may help to define the type and guide the choice of diagnostic procedures. Most tests are necessary only for severe constipation that does not respond to treatment.

Medical diagnostic procedures may include the following:
- Physical exam should include rectal exam and abdominal palpation to assess for obvious hard stool or impaction.
- Blood tests can identify hypothyroidism and excess parathyroid hormone.
- Abdominal x-ray may show large amounts of stool in the colon.
- Barium enema can indicate tumors or strictures causing obstruction.
- Colonic transit studies can show defects of the neuromuscular system.
- Defecography shows defecation process and abnormalities of anatomy.
- Anorectal manometry studies show malfunction of anorectal muscles.
- Colonic motility studies measures the pattern of colonic pressure.
- Colonoscope allows direct visualization of the lumen of the rectum and colon.

Bowel obstruction and infarction

Bowel obstruction occurs when there is a mechanical obstruction of the passage of intestinal contents because of constriction of the lumen, occlusion of the lumen, or lack of muscular contractions (paralytic ileus). Patients who have had any type of abdominal surgery are at highest risk for having a bowel obstruction due to adhesions. Symptoms include dehydration (the hallmark sign, leading to tachycardia, hypotension,decreased UOP) n/v, abdominal pain, distention (50% of patients), abdominal rigidity, diminished or no bowel sounds, severe constipation (obstipation). Respiratory distress from diaphragm pushing against pleural cavity may appear and patients may experience shock as plasma volume diminishes and electrolytes enter intestines from bloodstream. Sepsis may be present as bacteria proliferates in bowel and invade bloodstream. Upright chest and upright and supine abdominal xrays are inexpensive ways to confirm the diagnosis. Treatment includes surgical consultation, F&E replacement, NPO status, NGT for decompression in some, and pain management. Bowel infarction is ischemia of the intestines related to severely restricted blood supply. It can be the result of a number of different conditions, such as strangulated bowel or occlusion of arteries of the mesentery, and may follow untreated bowel obstruction. People present with acute abdomen and shock, and mortality rates are very high even with resection of infarcted bowel.

Intestinal perforation

Intestinal perforation is a complete rupture or penetration of the intestinal wall. There are a number of causes:
- Traumatic injuries, such as gunshot or knife wounds.
- NSAIDs and/or aspirin, especially in elderly with diverticulitis.
- Acute appendicitis.
- Peptic ulcer disease.
- Iatrogenic causes: laparoscopy, endoscopy, colonoscopy, radiotherapy
- Bacterial infections.
- Inflammatory bowel diseases, such as Crohn's disease or ulcerative colitis.
- Ingestion of toxic substances (acids) or foreign bodies (toothpicks).

The danger posed by infection after perforation varies depending upon the site. The stomach and proximal portions of the small intestine have little bacteria, but the distal portion of the small intestine contains aerobic bacteria, such as *E. coli*, as well as anaerobic bacteria. Symptoms include abdominal pain and distention and rigidity, fever, guarding and rebound tenderness, tachycardia and paralytic ileus with nausea and vomiting. Treatment is as for peritonitis, with antibiotics and surgical repair.

Acute abdominal trauma

Acute abdominal trauma may be blunt or penetrating:
- Blunt injuries from motor vehicle accidents (MVA), sports injuries, falls, and assaults are common causes of abdominal injury and comprise crush (compression), shear (tearing), and burst (sudden increased pressure). MVA often results in liver injury in the passenger with impact on that side and spleen injury in the driver with impact on the driver's side. Other injuries from blunt trauma include damage to the diaphragm, retroperitoneal hematomas, and intestinal injuries, including perforation.
- Penetrating wounds, on the other hand, are almost always related to gunshot wounds (high energy) or knife assaults (low energy). Gunshot wounds tend to cause more extensive damage than stab wounds, especially to the colon, liver, spleen and diaphragm. Interior injury may be extensive because the bullet damages tissue and may ricochet off of bone. Hemorrhage and peritonitis are common complications.

Gastric and intestinal injuries
Gastric injuries may result in perforation, primarily at the greater curvature. The risk increases if the person is injured with a full stomach after eating a meal and suffers blunt or penetrating force to the abdomen. Perforation results in severe pain, rigid abdomen, and bloody nasogastric drainage with peritonitis developing within hours, so early diagnosis and surgical repair must be done. Intestinal injuries may occur from blunt or penetrating trauma. Indications of rupture often appear 24-48 hours when the person presents with symptoms of peritonitis resulting from leakage of intestinal contents into the peritoneum. Symptoms may include distention, abdominal pain, absent bowel sounds, leukocytosis, fever, dyspnea, nausea and vomiting. Sepsis and abscess or fistula formation can occur. Treatment includes prompt antibiotic therapy, and surgical repair with peritoneal lavage. The abdominal wound may be left open to heal by secondary intention.

Hepatic injuries
Hepatic injury is the most common cause of death (mortality rates of 8-25%) from abdominal trauma and is often associated with multiple organ damage, so symptoms may be non-specific. Automobile accidents cause most blunt trauma. Elevation in liver transaminase levels indicates damage that may require CT examination with double contrast. Liver injuries are classified according to the degree of injury:
  I. Tears in capsule with hematoma.
  II. Laceration(s) of parenchyma (<3 cm).
  III. Laceration(s) of parenchyma (<3 cm).
  IV. Destruction of 25-75% of lobe from burst injury.
  V. Destruction of >75% of lobe from burst injury.
  VI. Avulsion [tearing away].

Hemodynamically stable patients are managed medically, but surgical repair may be necessary if the patient is unstable or bleeding. Hemorrhage is common complication of hepatic injury and may require ligation of hepatic arteries or veins. Treatment often includes intravenous fluids for fluid volume deficit as well as blood products (plasma, platelets) for coagulopathies.

Splenic injuries

The spleen is the most frequently injured solid organ in blunt trauma. Injuries to the spleen are the most common because it's not well protected by the rib cage and is very vascular. Symptoms may be very non-specific. Kehr sign (radiating pain in left shoulder) indicates intra-abdominal bleeding and Cullen sign (ecchymosis around umbilicus) indicates hemorrhage from ruptured spleen. Some may have right upper abdominal pain although diffuse abdominal pain often occurs with blood loss, associated with hypotension. Splenic injuries are classified according to the degree of injury:

1. Tear in splenic capsules or hematoma.
2. Laceration of parenchyma (<3 cm).
3. Laceration of parenchyma (>3cm).
4. Multiple lacerations of parenchyma or burst-type injury.

Treatment may be supportive if injury is not severe; otherwise, suturing of spleen may be needed. Because there is a risk of infection with splenectomy, every effort (bed rest, transfusion, reduced activity for at least 8 weeks) is done to avoid surgery because the spleen will often heal spontaneously.

Pancreatic injuries

Pancreatic injuries can result from motor vehicle accidents or assault with impact to the abdominal area, although it is not a common injury. Penetrating injuries (gunshot wounds and stabbings) are more common. Because of the location of the pancreas, impact compresses it against the vertebral column. Most people with pancreatic injury sustain other abdominal injuries as well, making diagnosis difficult. Symptoms may include diffuse abdominal or epigastric pain and well as vomiting of bile. Pancreatic injuries are classified according to degree of injury:

- Grade I: Minor contusion or laceration but ducts intact.
- Grade II: Major contusion or laceration but ducts intact and no tissue loss.
- Grade III: Distal transection or injury of parenchyma with ductal injury.
- Grade IV: Proximal transection or injury of parenchyma with probable ductal injury.
- Grade V: Massive disruption of the pancreatic head.

CT scans are most commonly used for diagnosis. Surgical exploration and repair of severe damage is the most common treatment. Pancreatitis and diabetes mellitus may be long-term sequelae. Treatment includes resting the bowel and nutritional support for Grade I and II blunt injury, and repair or possibly resection for penetrating and high grade injuries.

Nasogastric tubes, sump tubes, and Levin tubes

NG tubes are plastic or vinyl tubes inserted through the nose, down the esophagus, and into the stomach. Sump tubes are radiopaque with a vent lumen to prevent a vacuum from forming with high suction. Levin tubes have no vent lumen and are used only with low suction. NG tubes drain gastric secretions, allow sampling of secretions, or provide access to the stomach and upper GI tract. They are used for lavage after medication overdose, for decompression, and for instillation of medications or fluids. NG tubes are contraindicated with obstruction proximal to the stomach or gastric pathology, such as hemorrhage.

Tube-insertion length is estimated: earlobe to xiphoid + earlobe to nose tip + 15 cm.

Tube is inserted through naris with patient upright, if possible, and swallowing sips of water. Vasoconstrictors and topical anesthetic reduce gag reflex. Placement is checked with insufflation of air or aspiration of stomach contents and verified by xray. NG is secured and drainage bag provided. Tubes attached to continuous low or intermittent high suction must be monitored frequently.

PID

Pelvic inflammatory disease (PID) comprises infections of the upper reproductive system, often ascending from vagina and cervix, and includes salpingitis, endometritis, tubo-ovarian abscess, peritonitis, and perihepatitis. *Neisseria gonorrhoeae* and *Chlamydia trachomatis* are implicated in most cases but some infections are polymicrobial. Complications include increase in ectopic pregnancy and tubal factor infertility. Symptoms include lower abdominal pain, vaginal pain, discharge, or bleeding, dyspareunia, dysuria, fever, and nausea and vomiting.

Diagnostic studies include:
- Pregnancy test.
- Vaginal secretion testing, endocervical culture.
- CBC.
- Syphilis, HIV, and hepatitis testing.
- Transvaginal pelvic ultrasound.
- Endometrial biopsy.
- Laparoscopy for definitive diagnosis.

Treatments include:
- Broad spectrum antibiotics:
  - (Inpatient) Cefotetan 2 g IV every 12 hours or every 6 hours with doxycycline 100 mg every 12 hours.
  - (Outpatient) Ceftriaxone 250 mg IM x 1 dose with doxycycline 100 mg orally every 12 hours for 14 days with metronidazole 500 mg twice daily for 2 weeks for patients who had gynecological procedures recently.
- Laparoscopy to drain abscesses if symptoms do not improve 72 hours or less.
- Treatment specific to associated disorders (such as HIV or hepatitis).

Vulvovaginitis

Vulvovaginitis is inflammation of vulvar and vaginal tissues:
- Bacterial vaginosis (*Gardnerella vaginalis* or other bacteria).
- Fungal infections (usually *Candida albicans*).
- Parasitic infections (*Trichomonas vaginalis*).
- Allergic contact vaginitis (from soaps or other irritants).
- Atrophic vaginitis (postmenopause)

Symptoms include vaginal odor, swelling, discharge, or bleeding; pain and discomfort; or severe itching (common with *C. albicans).*

Diagnostic studies include physical exam and culture of discharge, pH testing with nitrazine paper: Greater than 4.5 is typical of bacterial and trichomonas infections. Less than 4.5 is typical of fungal infections.

Treatment includes:
- Bacterial infections: Metronidazole 500 mg orally twice daily for 7 days AND Metronidazole 0.75% gel intravaginally twice daily for 5 days AND Clindamycin 2% cream intravaginally at bedtime for 7 days.
- Fungal infections: Fluconazole 150 mg tablet in 1 dose **OR**
- Vaginal creams, tablets, or suppositories, such as butoconazole 2% cream for 3 days or tioconazole 6.5% ointment for 1 dose.
- Parasitic (trichomonas) Metronidazole 2 g orally in 1 dose.

Ovarian cyst

Ovarian cysts can grow within or on the ovaries:
- Functional: follicular cyst usually resolves in 1 to 3 months; corpus luteum usually resolves in a few weeks but cyst may grow to 4 inches, causing torsion and pain.
- Cystadenoma forma on exterior of ovary and may enlarge and cause pain.
- Endometrioma attaches to ovaries and causes pain during menses and sexual activity.
- Dermoid cyst may enlarge and cause pain.
- Polycystic ovaries may have multiple cysts.
- Ovarian cysts may cause problems if they rupture or hemorrhage and if they twist or become infected. Presenting symptoms include:
- Hypotension and hypovolemia if hemorrhage occurs, pain (often acute) and tenderness in lower abdomen on affected side and/or lower back pain, dysuria, and weight gain.

Diagnostic studies include:
- Pregnancy test to rule out ectopic pregnancy, ultrasound with Doppler flow.
- Treatment depends upon the type of cyst and complications:
- Emergency surgery for torsion.
- Antibiotics for infection.
- Hormone therapy may be useful for endometrioma.

Bartholin cyst

The Bartholin glands are small glands located on both sides of the vagina in the lips of the labia minora. The glands help to lubricate the vulvar area. A Bartholin cyst occurs when a duct to one gland becomes obstructed, usually because of infection or trauma, resulting in swelling and formation of a cyst (usually 1 to 3 cm but may be much larger with infection). Bartholin cyst is most common in women in their 20s. Blockage may result from tumors as well, but usually in women older than 40.

Symptoms of a Bartholin cyst include:
- Palpable mass on one side of the vagina (usually painless).
- Pain and tenderness and increasing size of lesion if infection and abscess occurs.

Treatment includes:
- Warm, moist compresses or sitz baths.
- Antibiotics for infection.
- Surgical incision and drainage may be necessary in some cases.

Phimosis and paraphimosis

Phimosis and paraphimosis are both restrictive disorders of the penis that occur in males who are uncircumcised or incorrectly circumcised. Phimosis is the inability to retract the foreskin proximal to the glans penis, sometimes resulting in urinary retention or hematuria. Treatments include:
- Dilating the foreskin with a hemostat (temporary solution).
- Circumcision.
- Application of topical steroids (triamcinolone 0.025% twice daily) from end of foreskin to glans corona for 4 to 6 weeks.

Paraphimosis occurs when the foreskin tightens above the glans penis and cannot be extended to normal positioning. This results in edema of the foreskin and circulatory impairment of the glans penis, sometimes progressing to gangrene, so immediate treatment is critical. Symptoms include pain, swelling, and inability to urinate. Treatments include:
- Compression of the glans to reduce edema (wrapping tightly with 2-inch elastic bandage for 5 minutes).
- Reducing edema by making several puncture wounds with 22 to 25 gauge needle.
- Local anesthetic and dorsal incision to relieve pressure.

Testicular torsion

Testicular torsion is a twisting of the spermatic cord within or below the inguinal canal, causing constriction of blood supply to the testis. Testicular torsion is most common at puberty but can occur at any age, sometimes precipitated by strenuous athletic participation or trauma, but it can also occur during sleep. Symptoms include acute onset of severe testicular pain and edema, although children may present with nonspecific abdominal discomfort initially. Diagnosis is based on clinical examination that demonstrates a firm scrotal mass. Color-flow duplex Doppler ultrasound may be helpful if diagnosis is not clear. Treatment includes:
- Manual detorsion (usually 1.5 rotations) with elective surgical repair. Right testicle is usually rotated counterclockwise and left, clockwise. Reduction of pain should occur. If pain increases with rotation, then rotation should be done in the opposite direction.
- Emergency surgical repair (if manual detorsion not successful).

Epididymitis and orchitis

Epididymitis, infection of the epididymis, is often associated with infection in a testis (epididymo-orchitis). In children, infection may be related to congenital anomalies that allow reflux of urine. In sexually active males 35 years or younger, it is usually related to STDs. In men older than 40, it is often related to urinary infections or benign prostatic hypertrophy with urethral obstruction. Symptoms include progressive pain in lower abdomen, scrotum, and/or testicle. Late symptoms include large tender scrotal mass. Diagnosis includes: Clinical examination. Pyuria. Urethral culture for STDs. Sonography. Orchitis alone is rare but occurs with mumps, other viral infections, and epididymitis. Ultrasound may be needed to rule out testicular torsion.

Treatment for both conditions depends upon the cause, but epididymitis usually resolves with antibiotics:
- Younger than 35 to 40 associated with STDs:
  - Ceftriaxone 250 mg IM and doxycycline 100 mg BID for 10 days.
- Older than 35 to 40 associated with other bacteria:
  - Ciprofloxacin 500 mg twice daily for 10 to 14 days.
  - Levofloxacin 250 mg daily for 10 to 14 days.
  - TMP/SMS DS twice daily for 10 to 14 days.

Prostatitis and benign prostatic hypertrophy

Prostatitis is an acute infection of the prostate gland, commonly caused by Escherichia coli, Pseudomonas aeruginosa, Staphylococcus aureus, or other bacteria. Symptoms include fever, chills, lower back pain, urinary frequency, dysuria, painful ejaculation, perineal discomfort. PSA will often be elevated in this patient population, unrelated to prostate cancer. Diagnosis is based on clinical findings of perineal tenderness and spasm of rectal sphincter. Treatments include Ciprofloxacin 500 mg orally twice daily for 1 month or TMP/SMX DS twice daily for 1 month. Most patients also have a urethral culture to check for STDs. Patients with suspected bacteremia should be admitted for monitoring.

Benign prostatic hypertrophy/hyperplasia usually develops after age 40. The prostate may slowly enlarge, but the surrounding tissue restrains outward growth, so the gland compresses the urethra. The bladder wall also goes through changes, becoming thicker and irritated, so that it begins to spasm, causing frequent urinations. The bladder muscle eventually weakens and the bladder fails to empty completely. Symptoms include urgency, dribbling, frequency, nocturia, incontinence, retention, and bladder distention. Diagnosis may include IVP, cystogram, and PSA. Treatment includes:
- Catheterization for urinary retention/bladder distention.
- Surgical excision.
- Avoid fluids close to bedtime, doube void, avoid caffeine and alcohol, alpha-adrenergic antagonists, and 5-alpha-reductase inhibitors.

Pyelonephritis

Pyelonephritis is a potentially organ-damaging bacterial infection of the parenchyma of the kidney. Pyelonephritis can result in abscess formation, sepsis, and kidney failure. Pyelonephritis is especially dangerous for those who are immunocompromised, pregnant, or diabetic. Most infections are caused by *Escherichia coli. Diagnostic* studies include urinalysis, blood and urine cultures. Patients may require hospitalization or careful follow-up. Symptoms vary widely but can include:
- Dysuria and frequency, hematuria, flank and/or low back pain.
- Fever and chills.
- Costovertebral angle tenderness.
- Change in feeding habits (infants).
- Change in mental status (geriatric)

Young women often exhibit symptoms more associated with lower urinary infection, so the condition may be overlooked.

Treatment includes:
- Analgesia.
- Antipyretics.
- Intravenous fluids
- Antibiotics: started but may be changed based on cultures.
    - Ceftriaxone or fluoroquinolone.
    - Monitor BUN. Normal 7-8 mg/dL (8-20 mg/dL >age 60). Increase indicates impaired renal function, as urea is end product of protein metabolism.

Cystitis

Urinary infections, cystitis, are common and often-chronic low-grade kidney infections develop over time, so observing for symptoms of urinary infections and treating promptly are very important.
- Changes in character of urine:
    - Appearance: The urine may become cloudy from mucus or purulent material. Hematuria may be present.
    - Color: Urine usually becomes concentrated and may be dark yellow/orange or brownish in color.
    - Odor: Urine may have a very strong or foul odor.
    - Output: Urinary output may decrease markedly.
- Pain: There may be lower back or flank pain from inflammation of the kidneys.
- Systemic: Fever, chills, headache, and general malaise often accompany urine infections. Some people suffer lack of appetite as well as nausea and vomiting. Fever usually indicates that the infection has affected the kidneys. Children may develop incontinence or loose stools and cry excessively.

Treatment:
- Increased fluid intake.
- Antibiotics.

Ureteral calculi

Renal and urinary calculi occur frequently, more commonly in males, and can relate to diseases (hyperparathyroidism, renal tubular acidosis, gout) and lifestyle factors, such as sedentary work. Calculi can form at any age, most composed of calcium, and can range in size from very tiny to >6mm. Those <4mm can usually pass in the urine easily. *Diagnostic* studies include clinical findings, UA, pregnancy test to rule out ectopic pregnancy, BUN and creatinine if indicated, ultrasound (for pregnant women and children), IV urography. Helical CT (non-contrast) is diagnostic. Symptoms occur with obstruction and are usually of sudden onset and acute:
- Severe flank pain radiating to abdomen and ipsilateral testicle or labium majorum, abdominal or pelvic pain (young children).
- Nausea and vomiting.
- Diaphoresis.
- Hematuria.

Treatment includes:
- Analgesia: opiates and NSAIDs.
- Instructions and equipment for straining urine.
- Antibiotics if concurrent infection.
- Extracorporeal shock-wave lithotripsy.
- Surgical removal: Percutaneous/standard nephrolithotomy.

Ruptured bladder

Bladder rupture can occur as the result of blunt or penetrating trauma from accidents or medical procedures. Prolonged labor can result in bladder necrosis that then ruptures. Sometimes ruptures occur with urinary retention causing overdistention. Bladder rupture may be associated with urethral injury. The 2 primary types of ruptures include:
- Intraperitoneal occurs when a full bladder bursts, usually with a 1-inch laceration in the posterior dome with urine spilling into the peritoneum. Higher incidence in children.
- Extraperitoneal with rupture of the bladder neck often associated with pelvic fractures.

Symptoms include:
- Hematuria, inability to urinate spontaneously.
- Abdominal pain and tenderness.
- Signs of peritonitis (with intraperitoneal rupture), including pain in shoulder (Kehr sign).

Diagnostic studies include:
- CT cystogram, cystogram, retrograde urethrogram if urethral damage suspected.

Treatments include:
- Extraperitoneal: Foley catheter if no urethral injury; otherwise, suprapubic catheter. Most heal without surgery.
- Intraperitoneal: Surgical exploration and repair.

Renal trauma

Most renal trauma is the result of blunt trauma associated with motor vehicle accidents, falls, sports injuries, and iatrogenic causes (endourologic procedures, biopsy), although gunshot wounds and stabbings also occur with increasing frequency. Various staging systems are used, but overall injuries are graded by severity:
- Contusion of cortex w/fracture(tear) of small confined area.
- Major fracture with perirenal hematoma and/or extravasation of urine.
- Multiple fractures with extensive bleeding.
- Severe vascular disruption decreasing perfusion of kidney.

Kidney injuries are often accompanied by other trauma (75%), so symptoms may be complex:
- Pain in abdominal or flank area.
- Hematuria.
- Abrasions or contusions in flank or abdominal area.
- Shock.

Delayed symptoms may occur: Hypertension and hydronephrosis

Treatment is usually nonoperative if the patient is hemodynamically stable, based on evaluation by CT, especially for blunt trauma. Gunshot wounds usually require:
- Surgical exploration.
- Bed rest.
- Monitoring of blood cell counts and vital signs.

Reducing infection risks associated with urinary catheters

Strategies for reducing infection risks associated with urinary catheters include:
- Using aseptic technique for both straight and indwelling catheter insertion.
- Limiting catheter use by establishing protocols for use, duration, and removal; training staff; issuing reminders to physicians; using straight catheterizations rather than indwelling; using ultrasound to scan the bladder; and using condom catheters.
- Utilizing closed-drainage systems for indwelling catheters.
- Avoiding irrigation unless required for diagnosis or treatment.
- Using sampling port for specimens rather than disconnecting catheter and tubing.
- Maintaining proper urinary flow by proper positioning, securing of tubing and drainage bag, and keeping drainage bag below the level of the bladder.
- Changing catheters only when medically needed.
- Cleansing external meatal area gently each day, manipulating the catheter as little as possible.
- Avoiding placing catheterized patients adjacent to those infected or colonized with antibiotic-resistant bacteria to reduce cross-contamination.

Removal of foreign bodies from genitourinary or gynecological orifices

Foreign bodies may be intentionally inserted into body orifices. Males, most often children, may insert items, such as paint brushes or ballpoint pens, into the urethra during sexual exploration. This may cause infection and hematuria with difficulty urinating. Diagnosis is by x-ray. Treatment may involve milking the urethra from proximal to distal end or removal by endoscope. In some cases, cystotomy may be necessary. Females, especially children and adolescents, may insert items, such as toilet paper, toys, or other items into the vagina during sexual exploration. More commonly, females may forget that a tampon or contraceptive sponge or cap is in place until they develop signs of infection or discharge. Treatment is a vaginal exam to remove the item, identification of any secondary infection, and then treatment of secondary infections as necessary. Items left in place for more than 48 hours pose a danger of infection with *Escherichia coli* or other anaerobic bacteria.

Chlamydia

Chlamydia is an STD caused by *Chlamydia trachomatis* and is often co-infected with gonorrhea. It may be transmitted by oral, anal, and vaginal sex. It is the most common STD in the United States. Symptoms of chlamydia include:
- Males: urethritis, epididymitis, proctitis, or Reiter syndrome (urethritis, rash, conjunctivitis). Many are asymptomatic.
- Females: Mild cervicitis with vaginal discharge and dysuria, but complications can lead to infertility and pelvic inflammatory disease (PID).

Diagnosis is most reliable from nucleic acid amplification test (NAAT) (*Amplicor, ProbeTEC*).

Treatment includes:
- Azithromycin 1 g orally in 1 dose **OR**
- Doxycycline 100 mg orally twice daily for 1 week.
- Avoidance of sexual contact for 1 week.
- Treatment of the infected person's sexual partner is very important to avoid reinfection after treatment.

Syphilis

Syphilis is caused by the spirochete *Treponema pallidum* and has increased in incidence over the last 10 years; it is associated with risk-taking behavior such as drug use. The disease has 3 phases, with an incubation period of about 3 weeks:
- Primary: chancre (painless) in areas of sexual contact, persisting 3 to 6 weeks.
- Secondary: General flu-like symptoms (sore throat, fever, headaches) and red papular rash on trunk, flexor surfaces, palms, and soles, and lymphadenopathy occur about 3 to 6 weeks after end of primary phase and eventually resolves.
- Tertiary (latent): Affects about 30% and includes CNS and cardiovascular symptoms 3 to 20 years after initial infection. Gummas (granulomatous lesions) may be widespread. Complications include dementia, meningitis, neuropathy, and thoracic aneurysm.

Diagnosis is by dark-field microscopy (primary or secondary) or serologic testing. The CDC provides treatment protocol for different populations.

Treatment includes:
- Primary, secondary, early tertiary: benzathine penicillin G 104 million units IM in 1 dose.
- Tertiary: benzathine penicillin G 2.4 million units IM weekly for 3 weeks.

Gonorrhea

Gonorrhea is caused by *Neisseria gonorrhoeae* and should be suspected with urinary infections. Symptoms include:
- Males: Dysuria and purulent discharge from the urethra, ependymitis, and prostatitis.
- Females: Many women are asymptomatic or may have lower abdominal pain, cystitis, or mucopurulent cervicitis, but untreated it can result in PID and chronic pain.

Rectal infections are common in women and homosexual males. Untreated, gonorrhea can become a systemic infection, resulting in petechial or pustular skin lesions, arthralgias, tenosynovitis, fever and malaise, and septic arthritis.

Diagnosis is by cervical or urethral culture or NAAT. Gram stains of urethral smears are more accurate for males than females. Cultures of multiple sites may be needed to confirm disseminated disease.

Treatment includes dual therapy:
- Ceftriaxone 250 mg IM in 1 dose AND azithromycin 1 g orally in 1 dose **OR**
- Ceftriaxone 250 mg IM in 1 dose AND doxycycline 100 mg twice daily for seven days

Genitourinary trauma

Genitourinary trauma may result from accidents or other force. Trauma of the vagina from vigorous consensual sex usually involves minor injuries to the posterior vaginal fornix. However, injuries related to sexual assault may be more severe, and bruising, tenderness, and lacerations should be plotted on a body diagram. Urethral injuries occur primarily in males, often indicated by blood at the meatus.

Blunt trauma, such as those that may occur with auto accidents or assault, may result in genitourinary trauma, with the kidneys and bladder the most common sites of injury. Hematuria is the most common indication of injury to the genitourinary tract but the amount of bleeding does not always correlate with injury in adults but does in children. Diagnostic studies depend on the suspected site of injury and are usually done if greater than 50 RBC/hpf, especially in children:
- Urethra: Retrograde urethrogram or cystogram.
- Kidney, ureter: CT with contrast.
- Bladder: Retrograde cystogram or CT retrograde cystogram.
- Venous injuries: Angiogram/venogram.
- Kidney pelvis: Retrograde pyelogram.

Assessment of rape and sexual abuse victims

Rape and sexual abuse victims (both male and female) should be treated sensitively and questioned privately. Examination should include:
- Assault history that includes what happened, when, where, and by whom. Questioning should determine if there is a possibility of drug-induced amnesia or activities, such as douching or showering, which might have destroyed evidence.
- Medical history to determine if there is a risk of pregnancy and when and if the last consensual sex occurred that might interfere with laboratory findings.
- Physical examination should include examination of the genitals, rectum, and mouth. The body should be examined for bruising or other injuries. Toluidine dye should be applied to the perineum before insertion of a speculum into the vagina to detect small vulvar lacerations.

Forensic evidence must be collected within 72 hours and requires informed consent and the use of a rape kit. Forensic evidence includes:
- Victim samples for control.
- Assailant-identifying samples
- Evidence of sexual activity.
- Evidence of force or coercion.

Nausea, vomiting, and HG during pregnancy

About 60% to 80% of pregnant woman suffer from nausea and vomiting (NV), especially during the first trimester, but only about 2% suffer severe (sometimes intractable) nausea and vomiting, known as hyperemesis gravidarum (HG), associated with weight loss, dehydration, hypokalemia, or ketonemia. Nausea and vomiting may be associated with numerous disorders, including cholelithiasis, pancreatitis, hepatitis, and ectopic pregnancy, especially when accompanied by abdominal pain. Diagnosis includes:
- Physical examination to rule out other disorders.
- CBC with serum electrolytes, BUN, creatinine, and urinalysis.
- Ketonuria is an indication of inadequate nutrition.

Treatment includes:
- IV fluids with glucose 5% in normal saline or Ringer's lactate.
- Oral fluids after nausea and vomiting controlled.
- Antiemetic drugs
- Acute treatment for NV and HG: promethazine, prochlorperazine, or chlorpromazine.
- Maintenance for NV: Doxylamine with pyridoxine, diphenhydramine, or cisapride.
- Maintenance for HG: Metoclopramide, trimethobenzamide, or ondansetron.

> ➤ **Review Video:** Nausea and Vomiting
> *Visit **mometrix.com/academy** and enter Code:* **631968**

Vaginal bleeding and abortion

Vaginal bleeding during the first trimester of pregnancy may indicate spontaneous abortion, ectopic pregnancy, gestational trophoblastic disease, or infection. All women of childbearing age with an intact uterus presenting with abdominal pain or vaginal bleeding should be assessed for pregnancy.

Abortion classifications:
- Threatened: Vaginal bleeding during first half of pregnancy without cervical dilatation.
- Inevitable: Vaginal bleeding with cervical dilatation.
- Incomplete: Incomplete loss of products of conception, usually between 6 and 14 weeks.
- Complete: Complete loss of products of conception, before 20 weeks.
- Missed: Death of fetus before 20 weeks without loss of products of conception within 4 weeks.
- Septic: Infection with abortion.

Diagnostic tests include:
- Pelvic examination. CBC, Rh factor, antibody screen, urinalysis, quantitative serum beta-hCG level.
- Ultrasound to rule out ectopic pregnancy.

Treatment includes:
- Suctioning of vaginal vault with Yankauer suction tip with pathologic examination of tissue. Evacuation of uterus for incomplete abortion.
- *RhoGAM* (50 to 150 mcg) for bleeding in unsensitized Rh-negative women.

Abruptio placenta and placenta previa

Abruptio placenta occurs when the placenta separates prematurely from the wall of the uterus. Symptoms include:

- Vaginal bleeding.
- Tender uterus with increased resting tone.
- Uterine contractions (hypertonic or hyperactive).
- Nausea and vomiting (in some patients).
- Dizziness.

Complications include fetal distress, hypotension, and disseminated intravascular coagulopathy (DIC), as well as fetal and/or maternal death. Fetal death is common with at least 50% separation.

Diagnosis includes:

- Ultrasound. CBC and type and crossmatch.
- Coagulation studies (50% have coagulopathy).

Treatment includes:

- Gynecological consultation.
- Crystalloids to increase blood volume.
- Fresh frozen plasma for coagulopathy.

Placenta previa occurs when the placenta implants over the cervical opening. Implantation may be complete (covering the entire opening), partial, or marginal (to the edge of the cervical opening). Symptoms include painless bleeding after 20th week of gestation. Diagnosis is per ultrasound. Vaginal examination with digit or speculum should be avoided. The condition may correct itself as the uterus expands, but bed rest may be needed. Emergency cesarean section is done for uncontrolled bleeding.

Hypertensive disorders during the second half of pregnancy

Hypertensive disorders of pregnancy comprise a continuum ranging from mild to severe:

- Hypertension: BP increased to at least 140/90, or 20 mm Hg increase in systolic or 10 mm Hg diastolic. May be chronic or transient without signs of preeclampsia or eclampsia.
- Preeclampsia: Hypertension associated with proteinuria (300 mg per 24 hours) and edema (peripheral or generalized) or increase of at least 5 pounds of weight in 1 week after 20th week of gestation. Severe preeclampsia is BP at least 160/110. Symptoms include headache, abdominal pain, and visual disturbances.
- Eclampsia: Preeclampsia with seizures occurring at 20th week of gestation to 1 month after delivery.
- HELLP syndrome (hemolysis, elevated liver enzymes [AST and ALT], and low platelets [less than 100,000]). Usually accompanied by epigastric or right upper quadrant pain.

Treatments include:

- Chronic hypertension: Methyldopa beginning with 250 mg every 6 hours.
- Preeclampsia, eclampsia, HELLP:
- Delivery of fetus (may be delayed with mild preeclampsia if fewer than 37 weeks gestation).
- Magnesium sulfate 4 to 6 g IV over 15 minutes initially and then 1 to 2 g per hour.
- Antihypertensive drugs.

Ectopic pregnancy

Ectopic pregnancy occurs when the fertilized ovum implants outside the uterus in an ovary, fallopian tube (the most common site), peritoneal cavity, or cervix. Early symptoms may include:
- Indications of pregnancy: amenorrhea, breast tenderness, nausea and vomiting. Positive Chadwick's sign (blue discoloration of cervix).
- Positive Hegar's sign (softening of isthmus). Bleeding may be the first indication as hormones fluctuate. Hormone hCG present in blood and urine.

Symptoms of rupture include:
- One-sided or generalized abdominal pain.
- Decreased hemoglobin and hematocrit.
- Hypotension with hemorrhage.
- Right shoulder pain because of irritation of the subdiaphragmatic phrenic nerve.

Diagnostic studies include:
- Vaginal exam.
- Pregnancy test.
- Transvaginal sonography (TVS) to rule out intrauterine pregnancy.
- hCG titers (increase more slowly with ectopic pregnancy)
- Progesterone level greater than 22 helps rule out ectopic pregnancy.

Treatments include:
- Methotrexate IM or IV if unruptured and 3.5 cm or less in size to inhibit growth and allow body to expel.
- Laparoscopic linear salpingostomy or salpingectomy.

Preterm labor and PROM

Preterm or premature labor occurs within weeks 20 to 37. Premature rupture of membrane (PROM) occurs when the membranes rupture before the onset of labor, and may lead to premature labor. There are numerous causes for PROM, including infections and digital pelvic exams. When a woman presents in labor, the estimated date of delivery should be obtained by questioning the date of the last menstrual period (LMP) and using a gestation calculator wheel or estimating with Nägele's rule: First day LMP minus 3 months plus 7 days = estimated date of delivery. Fetal viability is very low before 23 weeks of gestation but by 25 weeks, delaying delivery for 2 days can increase survival rates by 10%. Tocolytic drugs, which have many negative side effects, may be used to delay delivery in order to administer glucocorticoids, such as betamethasone or dexamethasone, to improve fetal lung maturity between weeks 24 to 36. Tocolytics include:
- Beta-adrenergics.
- Magnesium sulfates.
- Calcium channel blockers.
- Prostaglandin synthetase inhibitors.

Emergency delivery

Prolapsed umbilical cord, shoulder dystocia, and preterm delivery
Prolapsed umbilical cord occurs when the umbilical cord precedes the presenting fetal part or, in some cases, presents at the same time, so that pressure is applied to the cord, decreasing circulation to the fetus. Decelerations in fetal pulse less than 110 may indicate prolapse. Pulsations may be felt in the cord or may be absent, but relieving pressure on the cord by holding back the presenting part is critical for fetal survival. Oxygen should be administered and fetal heart rate monitored. Infusing the bladder with 350 to 500 mL of fluid (warm normal saline) while pressure is held against the presenting part may lift the fetal head and relieve pressure on the cord. Other methods include placing the woman in the Trendelenburg position or with knees to chest as medical personnel apply continued pressure to the presenting part while awaiting Caesarean section for delivery.

Breech presentation
Emergency delivery may occur when there are complications of pregnancy or a woman is in advanced labor with birth imminent. The delivery may proceed normally, but complications may require immediate intervention: breech presentation (common in premature births) is when the buttocks or lower extremities are the presenting part during delivery.

Types include:
- Complete: knees and hips both flexed with buttocks and feet presenting.
- Frank: hips flexed and knees extended with buttocks presenting.
- Footling or incomplete: hips and legs extended and one or both feet presenting. In some incomplete cases, the knees may present.

Complete and frank breech presentations may often be delivered vaginally as enough pressure is applied to adequately dilate the vagina, but the delivery should be spontaneous with medical staff keeping hands off until the umbilicus presents, then assisting with delivery of the legs and rotating the fetus to the sacrum anterior position and then gently turning to deliver the arms. Incomplete or footling presentations require caesarean sections.

Preterm infants
Emergency delivery often involves preterm infants, whose gestational age may not be clear upon delivery, so initial resuscitative efforts should be carried out until viability is determined. The infant should be dried and warmed immediately, such as by placing in a double-walled heated incubator or under a Plexiglas heat shield in single-walled incubators to prevent heat loss. Radiant warmers and plastic wrap over the infant may also be used. The head and neck must be well supported to prevent blockage of the trachea. A small roll should be placed under the shoulders and the head slightly elevated if child is in supine position, but the prone position splints the chest and decreases respiratory effort. Gentle nasopharyngeal suctioning may be needed to clear secretions. The infant should be evaluated with the Apgar scale and transferred to the neonatal ICU as necessary for further interventions. Apgar score below 4 requires resuscitations (8 to 10 is normal range).

Trauma during pregnancy

Trauma during pregnancy is one of the leading causes of death and injury to pregnant women. Automobile accidents, falls, and assault (often related to domestic abuse) can all result in death of the fetus. Complications of trauma may be uterine rupture, abruption, or uterine irritability, and onset of premature labor. Fetal-maternal hemorrhage may also occur. Direct injury to the fetus is common only in the late stages of pregnancy when blunt abdominal trauma with pelvic fracture

- 90 -

may cause fetal skull fracture or with gunshot wounds. Because fetal survival depends on maternal survival, initial resuscitation efforts are for the mother. After the airway is secured and IV (large bore) access is obtained, volume replacement is provided and any bleeding controlled. When the mother is stabilized, the gestational age of the fetus should be estimated and pelvic exam done. Radiologic exams should be done as indicated. All unsensitized Rh-negative (D-negative) women should receive *RhoGAM*. Tetanus prophylaxis should be given. Fetal assessment should include ultrasound and monitoring of fetal heart rate.

Postpartum hemorrhage

Most postpartum hemorrhage is excessive vaginal bleeding (greater than 500 mL for vaginal and greater than 1,000 mL for Caesarean section) occurring within 24 hours of delivery, related to uterine atony caused by failure of the uterus to contract adequately, uterine rupture or inversion, lacerations, or coagulopathies. It is more common after Caesarean section than vaginal delivery. Hemorrhage may be delayed in some cases, related to retained products of conception, uterine polyps, or coagulopathies. Careful history and examination to determine cause of bleeding is necessary.

Symptoms include:
- Excessive bleeding.
- Hypotension and tachycardia.
- Decreased hematocrit.
- Pain and/or edema in vagina/perineum.

Treatment includes:
- Stabilizing patient.
- Two IV lines (large bore) inserted.
- Laboratory testing for CBC, clotting, and type and crossmatch.
- Vaginal exam with speculum to identify and repair lacerations.
- Oxytocin or methylergonovine maleate for uterine atony.
- Ultrasound to check for retained products of conception.
- Obstetric consultation for uterine inversion (observed as mass in vagina).
- Fresh frozen plasma for coagulopathies.

Newborn resuscitation

Newborn resuscitation is indicated for pulse rate less than 100 or obvious respiratory distress. Resuscitation is common for birth weights less than 1,500 g. Survival is rare at 22 weeks but increases with each week of gestation. Resuscitation includes:
- Maintain body temperature by placing on warm sterile surface.
- Clear airway with gentle suction and evaluate for respirations.
- Initiate positive pressure ventilation with 100% oxygen.
- Suctioning of the trachea if meconium staining associated with depression of the infant.
- Stimulation. (often covered with drying and warming the infant)
- Cardiac massage if heart rate less than 60 bpm, depressing sternum one-third of the distance to the vertebrae (1 ventilation per 3 compressions).

- Insertion of umbilical venous catheter for administration of medications that include:
  - Epinephrine 0.1 to 0.3 mL/kg (1:10,000 solution) IV or 2 to 2.5 times this dose down an endotracheal tube to stimulate heart.
  - Normal saline or Ringer's lactate to expand volume.

Resuscitative efforts may be discontinued after 10 minutes without heartbeat or respiratory effort. Infants that were able to be resuscitated are at risk for the following complications: hypothermia, apnea, seizures, encephalopathy, hypoglycemia, hypotension, pulmonary issues, feeding issues, and electrolyte imbalances.

Psychosocial and Medical Emergencies

Child Abuse

Children rarely admit to being abused and, in fact, deny it and attempt to protect the abusing parent, so the nurse must rely on physical and behavioral signs to determine if there is cause to suspect abuse:

- Behavioral indicators: The child may be overly compliant or fearful with obvious changes in demeanor when a parent/caregiver is present. Some children act out with aggression toward other children or animals. Children may become depressed or suicidal or present with sleeping or eating disorders. Behavior may become increasingly self-destructive as the child ages.
- Physical indicators: The type, location, and extent of injuries can raise suspicion of abuse. Head and facial injuries and bruising are common as are bite or burn marks. There may be hand prints or grab marks, or unusual bruising, such as across the buttocks. Any bruising, swelling, or tearing of the genital area or STDs are cause for concern.

About 5 million cases of suspected child abuse are reported in the United States each year. In accordance with the Child Abuse Prevention and Treatment and Adoption Act Amendments (1996) and the Model Child Protection Act, all states have instituted mandatory reporting of child abuse. The nurse should be knowledgeable about the statutes in the state of practice, but medical personnel are mandatory reporters and must report the following:

- Child abuse or neglect that places the child in risk of harm (physical or emotional), death, or exploitation.
- Sexual abuse, including rape, molestation, prostitution, incest, or coercion to engage in any type of sexually explicit behavior.
- While some statutes mandate reporting of suspicion, others mandate more knowledge; however, there is criminal and civil liability involved if child abuse is not reported and most states provide immunity for reporters, so the best course is to report suspicions to child protective services or the police, according to the state requirements.

Intimate partner violence and abuse

Intimate partner violence and abuse (IPVA) is a pattern of coercive behaviors that can include violent injuries, psychological abuse, sexual assault, stalking, isolation, and threats. Routine screening should be conducted for adolescent and adult women seen in the ED. Signs of IPVA include:

- Abusive injuries: bite marks, cigarette burns, neck bruises, black eyes.
- Defensive injuries: forearm bruises/fractures.
- Central injuries: head, thorax, and abdomen.
- Mismatch between injuries and history.
- Signs of injuries in various states of healing.
- Delayed reporting of injuries.
- Multiple ED visits with various complaints.
- Suicide attempts.
- Unwanted pregnancy or STDs.
- Fear of partner or controlling behavior by partner.

Screening guidelines should be followed carefully and safety assessment completed with documentation, indicating if patient volunteered a statement about abuse. Victim should be supported and validated with referral to IPVA experts. Each state has specific laws that must be followed in related to IPVA, and staff must be aware of these laws and police response.

Elder abuse

The many different types of elder abuse include physical (such a hitting or improperly restraining), sexual, psychological, financial, and neglect. Elder abuse may be difficult to diagnose, especially if the person is cognitively impaired, but symptoms can include fearfulness, disparities in reports of injuries between patient and caregiver, evidence of old or repeated injuries, poor hygiene and dental care, decubital ulcers, malnutrition, undue concern with costs on caregiver's part, unsupportive attitude of caregiver, and caregiver's reluctance or refusal to allow patient to communicate privately with ED staff. Self-abuse can also occur when patients are not able to adequately care for themselves.

Diagnosis of elder abuse includes assessment, and careful history and physical exam, including directly questioning patient about abuse.

Treatment includes attending to injuries or physical needs, which can vary widely, and referral to adult protective services as indicated. Reporting laws regarding elder abuse vary somewhat from one state to another, but all states have laws regarding elder abuse and 42 require mandatory reporting by heath workers.

Neglect

While some children may not be physically or sexually abused, they may suffer from profound neglect or lack of supervision that places them at risk. Indicators include:
- Appearing dirty and unkempt, sometimes with infestations of lice, and wearing ill-fitting torn clothing and shoes.
- Being tired or sleepy during the daytime.
- Having untended medical or dental problems, such as dental caries.
- Missing appointments and not receiving proper immunizations.
- Being underweight for stage of development.

Neglect can be difficult to assess, especially if the ED is serving a homeless or very poor population. Home visits may be needed to ascertain if there is adequate food, clothing, or supervision, and this may be beyond the care provided by the ED. Suspicions should be reported to child protective services so that social workers can assess the home environment.

Panic attacks

Panic attacks are short episodes (peaking in 5 to 10 minutes) of intense anxiety that can result in a wide variety of symptoms that include:
- Dyspnea.
- Palpitations.
- Hyperventilation.
- Nausea and vomiting.

- Intense fear or anxiety.
- Pain and pressure in the chest.
- Dizziness and fainting.
- Tremors

Panic attacks may be associated with agoraphobia, depression, or IPVA, so a careful history is important. Typically, patients believe they are dying or having a heart attack and require reassurance and treatment, such as diazepam or lorazepam, in the ED for the acute episode, In severe cases, ASA may be given and EKG done to rule out cardiac abnormalities. Patients should be referred for psychiatric evaluation for ongoing medications, such as SSRIs (sertraline, paroxetine, fluoxetine), to prevent recurrence. Panic attacks become chronic panic disorders if they are recurrent followed by at least a month of fear of another attack.

Bereavement

Bereavement occurs after the death of family, friend, or someone to whom a person identifies closely. It is a time of mourning and is part of the natural grieving process, but some people are not able to move past the grieving process and may suffer signs related to depression, such as poor appetite, insomnia, and other symptoms, such as chest pain, that may mimic physical illnesses. Some may enter a stage of denial or anger that interferes with their daily activities and work. People suffering bereavement may present in the ED with vague and varied complaints. A careful history is important. Treatment varies according to the needs of the individual. In some cases, SSRIs (such as fluoxetine) may provide temporary relief, but the patient should be referred for psychological counseling, bereavement services, or psychiatric care, depending upon the severity of symptoms.

Bipolar disorder

Bipolar disorder causes severe mood swings between hyperactive states and depression, accompanied by impaired judgment because of distorted thoughts. The hypomanic stage may allow for creativity and good functioning in some people, but it can develop into more severe mania, which may be associated with psychosis and hallucinations with rapid speech and bizarre behavior, and then into periods of profound depression. While most cases are diagnosed in late adolescence, there is increasing evidence that some children present with symptoms earlier; especially at risk are children with a bipolar parent. Bipolar disorder is associated with high rates of suicide, so early diagnosis and treatment is critical. Symptoms may be relatively mild or involve severe rapid cycling between mania and depression.

Treatment includes both medications (usually given continually) to prevent cycling and control depression, and psychosocial therapy, such as cognitive therapy, to help control disordered thought patterns and behavior. Psychiatric referral should be made.

Eating disorders

Anorexia nervosa

Eating disorders are a profound health risk and can lead to death, especially for adolescent girls, although boys also have eating disorders, often presenting as excessive exercise. Anorexia nervosa is characterized by profound fear of weight gain and severe restriction of food intake, often accompanied by abuse of diuretics and laxatives, which can cause electrolyte imbalances as well as kidney and bowel disorders and delay or cessation of menses. Symptoms include growth retardation, amenorrhea (missing 3 consecutive periods), unexplained and sometimes precipitous weight loss (at least 15% below normal weight), dehydration, loss of appetite, hypoglycemia, hypercholesterolemia, or carotenemia with yellowing of skin, emaciated appearance, osteoporosis, bradycardia, and food obsessions and rituals. Diagnosis includes complete history, physical, and psychological exam with CBC and chemical panels to rule out other disorders. Treatment includes volume and electrolyte replacement initially with referral to psychiatric care for long-term management of the disorder and nutritional plans

Bulimia nervosa
Bulimia nervosa includes binge eating followed by vomiting (at least 2 times monthly for at least 3 months), often along with diuretics, enemas, and laxatives. Some may engage in periods of fasting or excessive exercise rather than vomiting to offset the effects of binging. Gastric acids from purging can damage the throat and teeth. While bulimics may maintain a normal weight, they are at risk for severe electrolyte imbalances that can be life-threatening. Binge eating affects 2% to 5% of females and includes grossly overeating, often resulting in obesity, depression, and shame.

Symptoms include hypokalemia, metabolic acidosis, fluctuations of weight, dental caries and loss of enamel, knuckle scars (from contact with teeth while inducing vomiting), parotid and submandibular gland enlargement, and insulin-dependent diabetes.

Diagnosis includes complete history, physical, and psychological exam with CBC and chemical panels to rule out other disorders.

Treatment includes volume and electrolyte replacement initially with referral to psychiatric care for long-term management of the disorder and nutritional plans, as well as SSRIs, naltrexone, and ondansetron.

Management of patients with violent behavior

Patients may exhibit violent behavior for a number of reasons, including metabolic disorders (hypoglycemia), neurological disorders (brain tumor), psychiatric disorders (schizophrenia), or substance abuse (drugs and alcohol). Patients who make threats or have a history of violent behavior should be approached with caution. Diagnosis includes history, physical exam, CBC and chemistry panel, toxicology screening, ECG, and, in some cases, CT scans or lumbar punctures. Violent behavior tends to escalate from anxiety to defensiveness to aggression, so identifying these signs and providing support through information, setting limits, using restraints, and seclusion can avoid injuries. Handcuffs should not be removed in the ED, and patients who are so violent they must be restrained should not be allowed to leave the ED against medical advice.

Medical treatment includes:
- Antipsychotic drugs: haloperidol 5 mg IM (1 to 2 mg for elderly patients).
- Benzodiazepines: Lorazepam 2 to 4 mg IM/IV (often in conjunction with antipsychotic drugs).
- Hypnotics: Droperidol 2.5 mg IM/IV.

Mental status

Assessment of mental status helps to differentiate between functional and organic disorders. The patient should be questioned and observed carefully. Areas of assessment include:
- Behavior, including spontaneous or abnormal behavior.
- Affect appropriateness.
- Orientation to place, time, person, and events.
- Language comprehension.
- Memory recall of historical, recent, and current events.
- Ability to concentrate.
- Level of consciousness.
- Disordered thought processes, such as paranoia, delusions, threats of violence or suicide.
- Sensory, including visual hallucinations (usually a sign of organic disease).
- Neurological exam.
- Physical examination, including assessment of the head for trauma.
- Laboratory tests, including toxicology and blood alcohol levels, and referral to appropriate clinical specialists, such as neurosurgeons, internists, or psychiatrists, may be indicated depending upon the outcome of the mental status assessment.

Those who pose a danger to themselves or others should be hospitalized for further testing and treatment.

Shaken baby/shaken impact syndrome

Shaken baby syndrome is believed to be the result of vigorous shaking of an infant, causing acute subdural hematoma with subarachnoid and retinal hemorrhages. It is believed that the shaking of the brain causes coup and contrecoup damage, as well as damaging vessels and nerves with resultant cerebral edema. Some authorities, however, believe that the extent of injuries typically seen with these infants precludes just shaking and that they must also suffer blunt impact, as the injuries are more compatible with the head striking against a solid surface with great force, so the newer terminology is shaken impact syndrome, which includes shaking AND impact. Symptoms include:
- Mortality rate of about 50%.
- Severe residual problems that may include vision and hearing defects, seizures, intellectual disability or impaired cognition, paralysis, or coma.
- Sometimes children may not exhibit obvious neurological symptoms immediately after trauma but have learning disabilities and behavioral disorders that appear in school.

Treatment includes:
- Stabilizing patient.
- Neurosurgical consult.

Suicidal patients

Patients may attempt suicide for many reasons, including severe depression, social isolation, situational crisis, bereavement, or psychotic disorder (schizophrenia). Suicidal patients should be referred for psychiatric evaluation. If a person attempts suicide, he/she should be hospitalized and assessed for continued risk after initial treatment, which depends upon the type of suicide attempt.

Suicidal indications include:
- Depression or dysphoria.
- Hostility to others.
- Problems with peer relationships, and lack of close friends.
- Post-crisis stress (divorce, death in family, graduation, college).
- Withdrawn personality,
- Quiet, lonely appearance, behavior.
- Change in behavior (drop in grades, wearing black clothes, unkempt appearance, sleeping excessively, or not sleeping).
- Co-morbid psychiatric problems (bipolar, schizophrenia).
- Drug abuse.

Risks for repeat attempt include:
- Violent suicide attempt (knives, gunshots).
- Suicide attempt with low chance of rescue.
- Ongoing psychosis or disordered thinking.
- Ongoing severe depression and feeling of helplessness.
- History of previous suicide attempts.
- Lack of social support system.

Acute latex sensitivity

Latex sensitivity is increasing in frequency, especially among those who are exposed to latex regularly through work, such as rubber industry workers, or who have repeated contact with the health care system. Children with myelomeningocele have a high incidence. Latex sensitivity may manifest as 3 different types of reactions:
- Irritant (nonimmune): erythematous irritation from contact.
- Contact dermatitis (type 4): dry erythema beyond area of contact with pruritus, weeping, and blistering, and results from chemicals (thiurams and thiazoles) used in production of latex.
- IgE (type I) (immune reaction): Response to proteins in latex with urticaria, rhinitis, angioedema, asthma, laryngeal edema, anaphylactic shock, and death.

Treatment for type I reaction includes:
- Establish patent airway and intubate if necessary for ventilation.
- High-flow oxygen (100%).
- Monitor vital signs.
- Administer epinephrine autoinjector or solution.
- Albuterol per nebulizer for bronchospasm.
- IV fluids to provide bolus of fluids for hypotension.
- Diphenhydramine if shock persists.
- Methylprednisolone if no response to other drugs.

DIC

Disseminated intravascular coagulation (DIC) (consumption coagulopathy) is a secondary disorder that is triggered by another, such as trauma, congenital heart disease, necrotizing enterocolitis, sepsis, and severe viral infections. DIC triggers both coagulation and hemorrhage through a complex series of events that includes trauma that causes tissue factor (transmembrane glycoprotein) to enter the circulation and bind with coagulation factors, triggering the coagulation cascade. This stimulates thrombin to convert fibrinogen to fibrin, causing aggregation and destruction of platelets and forming clots that can be disseminated throughout the intravascular system. These clots increase in size as platelets adhere to the clots, causing blockage of both the microvascular systems and larger vessels, and this can result in ischemia and necrosis. Clot formation triggers fibrinolysis and plasmin to breakdown fibrin and fibrinogen, causing destruction of clotting factors, resulting in hemorrhage. Both processes, clotting and hemorrhage, continue at the same time, placing the patient at high risk for death, even with treatment.

The onset of symptoms of DIC may be very rapid or a slower chronic progression from a disease. Those who develop the chronic manifestation of the disease usually have fewer acute symptoms and may slowly develop ecchymosis or bleeding wounds. Symptoms include:
- Bleeding from surgical or venous puncture sites.
- Evidence of GI bleeding with distention, bloody diarrhea.
- Hypotension and acute symptoms of shock.
- Petechiae and purpura with extensive bleeding into the tissues.
- Laboratory abnormalities:
  ○ Prolonged prothrombin and partial prothrombin times.
  ○ Decreased platelet counts and fragmented RBCs.
  ○ Decreased fibrinogen.

Treatment includes:
- Identifying and treating underlying cause.
- Replacement blood products, such as platelets and fresh frozen plasma.
- Anticoagulation therapy (heparin) to increase clotting time.
- Cryoprecipitate to increase fibrinogen levels.
- Coagulation inhibitors and coagulation factors.

Autotransfusion

Autotransfusion (autologous blood transfusion) is collecting of the patient's blood and re-infusing it. This is life-saving if other donor blood is not available. Blood in trauma cases is usually collected from a body cavity, such as pleural (hemothorax with $\geq$1500 mL blood) or peritoneal space (rare). Autotransfusion is contraindicated if malignant lesions are present in area of blood loss, contamination of pooled blood, or wounds >4-6 hours old. Commercial collection/transfusion kits (Pleur-Evac®, Thora-Klex®) are available but blood can be collected through the chest tube into a sterile bottle, which is then disconnected and connected to IV tubing for infusion, **OR** the blood in the bottle may be transferred to a blood collection bag for use. Commercial kits use either a chest tube or suction tube to withdraw blood and provide specific procedures. Blood is filtered. Heparin is not routinely used but citrate phosphate dextrose (CPD) (25-70 mL/500 mL blood) is often added to the aspirant to prevent clotting. Complications from autotransfusion are rare.

IO infusion

Intraosseous (IO) infusion is an alternative to IV access for neonates, pediatric emergencies, and adult emergencies when rapid temporary access is necessary or when peripheral or vascular access cannot be achieved. It is often used in pediatric cardiac arrest. Because yellow marrow replaces red marrow, access in those older than 5 is more difficult.

Preferred sites include:
- 0 to 5: proximal tibia (preferred).
- Older children and adults: medial malleolus. The sternum can support higher infusion rates.
- Other sites include the distal femur, clavicle, humerus, and ileum.

IO infusion is used to administer fluids and anesthesia and to obtain blood samples. Equipment requires a special needle (13 to 20 gauge) as standard needles may bend. The bone injection gun (BIG) with a loaded spring facilitates insertion. The First Access for Shock and Trauma (FAST) needle is intended for use in the sternum of adults and prevents accidental puncture of the thoracic cavity. Knowledge of bony landmarks and correct insertion angle and site are important. Position is confirmed by aspiration of 5 to 10 mL of blood and marrow before infusion.

Acute adrenal insufficiency

Acute adrenal insufficiency (adrenal crisis) is a sudden, life-threatening condition resulting from an exacerbation of primary chronic adrenal insufficiency (Addison's disease), often precipitated by sepsis, surgical stress, adrenal hemorrhage related to septicemia, anticoagulation complications, and cortisone withdrawal related to decreased dose or inadequate dose to compensate for stress. Acute adrenal insufficiency may occur in those who do not have Addison's disease, such as those who have received cortisone for various reasons, usually a minimum of 20 mg daily for at least 5 days. Symptoms include:
- Fever
- Nausea and vomiting.
- Abdominal pain.
- Weakness and general fatigue.
- Disorientation, confusion.
- Hypotensive shock.
- Dehydration.
- Electrolyte imbalance with hyperkalemia, hypercalcemia, hypoglycemia and hyponatremia.

Treatment includes:
- IV fluids in large volume
- Glucocorticoid
- 50% dextrose if indicated (hypoglycemia)
- Mineralocorticoid may be needed after intravenous solutions.
- The precipitating cause must be identified and treated as well.

SIADH

Syndrome of inappropriate secretion of antidiuretic hormone (SIADH) is related to hypersecretion of the posterior pituitary gland. This causes the kidneys to reabsorb fluids, resulting in fluid retention, and triggers a decrease in sodium levels (dilutional hyponatremia), resulting in production of only concentrated urine. This syndrome may result from central nervous systems disorders, such as brain trauma, surgery, or tumors. It may also be triggered by other disorders, such as tumors of various organs, pneumothorax, acute pneumonia, and other lung disorders. Some medications (vincristine, phenothiazines, tricyclic antidepressants, and thiazide diuretics) may also trigger SIADH.

Symptoms include:
- Anorexia with nausea and vomiting
- Irritability
- Stomach cramps
- Alterations of personality.
- Increasing neurological dysfunction, including stupor and seizures, related to progressive sodium depletion.

Treatment includes:
- Identifying and treating underlying cause. (d/c causative drug)
- Urine specific gravity
- Correct fluid volume excess and electrolytes
- Monitor UOP
- Seizure precautions

With SIADH expect low serum sodium and serum osmolality with high urine osmolality.

Addison disease

Adrenocortical insufficiency (Addison disease) is caused by damage to the adrenal cortex. It is related to a variety of causes, such as autoimmune disease or genetic disorders, but it may relate to destructive lesions or neoplasms. Without treatment, the condition is life-threatening. Symptoms may be vague and the condition undiagnosed until 80% to 90% of the adrenal cortex has been destroyed:
- Chronic weakness and fatigue.
- Abdominal distress with nausea and vomiting.
- Salt or licorice craving, resulting from deficiency of aldosterone.
- Pigmentary changes in skin and mucous membranes, hyperpigmentation.
- Hypotension.
- Hypoglycemia.
- Recurrent seizures (more common in children).

Treatment:
- Hormone replacement therapy with glucocorticoids (cortisol) and mineralocorticoids (aldosterone) may be taken orally or monthly parenteral injections or subcutaneous implantation of desoxycorticosterone acetate every 9 to 12 months.
- During times of stress or illness, the demand for glucocorticoids may increase and dosages up to 3 times the normal dosage may be needed to prevent an acute crisis.

> **Review Video:** Addison's Disease
> *Visit **mometrix.com/academy** and enter **Code:** 813552*

Hyperthyroidism

Hyperthyroidism (thyrotoxicosis) usually results from excess production of thyroid hormones (Graves' disease) from immunoglobulins providing abnormal stimulation of the thyroid gland. Other causes include thyroiditis and excess thyroid medications. Symptoms include:
- Hyperexcitability
- Tachycardia (90-160) and atrial fibrillation.
- Increased systolic (but not diastolic) BP.
- Poor heat tolerance, skin flushed and diaphoretic.
- Dry skin and pruritus (especially in the elderly).
- Hand tremor, progressive muscular weakness.
- Exophthalmos (bulging eyes).
- Increased appetite and intake but weight loss.

Treatment includes:
- Radioactive iodine to destroy the thyroid gland. Propranolol may be used to prevent thyroid storm. Thyroid hormones are given for resultant hypothyroidism.
- Antithyroid medications, such as Propacil® or Tapazole® to block conversion of T4 to T3.
- Surgical removal of thyroid is used if patients cannot tolerate other treatments or in special circumstances, such as large goiter. Usually one-sixth of the thyroid is left in place and antithyroid medications are given before surgery.

> **Review Video:** 7 Symptoms of Hyperthyroidism
> *Visit **mometrix.com/academy** and enter Code:* **923159**

> **Review Video:** Grave's Disease
> *Visit **mometrix.com/academy** and enter Code:* **516665**

> **Review Video:** Thyroid and Antithyroid
> *Visit **mometrix.com/academy** and enter Code:* **666133**

Thyrotoxic storm

Thyrotoxic storm is a severe type of hyperthyroidism with sudden onset, precipitated by stress, such as injury or surgery, in those un-treated or inadequately treated for hyperthyroidism. If not promptly diagnosed and treated, it is fatal. Incidence has decreased with the use of antithyroid medications but can still occur with medical emer-gencies or pregnancy. Diagnostic findings are similar to hyper-thyroidism, and include increased T3 uptake and decreased TSH.

Symptoms include:
- Increase in symptoms of hyperthyroidism.
- Increased temperature >38.5°C.
- Tachycardia >130 with atrial fibrillation and heart failure.
- Gastrointestinal disorders, such as nausea, vomiting, diarrhea, and abdominal discomfort.
- Altered mental status with delirium progressing to coma.

Treatment includes:
- Controlling production of thyroid hormone through antithyroid medications, such as propylthiouracil and methimazole.
- Inhibiting release of thyroid hormone with iodine therapy (or lithium).
- Controlling peripheral activity of thyroid hormone with propranolol.
- Fluid and electrolyte replacement.
- Glucocorticoids, such as dexamethasone.
- Cooling blankets.
- Treatment of arrhythmias as needed with antiarrhythmics and anticoagulation.

Hypothyroidism

Hypothyroidism occurs when the thyroid produces inadequate levels of thyroid hormones. Conditions may range from mild to severe myxedema. There are a number of causes:
- Chronic lymphocytic thyroiditis (Hashimoto's thyroiditis).
- Excessive treatment for hyperthyroidism
- Atrophy of thyroid.
- Medications, such as lithium, iodine compounds
- Radiation to the area of the thyroid.
- Diseases that affect the thyroid, such as scleroderma
- Iodine imbalances.

Symptoms may include chronic fatigue, menstrual disturbances, hoarseness, subnormal temperature, low pulse rate, weight gain, thinning hair, thickening skin. Some dementia may occur with advanced conditions. Clinical findings may include increased cholesterol with associated atherosclerosis and coronary artery disease. Myxedema may be characterized by changes in respiration with hypoventilation and CO_2 retention resulting in coma. Treatment involves hormone replacement with synthetic levothyroxine (Synthroid®) based on TSH levels, but this increases the oxygen demand of the body, so careful monitoring of cardiac status must be done during early treatment to avoid myocardial infarction while reaching euthyroid (normal) level.

Febrile seizure

Febrile seizure is a generalized seizure associated with fever (usually more than 38.8°C [101.8°F]) from any type of infection (upper respiratory tract, urinary) but without intracranial infection or other cause, occurring between 6 months and 5 years of age. Careful clinical examination must be conducted to rule out more serious disorders. Laboratory tests are conducted in relation to symptoms. Lumbar puncture is not usually indicated unless intracranial infection is suspected. Seizures usually last less than 15 minutes and are without subsequent neurological deficit.

Treatment includes:
- Fever control: acetaminophen 10 to 15 mg/kg every 4 hours **OR** ibuprofen 10 mg/kg every 6 to 8 hours.
- Tepid water bath (NOT alcohol).
- Repeat seizures or history of febrile seizures: Phenobarbital 15 mg/kg IV and 4 to 6 mg/kg each day until improvement.
- Antiepileptic drugs (AEDs) are usually not advised unless seizures are complex, child is younger than 6 months, or there is a preexisting neurological disorder: diazepam 0.2 to 0.5 mg/kg every 8 hours during fever. (May cause lethargy.)

- 103 -

Fibromyalgia

Fibromyalgia is a complex syndrome of disorders that include fatigue, chronic generalized muscle pain, and focal areas of tenderness persisting for at least 3 months. The cause of fibromyalgia is not clear and has only recently been recognized as a distinct disorder. Diagnosis is by clinical exam and ruling out joint and muscle inflammation that could be cause of the pain. On clinical exam there are specific tender points usually at multiple areas. Symptoms include:

- Fatigue.
- Pain and stiffness unresponsive to treatment, persisting for months.
- Sleep disorders.
- Irritable bowel syndrome.
- Stiffness in neck and shoulders associated with headache and pain in face.
- Sensitivity to odor, noises, and lights.
- Mood disorders, such as depression, anxiety.
- Dysmenorrhea.
- Paresthesia in hands and feet.

Treatment includes:
- Analgesia: acetaminophen, tramadol, or NSAIDs.
- Antidepressants, such as amitriptyline, nortriptyline, or fluoxetine. Duloxetine and venlafaxine have been shown to reduce pain.
- Antiseizure medication: Pregabalin is the first FDA-approved treatment for the pain of fibromyalgia.
- Referral for physical therapy and/or cognitive therapy.

Diabetes mellitus

Diabetes mellitus, often simply referred to as diabetes, is a group of metabolic diseases which are characterized by dysfunctional use or production of insulin, resulting in elevated blood glucose levels. Diabetes mellitus is the most common metabolic disorder in children, affecting about 1.5 million children and adolescents with 70% to 85% with type I and the rest with type II. The peak age of onset for both types is 10 to 12 in girls and 12 to 14 in boys.

Type I: Immune-mediated form with insufficient insulin production because of destruction of pancreatic beta cells.
- Symptoms include:
  - Pronounced polyuria and polydipsia.
  - Short onset.
  - May be overweight, or have recent weight loss.
  - Ketoacidosis present on diagnosis.
- Treatment:
  - Insulin as needed to control blood sugars.
  - Glucose monitoring 1 to 4 times daily.
  - Diet control with carbohydrate control.
  - Exercise.

Type II: Insulin-resistant form with defect in insulin secretion.
- Symptoms include:
  - Long onset.
  - Obese with no weight loss or significant weight loss.
  - Mild or absent polyuria and polydipsia.
  - May have ketoacidosis or glycosuria without ketonuria.
  - Androgen-mediated problems such a hirsutism and acne.
  - Hypertension.
- Treatment:
  - Oral medications or insulin to control blood sugars.
  - Glucose monitoring.
  - Diet control with carbohydrate control.
  - Exercise.

DKA

Diabetic ketoacidosis (DKA) is a complication of diabetes mellitus. Inadequate production of insulin results in glucose being unavailable for metabolism, so lipolysis (breakdown of fat) produces free fatty acids (FFAs) as an alternate fuel source. Glycerol in both fat cells and the liver is converted to ketone bodies (beta-hydroxybutyric acid, acetoacetic acid, and acetone), which are used for cellular metabolism less efficiently than glucose. Excess ketone bodies are excreted in the urine (ketonuria) or exhalations. The ketone bodies lower serum pH, leading to ketoacidosis. Symptoms include:
- Kussmaul respirations: hyperventilation to eliminate buildup of carbon dioxide, associated with "ketone breath."
- Fluid imbalance, including loss of potassium and other electrolytes from cellular death, resulting in dehydration and diuresis with excess thirst.
- Cardiac arrhythmias, related to potassium loss, can lead to cardiac arrest.
- Hyperglycemia, with glucose levels above normal. Normal values:
  - Neonate: 40 to 60 mg/dL.
  - Younger than 12 months: 50 to 90 mg/dL.
  - Older than 12 months: 60 to 100 mg/dL.

Treatment includes:
- Insulin therapy by continuous infusion initially.
- Electrolyte replacement.

HHS

Hyperosmolar hyperglycemic state (HHS, also known as nonketotic hyperglycemia) occurs in people without history of diabetes or with mild type 2 diabetes but with insulin resistance resulting in persistent hyperglycemia, which causes osmotic diuresis. Fluid shift from intracellular to extracellular spaces to maintain osmotic equilibrium, but the increased glucosuria and dehydration results in hypernatremia and increased osmolarity. This condition is most common in those 50-70 years old and often is precipitated by an acute illness, such as a stroke, medications such as thiazides, or dialysis treatments. HNNS differs from ketoacidosis because, while the insulin level is not adequate, it is high enough to prevent the breakdown of fat. Onset of symptoms often occurs over a few days. Symptoms include:
- Polyuria.
- Dehydration.

- Hypotension & Tachycardia.
- Blood glucose: >600 mg/dL.
- Serum osmolality >350 mOsm/L
- Increased BUN and creatinine
- Changes in mental status, seizures, hemiparesis.

Treatment is similar to that for ketoacidosis:
- Insulin
- Intravenous fluids and electrolytes.
- Correct blood glucose and other labs.

Expect increased serum sodium, serum osmolality and urine osmolality.

Acute hypoglycemia

Acute hypoglycemia (hyperinsulinism) may result from pancreatic islet tumors or hyperplasia, increasing insulin production, or from the use of insulin to control diabetes mellitus. Hyperinsulinism can cause damage to the central nervous and cardiopulmonary systems, interfering with functioning of the brain and causing neurological impairment. Causes may include:
- Genetic defects in chromosome 11 (short arm)
- Severe infections, such as Gram-negative sepsis, endotoxic shock.
- Toxic ingestion of alcohol or drugs, such as salicylates.
- Too much insulin for body needs.
- Too little food or excessive exercise.

Symptoms include:
- Blood glucose <50-60 mg/dL.
- Central nervous system: seizures, altered consciousness, lethargy, and poor feeding with vomiting, myoclonus, respiratory distress, diaphoresis, hypothermia, and cyanosis.
- Adrenergic system: diaphoresis, tremor, tachycardia, palpitation, hunger, and anxiety.

Treatment depends on underlying cause and includes:
- Glucose/Glucagon administration to elevate blood glucose levels.
- Diazoxide (Hyperstat®) to inhibit release of insulin.
- Somatostatin (Sandostatin®) to suppress insulin production.
- Careful monitoring.

ATN

Acute tubular necrosis (ATN) occurs when a hypoxic condition causes renal ischemia that damages tubular cells of the glomeruli so they are unable to adequately filter the urine, leading to acute renal failure. Causes include hypotension, hyperbilirubinemia, sepsis, surgery (especially cardiac or vascular), and birth complications. ATN may result from nephrotoxic injury related to obstruction or drugs, such as chemotherapy, acyclovir, and antibiotics, such as sulfonamides and streptomycin. Symptoms may be non-specific initially and can include life-threatening complications. Symptoms include:
- Lethargy.
- Nausea and vomiting.
- Hypovolemia with low cardiac output and generalized vasodilation.

- Fluid and electrolyte imbalance leading to hypertension, CNS abnormalities, metabolic acidosis, arrhythmias, edema, and congestive heart failure.
- Uremia leading to destruction of platelets and bleeding, neurological deficits, and disseminated intravascular coagulopathy (DIC).
- Infections such as pericarditis and sepsis.

Treatment includes:
- Identifying and treating underlying cause, discontinuing nephrotoxic agents.
- Supportive care.
- Loop diuretics (in some cases), such as Lasix®.
- Antibiotics for infection (can include pericarditis and sepsis).
- Kidney dialysis.

Hemodialysis arteriovenous fistula

The arteriovenous fistula is the preferred type of vascular access for long-term hemodialysis. The fistula is created by surgically connecting and artery and vein, most commonly the radial-cephalic (Brescia-Comino forearm fistula), although the brachial-cephalic may be used. The venous portion dilates and hypertrophies over time so it can be used for repeated treatments. The fistula should be used only for hemodialysis except in cases of severe emergency. Access procedure:
- Ascertain patency by auscultating the fistula to ascertain bruit and palpate for thrill over anastomosis site.
- Cleanse tissue with povidone-iodine.
- Choose the smallest needle necessary and puncture 1 to 2 cm from anastomosis on venous side. Two needles are inserted for dialysis. The distal needle is to draw blood into the hemodialysis machine and the proximal needle returns blood.
- Apply local pressure for 5 minutes after removal of needle.

Anemia

Anemia results in a decrease in oxygen transportation and decreased perfusion throughout the body, causing the heart to compensate by increasing cardiac output. As the blood becomes less viscous, there is decreased peripheral resistance, so more blood is pumped to the heart, and this increased flow can cause turbulence that results in a heart murmur and, if severe or prolonged, heart failure. Anemia is commonly caused by hemorrhage, hemolysis, hematopoiesis, or dietary iron deficiency in women who are menstruating. Children can tolerate low oxygen levels better than adults; however, growth and sexual development may be delayed with chronic anemia.

Symptoms include:
- General malaise and weakness, poor feeding/anorexia.
- Pallor, shortness of breath on exertion.
- Headache, dizziness, apathy, depression, decreased attention span, slowed thought processes.
- Shock symptoms (with severe blood loss): tachycardia, hypotension, poor peripheral circulation, and pallor.

Treatment:

- Treatment of underlying cause.
- Blood or blood components as indicated.
- Supportive care: oxygen, IV fluids.
- Referral for splenectomy (hemolytic anemias).

Sickle cell disease

Sickle cell disease is a recessive genetic disorder of chromosome 11, causing hemoglobin to be defective so that red blood cells (RBCs) are sickle-shaped and inflexible, resulting in their accumulating in small vessels and causing painful blockage. While normal RBCs survive 120 days, sickled cells may survive only 10 to 20 days, stressing the bone marrow that cannot produce fast enough and resulting in severe anemia. There are 5 variations of sickle cell disease, with sickle cell anemia the most severe. Different types of crises occur (aplastic, hemolytic, vaso-occlusive, and sequestrating), which cause infarctions in organs, severe pain, damage to organs, and rapid enlargement of liver and spleen Complications include anemia, acute chest syndrome, congestive heart failure, strokes, delayed growth, infections, pulmonary hypertension, liver and kidney disorders, retinopathy, seizures, and osteonecrosis. Sickle cell disease occurs almost exclusively in African Americans in the United States, with 8% to 10% carriers. Treatment for sickle cell disease includes:

- Prophylactic penicillin for children from 2 months to 5 years to prevent pneumonia.
- IV fluids to prevent dehydration.
- Analgesics (morphine) during painful crises.
- Folic acid for anemia.
- Oxygen for congestive heart failure or pulmonary disease.
- Blood transfusions with chelation therapy to remove excess iron **OR** erythropheresis, in which red cells are removed and replaced with healthy cells, either autologous or from a donor.
- Hematopoietic stem cells transplantation is the only curative treatment, but immunosuppressive drugs must be used and success rates are only about 85%, so the procedure is only used on those at high risk. It requires ablation of bone marrow, placing the patient at increased risk.
- Partial chimerism uses a mixture of the donor and the recipient's bone marrow stem cells and does not require ablation of bone marrow. It is showing good success.

> ➤ **Review Video:** Sickle Cell Disease
> *Visit **mometrix.com/academy** and enter **Code: 603869***

Polycythemia vera

Polycythemia vera is a condition in which there is abnormal production of blood cells in the bone marrow. Erythrocytes (red blood cells) are primarily affected. The disease is more common in men older than 40 years. Polycythemia may be primary or secondary, related to conditions causing hypoxia. The blood increases in viscosity, resulting in a number of symptoms:

- Dizziness, headache, weakness, and fatigue.
- Dyspnea, especially when supine.
- Flushing of skin/skin discoloration (blue-tinged)/red lesions.
- Itching after warm bath.
- Left upper abdominal fullness and splenomegaly.

- Phlebitis from blood clots.
- Vision disturbances.
- Complications include stroke, hemorrhage, and heart failure.

Diagnosis includes:
- CBC with differential, chemistry panel, bone marrow biopsy, Vitamin B12 level.
- Red cell mass more than 25% above normal.

Treatment includes:
- Phlebotomy to remove 500 mL (lesser amounts for children) of blood to decrease blood viscosity, repeated weekly until hematocrit stable (less than 45%).
- Referral for chemotherapy to suppress marrow production: hydroxyurea.
- Interferon to decrease need for phlebotomy.

Von Willebrand disease

Von Willebrand disease is a group of congenital bleeding disorders (inherited from either parent) affecting 1% to 2% of the population, associated with deficiency or lack of vW factor (vWF), a glycoprotein that is synthesized, stored, and secreted by vascular endothelial cells. This protein interacts with thrombocytes to create a clot and prevent hemorrhage; however, with von Willebrand disease, this clotting mechanism is impaired. There are 3 types:
- Type I: Low levels of vWF and also sometimes factor VIII. (Dominant inheritance.)
- Type II: Abnormal vWF (subtypes a, b) may increase or decrease clotting. (Dominant inheritance.)
- Type III: Absence of vWF and less than 10% factor VIII. (Recessive inheritance.)

Symptoms vary in severity and include:
- Bruising
- Menorrhagia
- Recurrent epistaxis
- Hemorrhage

Treatment includes:
- Desmopressin acetate parenterally or nasally to stimulate production of clotting factor (mild cases).
- Severe bleeding: factor VIII concentrates with vWF, such as *Humate-P*.

Hemophilia

Hemophilia is an inherited disorder in which the person lacks adequate clotting factors. There are 3 types:
- Type A: lack of clotting factor VIII (90% of cases)
- Type B: lack of clotting factor IX
- Type C: lack of clotting factor XI (affects both sexes, rarely occurs in the United States).

Both Type A and B are usually X-linked disorders, affecting only males. The severity of the disease depends on the amount of clotting factor in the blood. Symptoms include:
- Bleeding with severe trauma or stress (mild cases).
- Unexplained bruises, bleeding, swelling, joint pain.

- Spontaneous hemorrhage (severe cases), often in the joints but can be anywhere in the body.
- Epistaxis, mucosal bleeding.
- First symptoms often occur during infancy when the child becomes active, resulting in frequent bruises.

Treatment includes:
- Desmopressin acetate parenterally or nasally to stimulate production of clotting factor (mild cases).
- Infusions of clotting factor from donated blood or recombinant clotting factors (genetically engineered), utilizing guidelines for dosing.
- Infusions of plasma (Type C).

Idiopathic thrombocytopenia purpura

Idiopathic thrombocytopenia purpura is an autoimmune condition in which the thrombocyte (platelet) count is below normal (less than 150,000/mm^3) but the other blood values are normal, resulting in purple bruises and petechiae on the skin and mucous membranes from superficial bleeding. The acute form (lasts less than 6 months) occurs primarily in children after viral infections or live virus vaccination. The chronic form (lasts more than 6 months) is more common in adults (primarily female) but can occur at any age, and the cause is unknown. Other symptoms include menorrhagia, epistaxis, GI bleeding, and bleeding gums. Retinal and cerebral hemorrhage (rare) may occur. Diagnosis includes: CBC and platelet count.

Treatment includes:
- Corticosteroids to increase platelet count.
- IV immune globulin for severe bleeding, platelet counts less than 50,000 (adults) or platelet count less than 20,000 (pediatrics).
- Hemorrhage: volume replacement if indicated as for hypovolemic shock.

Treatment for chronic disease:
- Thrombopoiesis-stimulating agents (romiplostim, eltrombopag), glucocorticoids, and immunosuppressive agents (rituximab).

AIDS

AIDS is a progression of infection with human immunodeficiency virus (HIV). AIDS is diagnosed when the following criteria are met:
- HIV infection.
- CD4 count less than 200 cells/mm^3.
- AIDS defining condition, such as opportunistic infections (cytomegalovirus, tuberculosis), wasting syndrome, neoplasms (Kaposi sarcoma), or AIDS dementia complex.

Because there is such a wide range of AIDS defining conditions, the patient may present with many types of symptoms, depending upon the diagnosis, but more than half of AIDS patients exhibit:
- Fever.
- Lymphadenopathy.
- Pharyngitis.
- Rash.

- Myalgia/Arthralgia.
- It is important to review the following:
- CD4 counts, to determine immune status.
- WBC and differential for signs of infection.
- Cultures to help identify any infective agents.
- CBC to evaluate for signs of bleeding or thrombocytopenia.

Treatment aims to cure or manage opportunistic conditions and control underlying HIV infection through highly active anti-retroviral therapy (HAART), 3 or more drugs used concurrently.

Hodgkin's disease

Hodgkin disease (lymphoma) is cancer originating in the lymphatic system, resulting in impairment of the immune system. The cancer eventually spreads outside the lymphatic system to other organs. With HD, the lymphatic system produces large abnormal B cells (Reed-Sternberg cells), impairing the ability of the body to produce antibodies. Diagnosis may include biopsy of enlarged nodes, CBC, radiographs, CT scan, MRI, gallium scan to show spread of HD, PET scan, and bone marrow biopsy. Symptoms include:
- Painless, enlarged lymph nodes (neck, axillary, clavicular, and femoral areas), sometimes to greater than 1 inch in diameter, with enlargement progressing from one nodal group to another.
- Fever with chills and night sweats.
- Anorexia.
- Pruritus, weakness and fatigue, opportunistic infections.
- Other symptoms relate to the area affected by the lymphoma, such as chest pain, cough and dyspnea, or abdominal pain and swelling.

Treatment includes:
- Stabilizing patient
- Treating opportunistic infections
- Referral to oncology/radio-therapy for radiation and chemotherapy

Leukemia

Leukocytes are white blood cells (WBCs). Normal total values vary according to age:
- Neonate: 9,000 to 30,000/mm³.
- 1 month: 5,000 to 19,500/mm³.
- 1 to 3 years: 6,000 to 17,500/mm³.
- 8 to 13 years: 4,500 to 13,500/mm³.
- Older than 18 years: 4,500 to 11,000/mm³.

The differential is the percentage of each type of WBC out of the total. The differential will shift with infection or allergies, but should return to normal values:
- Myelocytes: 0%.
- Neutrophils (bands): 3% to 5%.
- Neutrophils (segs): 54% to 62%.
- Lymphocytes: 25% to 33%.

- Monocytes: 3% to 7%.
- Eosinophils: 1% to 3%.
- Basophils: 0.5% to 1%.

Leukemia occurs when one type of WBC proliferates with immature cells, with the defect occurring in the hematopoietic stem cell, either lymphoid (lympho-) or myeloid (myelo-). Usually leukemias classified as blast cell or stem cell refers to lymphoid defects. With acute leukemia, WBC count remains low because the cells are halted at the blast stage and the disease progresses rapidly. Chronic leukemia progresses more slowly and most cells are mature.

> **Review Video:** Leukemia
*Visit **mometrix.com/academy** and enter **Code: 940024***

Common childhood leukemias
AML and ALL are the 2 most common types of leukemias that affect children.
- Acute myeloid leukemia (*AML*) is also referred to as granulocytic, myelocytic, monocytic, myelogenous, monoblastic, and monomyeloblastic leukemia. It is caused by a defect in the stem cells that differentiate into all myeloid cells. It affects all ages, occurring in children and adults, and often has a genetic component. Survival rates with adequate treatment are about 50%.
- Acute lymphocytic leukemia (*ALL*) is also referred to as lymphatic, lymphocytic, lymphoblastic, or lymphoblastoid leukemia, and is caused by a defect in the stem cells that differentiate into lymphocytes. This is the most common type of childhood leukemia, peaking between ages 2 to 5. The cause is not known. There are a number of different types of ALL, and treatment and survival relate to the type. Overall survival rates with adequate treatment are about 80%.

Some rare forms of leukemia are named for the cells involved, such as basophilic leukemia.

Physiological consequences
Leukemia is a condition in which the proliferating cells compete with normal cells for nutrition. Leukemia affects all cells because the abnormal cells in the bone marrow depress the formation of all elements, resulting in several consequences, regardless of the type of leukemia:
- Decrease in production of erythrocytes (RBCs), resulting in anemia.
- Decrease in neutrophils, resulting in increased risk of infection.
- Decrease in platelets, with subsequent decrease in clotting factors and increased bleeding.
- Increased risk of physiological fractures because of invasion of bone marrow that weakens the periosteum.
- Infiltration of liver, spleen, and lymph glands, resulting in enlargement and fibrosis
- Infiltration of the CNS, resulting in increased intracranial pressure, ventricular dilation, and meningeal irritation with headaches, vomiting, papilledema, nuchal rigidity, and coma progressing to death.
- Hypermetabolism that deprives cells of nutrients, resulting in anorexia, weight loss, muscle atrophy, and fatigue.

Treatment

Leukemia treatment depends upon the protocol established for each type of leukemia. Combined drugs are usually more effective than single. Chemotherapy usually includes 3 stages:

- Induction therapy: The purpose is to induce remission to the point that the bone marrow is clear of disease and blood cell counts are normal. Chemotherapy is usually given for about 4 to 6 weeks, followed by transplantation or the next stage of chemotherapy. The chemotherapy is potent and suppresses blood elements, leaving the body at risk for serious infections and hemorrhage, so supportive care is critical.
- Consolidation therapy: The goal is to kill any cells that may have escaped the induction stage. This stage lasts 4 to 8 months. Intrathecal chemotherapy may be coadministered as a prophylaxis to prevent CNS involvement.
- Maintenance therapy: Treatment may continue for another 2 to 3 years, but with less intense chemotherapy to maintain remission. Weekly blood cell counts monitor progress and side effects.

Sometimes after the 3 stages of chemotherapy are completed, the patient will relapse and leukemic cells return. In that case, reinduction is carried out, usually using a different arsenal of drugs. Many drugs in use now, especially for relapses, are those in clinical trials. Clinical trials are ongoing for many chemotherapeutic agents to determine the best combination of drugs and duration of treatment. Other treatments may be instituted, depending on the severity of the disease:

- Intrathecal chemotherapy is administered into the spinal fluid for treatment of infiltration of the CNS.
- Radiation to the brain may be indicated in addition to intrathecal chemotherapy with severe disease but poses danger to brain development.
- "Bone marrow" or cord blood transplant, also known as hematopoietic stem cell transplantation (HCST), may be done if chemotherapy fails or after the first remission for AML, which has a lower cure rate.

Anaphylaxis syndrome

Anaphylaxis syndrome is a sudden acute systemic immunoglobulin E (IgE) or nonimmunoglobulin E (non-IgE) inflammatory response affecting the cardiopulmonary and other systems.

- IgE-mediated response (anaphylactic shock) is an antibody-antigen reaction against an allergen, such as milk, peanuts, latex, insect bites, or fish. This is the most common type.
- Non-IgE–mediated response (anaphylactoid reaction) is a systemic reaction to infection, exercise, radiocontrast material, or other triggers. While the response is almost identical to the other type, it does not involve IgE.

Typically, with IgE-mediated response, an antigen triggers release of substances, such as histamine and prostaglandins, which affect the skin, cardiopulmonary, and GI systems. Histamine causes initial erythema and edema by inducing vasodilation. Each time the patient has contact with the antigen, more antibodies form in response, so allergic reactions worsen with each contact. In some cases, initial reactions may be mild, but subsequent contact can cause severe life-threatening response.

Anaphylaxis syndrome may present with a few symptoms or a wide range that encompasses cardiopulmonary, dermatological, and gastrointestinal responses. Symptoms include:
- Severe generalized edema and angioedema. Lips and tongue may swell.
- Sudden onset of weakness, dizziness, confusion.
- Urticaria
- Increased permeability of vascular system and loss of vascular tone.
- Severe hypotension leading to shock.
- Laryngospasm/bronchospasm with obstruction of airway causing dyspnea and wheezing.
- Nausea, vomiting, and diarrhea.
- Seizures, coma and death.

Treatments include:
- Establish patent airway and intubate if necessary for ventilation.
- Provide oxygen at 100% high flow.
- Monitor VS.
- Administer epinephrine (Epi-pen® or solution).
- Albuterol per nebulizer for bronchospasm.
- Intravenous fluids to provide bolus of fluids for hypotension.
- Diphenhydramine if shock persists.
- Methylprednisolone if no response to other drugs.

Severe infections

There are a number of terms used to refer to severe infections and often used interchangeably, but they are part of a continuum:
- Bacteremia is the presence of bacteria in the blood but without systemic infection.
- Septicemia is a systemic infection caused by pathogens (usually bacteria or fungi) present in the blood.
- Systemic inflammatory response syndrome (SIRS), a generalized inflammatory response affecting many organ systems, may be caused by infectious or non-infectious agents, such as trauma, burns, adrenal insufficiency, pulmonary embolism, and drug overdose. If an infectious agent is identified or suspected, SIRS is an aspect of sepsis. Infective agents include a wide range of bacteria and fungi, including *Streptococcus pneumoniae* and *Staphylococcus aureus*. SIRS includes 2 of the following:
  - Elevated (>38°C) or subnormal rectal temperature (<36°C).
  - Tachypnea or $PaCO_2$ <32 mm Hg.
  - Tachycardia.
  - Leukocytosis (>12,000) or leukopenia (<4000).

Infections can progress from bacteremia, septicemia, and SIRS to the following:
- Sepsis is presence of infection either locally or systemically in which there is a generalized life-threatening inflammatory response (SIRS). It includes all the indications for SIRS as well as one of the following:
  - Changes in mental status.
  - Hypoxemia (<72 mm Hg) without pulmonary disease.
  - Elevation in plasma lactate.
  - Decreased urinary output <5 mL/kg/wt for >1 hour.

- Severe sepsis includes both indications of SIRS and sepsis as well as indications of increasing organ dysfunction with inadequate perfusion and/or hypotension.
- Septic shock is a progression from severe sepsis in which refractory hypotension occurs despite treatment. There may be indications of lactic acidosis.

Multi-organ dysfunction syndrome *(MODS)* is the most common cause of sepsis-related death. Cardiac function becomes depressed, acute respiratory distress syndrome (ARDS) may develop, and renal failure may follow acute tubular necrosis or cortical necrosis. Thrombocytopenia appears in about 30% of those affected and may result in disseminated intravascular coagulation (DIC). Liver damage and bowel necrosis may occur.

> ➤ **Review Video:** Multiple Organ Dysfunction System
> *Visit **mometrix.com/academy** and enter **Code:** 394302*

Septic shock

Septic shock is caused by toxins produced by bacteria and cytokines that the body produces in response to severe infection, resulting in a complex syndrome of disorders. Symptoms are wide-ranging:
- Initial: Hyper- or hypothermia, increased temperature (above 38°C) with chills, tachycardia with increased pulse pressure, tachypnea, alterations in mental status (dullness), hypotension, hyperventilation with respiratory alkalosis ($PaCO_2 \leq 30$ mm Hg), increased lactic acid, and unstable BP, and dehydration with increased urinary output.
- Cardiovascular: Myocardial depression and dysrhythmias.
- Respiratory: Adults respiratory distress syndrome (ARDS).
- Renal: acute renal failure (ARF) with decreased urinary output and increased BUN.
- Hepatic: Jaundice and liver dysfunction with an increase in transaminase, alkaline phosphatase and bilirubin.
- Hematologic: Mild or severe blood loss (from mucosal ulcerations), neutropenia or neutrophilia, decreased platelets, and DIC.
- Endocrine: Hyperglycemia, hypoglycemia (rare).
- Skin: cellulitis, erysipelas, and fasciitis, acrocyanotic and necrotic peripheral lesions.

Septic shock is most common in newborns, those >50, and those who are immunocompromised. There is no specific test to confirm a diagnosis of septic shock, so diagnosis is based on clinical findings and tests that evaluate hematologic, infectious, and metabolic states: CBC, DIC panel, electrolytes, liver function tests, BUN, creatinine, blood glucose, ABGs, urinalysis, ECG, radiographs, blood and urine cultures. Treatment must be aggressive and includes:
- Oxygen and endotracheal intubation as necessary.
- IV access with 2-large bore catheters and central venous line.
- Rapid fluid administration at 0.5L NS or isotonic crystalloid every 5-10 minutes as needed (to 4-6 L).
- Monitoring urinary output to optimal >30mL/hr.
- Inotropic agents (dopamine, dobutamine, norepinephrine) if no response to fluids or fluid overload.
- Empiric IV antibiotic therapy (usually with 2 broad spectrum antibiotics for both gram-positive and gram-negative bacteria) until cultures return and antibiotics may be changed.
- Hemodynamic and laboratory monitoring.
- Removing source of infection (abscess, catheter).

Hypovolemic shock/volume deficit

Hypovolemic shock occurs when there is inadequate intravascular fluid.
- The loss may be *absolute* because of an internal shifting of fluid, or an external loss of fluid, as occurs with massive hemorrhage, thermal injuries, severe vomiting or diarrhea, and injuries (such as ruptured spleen or dissecting arteries) that interfere with intravascular integrity.
- Hypovolemia may also be *relative* and related to vasodilation, increased capillary membrane permeability from sepsis or injuries, and decreased colloidal osmotic pressure that may occur with loss of sodium and some disorders, such as hypopituitarism and cirrhosis.

Hypovolemic shock is classified according to the degree of fluid loss:
- Class I: <750 ml or ≤15% of total circulating volume (TCV).
- Class II: 750-100 ml or 15-30% of TCV.
- Class III: 1500-2000 ml or 30-40% of TCV.
- Class IV: >2000 ml or >40% of TCV.

Hypovolemic shock occurs when the total circulating volume of fluid decreases, leading to a fall in venous return that in turn causes a decrease in ventricular filling and preload, indicated by ↓ in right atrial pressure (RAP) and pulmonary artery occlusion pressure (PAOP). This results in a decrease in stroke volume and cardiac output. This in turn causes generalized arterial vasoconstriction, increasing afterload (↑ systemic vascular resistance), causing decreased tissue perfusion. Symptoms include:
- Anxiety.
- Pallor.
- Cool and clammy skin.
- Delayed capillary refill
- Cyanosis.
- Hypotension.
- Increasing respirations.
- Weak, thready pulse.

Treatment is aimed at identifying and treating the cause of fluid loss and reestablishing an adequate intravascular volume of fluid through administration of blood, blood products, autotransfusion, colloids (such as plasma protein fraction), and/or crystalloids (such as normal saline). Oxygen may be given and intubation and ventilation may be necessary. Medications may include vasopressors, such as dopamine.

Rapid fluid resuscitation
Rapid fluid resuscitation is used to treat hypovolemic shock and prevents irreversible organ injury and death. High flow rates have increased with new equipment and techniques. Isotonic fluids may be infused at rates greater than 800 mL/ min, crystalloids greater than 500 mL/min, and blood greater than 800 mL/min. The minimum internal diameter (ID) of the equipment should be maintained through the length (including catheter tip) and must be considered to ensure maximum flow rates. Y-type IV tubing setups must be used to eliminate time lost in changing IV bags. External pressure devices, especially air pressure devices, should provide constant pressure on the IV bag. Blood warmers (or mixing cold RBCs 1:1 with warmed NS 70°C) are necessary to avoid

hypothermia and hemolysis. Rapid percutaneous insertion of catheter (14-gauge) or cutdown should be done to ensure ID of at least 3.66 mm. Infusion may be started with a smaller gauge catheter while cutdown or larger gauge catheter is inserted.

Distributive shock

Distributive shock occurs with adequate blood volume but inadequate intravascular volume because of arterial/venous dilation that results in decreased vascular tone and hypoperfusion of internal organs. Cardiac output may be normal or blood may pool, decreasing cardiac output. Distributive shock may result from anaphylactic shock, septic shock, neurogenic shock, and drug ingestions. Symptoms include:
- Hypotension (systolic <90mm Hg or <40mm Hg from nor-mal), tachypnea, tachycardia (>90) (may be lower if patient receiving β-blockers.
- Skin initially warm, later hypoperfused.
- Hyper- or hypothermia (>38°C or <36°C).
- Hypoxemia.
- Alterations in mentation.
- Decreased Urinary output.
- Symptoms related to underlying cause.

Treatment includes treating underlying cause and stabilizing hemodynamics:
- Septic shock or anaphylactic therapy and monitoring as indicated.
- Oxygen with endotracheal intubation if necessary.
- Rapid fluid administration at 0.25-0.5L NS or isotonic crystalloid every 5-10 minutes as needed to 2-3 L.
- Inotropic agents (dopamine, dobutamine, norepinephrine) if necessary.

MODS

Multi-organ dysfunction syndrome (MODS)is progressive deterioration and failure of 2 or more organ systems with mortality rates of 45-50% with 2 organ systems involved and up to 80-100% if there are ≥3 systems failing. Trauma patients and those with severe conditions, such as shock, burns, and sepsis, are particularly vulnerable, especially in those >65. MODS may be primary or secondary:
- Primary MODS relates to direct injury/disorder of the organ systems, resulting in dysfunction, such as with thermal injuries, traumatic pulmonary injuries, and invasive infections.
- Secondary MODS relates to dysfunction of organ systems not directly involved in injury/disorder but developing as the result of a systemic inflammatory response syndrome (SIRS) as the patient's immune and inflammatory responses become dysregulated. In some patients, failure of organ systems is sequential, usually progressing from the lungs, the liver, the gastrointestinal system, and the kidneys to the heart. However, in other cases, various organ systems may fail at the same time.

Maxillofacial, Ocular, Orthopedic and Wound Emergencies

Peritonsillar abscess

Peritonsillar abscess (PTA), which usually derives from tonsillitis, progresses from cellulitis to abscess between the palatine tonsil and capsule. It is often polymicrobial. It usually occurs bilaterally between the ages of 20 to 30. Complications include obstruction of airway, rupture with aspiration of purulent material, septicemia, endocarditis, and epiglottitis. The infection is often polymicrobial. Symptoms include fever, pain, hoarseness, muffling of voice, dysphagia, tonsillar edema, erythema, exudate, and edema of palate with displacement of uvula.

Diagnosis:
- Aspiration of purulent material (usually diagnostic).
- CT with contrast, ultrasound.
- On exam: displacement of the uvula, with enlarged tonsils.

Treatments include:
- Needle aspirations (often multiple) with needle penetrating 1 cm or less to avoid carotid artery.
- Abscess incision and drainage if aspiration not successful.
- IV volume replacement.

Antibiotics: IV ampicillin-sulbactam or clindamycin until culture results come back and in areas with high rates of CA-MRSA vancomycin may be added. Once the patient shows signs of clinical improvement, they may switch to oral antibiotics (needing 14 days total).

Bell's palsy

Bell's palsy is caused by inflammation of cranial nerve VII, usually from a herpes simplex I or II infection, and generally affects only one side of the paired nerves. Onset is generally sudden, and symptoms peak by 48 hours with a wide range of presentation. Symptoms usually subside within 2 to 6 months but may persist 1 year:
- Mild weakness on one side of face to complete paralysis with distortion of features.
- Drooping of eyelid and mouth.
- Tearing in affected eye.
- Taste impairment.

Diagnosis includes:
- Neurological, eye, parotid gland, and ear exam to rule out other cranial nerve involvement or conditions.

Treatment includes:
- Artificial tears during daytime with lubricating ophthalmic ointment and patch at night to protect eye.
- Prednisone 60 mg daily for 5 days with tapering over 5 days
- For severe cases use Prednisone AND Acyclovir 400 mg 5 times daily for 7 days.

- 118 -

Temporal arteritis

Temporal arteritis (TA) also called giant cell arteritis is inflammation of the blood vessels of the head, especially the temporal artery, and the thoracic aorta and branches. TA is commonly associated with polymyalgia rheumatica (30% or less of patients) but can occur with other systemic disorders such as lupus erythematous, Sjögren syndrome, and rheumatoid arthritis. TA is a progressive disorder that can result in blindness and is most common in those older than 50.

Symptoms include:
- New onset of headaches.
- Vision fluctuations, including decreased visual acuity and loss of vision.
- Intermittent claudicating pain in jaw, tongue, and upper extremities.
- Fever.

Diagnosis includes:
- Temporal artery biopsy (definitive).
- ESR greater than 50 mm/h (may be normal in about 20%).
- CRP greater than 2.45 mg/dL.

Treatment should begin immediately if the diagnosis is suspected to prevent blindness:
- Prednisone 60 mg daily.

Trigeminal neuralgia

Trigeminal neuralgia (tic douloureux) is a neurological condition in which blood vessels press on the trigeminal nerve as it leaves the brainstem causing severe pain on one side of the face or jaw. The shock-like pains may involve a small area or half the face and in rare cases both sides of the face at different times. The pain lasts from seconds to 2 minutes and is extremely debilitating and may be precipitated by movement, vibration, or contact with the face or mouth. Trigeminal neuralgia is most common in women older than 50. Patients may go through periods of remission and recurrences. Diagnosis is by history and neurological exam. Treatment includes:
- Carbamazepine is the drug of choice and usually controls pain initially, but the effects may decrease over time.
- Phenytoin or oxcarbazepine may be used in place of carbamazepine.
- Baclofen (muscle relaxant) potentiates other drugs.
- Surgical procedures may be done if no response to medications.

Removing a foreign body from the ear

Foreign bodies in the ear (most often in children) can be organic or inorganic materials or insects. Careful history should be done to determine the type of foreign body before attempting removal. Children may require conscious sedation or general anesthesia for deep insertions. Irrigations should not be done if tympanic membrane is ruptured or cannot be visualized.

Procedure:
- Examine ear to determine if tympanic membrane is intact.
- Drown insects with lidocaine 2% solution and then suction.
- Irrigate small nonorganic particles with pulsatile flow aimed at wall of the canal.

- Use cerumen loops, right-angle hooks, and/or alligator forceps to grasp and remove item.
- Carefully examine the ear canal after removal of the item for lacerations or abrasions.
- Topical antibiotic if extensive cutaneous abrasion or laceration or for organic material.

Removing foreign bodies from the eye

Foreign bodies in the eye should be assessed carefully with slit lamp with corneal examination using optical sectioning before attempting removal of the foreign body. Foreign bodies that penetrate the cornea full-thickness should not be removed in the ED, but superficial foreign bodies can safely be removed.

Procedure:
- Apply topical anesthetic to both eyes (to suppress blinking in the unaffected eye).
- Eye held open by hand or with wire eyelid speculum.
- Foreign body is carefully removed with small gauge needle or moistened cotton swab.
- Rust ring from metallic objects should be removed with ophthalmic burr (if not over pupil), and patient referred to ophthalmologist for further rust ring removal within 24 hours.
- Eyelid everted and examined carefully for further foreign bodies.
- Abrasions treated as indicated.

Removing a foreign body from the nares

Children may insert various organic and inorganic foreign bodies in the nose. In most cases, this is observed, but persistent unilateral obstruction of nose, foul discharge, or epistaxis is suggestive of foreign body. Small or uncooperative children may need to be restrained with conscious sedation or papoose board.

Procedure:
- Vasoconstrictor/topical anesthetic applied: 1 mL of phenylephrine with 3 mL of lidocaine 4%.
- Aerosolized racemic epinephrine may be used for decongestion, to loosen foreign body.
- Examine nares with speculum.

Removal techniques:
- Positive pressure: Blowing nose on command. For small children, block opposite nares and have caregiver blow puff of air in mouth, forcing item out of nares.
- Suction with catheter.
- Use alligator or bayonet forceps to grasp item.
- Pass a curette behind item, rotate, and the use to pull item out.
- Pass Fogarty vascular catheter past item, inflate balloon, pull catheter back out.

Ludwig angina

Ludwig angina is cellulitis, usually caused by *Streptococcus* or *Staphylococcus,* of the submandibular spaces and lingual space that can result in obstruction of the airway as the swelling in the mouth floor pushes the tongue superior and posterior. Symptoms include:
- Evidence of poor dental hygiene and odontogenic abscess (usually from lower third molars or surrounding gums) that has spread into soft tissue.
- Dysphagia.

- Odynophagia, trismus, edema of the upper neck (midline)
- Erythema, stridor and cyanosis (late signs of obstruction)
- Changes in mental status.

Diagnosis includes:
- Examination of the head and neck to observe for swelling of the upper neck, floor of mouth, and tongue.
- CT scan.
- Culture (treatment should, however, begin immediately).

Treatments include:
- Nasotracheal intubation (with fiberoptic tube if necessary) and ventilation if respiratory obstruction.
- IV antibiotics, such as penicillin or clindamycin.
- Referral to surgeon for incision and drainage as indicated.

Otitis externa

Otitis externa (OE) is infection of the external ear canal, either bacterial or mycotic. Common pathogens include bacteria, *Pseudomonas aeruginosa*, *Staphylococcus aureus,* and fungi, *Aspergillus* and *Candida.* OE is often caused by chlorine in swimming pools killing normal flora and allowing other bacteria to multiply. Fungal infections may be associated with immune disorders, diabetes, and steroid use. Symptoms include:
- Pain, swelling, and exudate.
- Itching (pronounced with fungal infections).
- Red pustular lesions.
- Black spots over tympanic membrane (fungus).

Diagnosis: On exam, tenderness when touched on tragus or when the auricle is pulled, erythema, and history.

Treatment includes:
- Irrigate ear with Burow's solution or saline to clean and remove debris or foreign objects.
- Bacteria: Antibiotic ear drops, such as ciprofloxacin and ofloxacin. If impetigo, flush with hydrogen peroxide 1:1 solution and apply mupirocin twice daily for 5 to 7 days. Lance pointed furuncles.
- Fungus: Solution of boric acid 5% in ethanol; clotrimazole-miconazole solution with/without steroid for 5 to 7 days.
- Analgesics as needed.

Otitis media

Otitis media, inflammation of the middle ear, usually follows upper respiratory tract infections or allergic rhinitis. The eustachian tube swells and prevents the passage of air. Fluid from the mucous membranes pools in the middle ear, causing infection. Common pathogens include *Streptococcus pneumoniae, Haemophilus influenzae,* and *Moraxella catarrhalis.*

Some genetic conditions, such as trisomy 21 and cleft palate, may include abnormalities of the eustachian tube, increasing risk. There are 4 forms:

- Acute: 1 to 3 weeks with swelling, redness, and possible rupture of the tympanic membrane, fever, pain (ear pulling), and hearing loss.
- Recurrent: 3 episodes in 6 months or 4 to 6 in 12.
- Bullous: Acute infection with ear popping pressure in middle ear, pain, hearing loss, and bullae between layers of tympanic membrane, causing bulging.
- Chronic: Persists at least 3 months with thick retracted tympanic membrane, hearing loss, and drainage.

Diagnosis: Distinguishing features on assessment of acute otitis media include a bulging or perforated tympanic membrane, signs of inflammation, or purulent fluid present.

Treatment:

- Many cases of AOM resolve spontaneously, so observation with the ability to initiate antibiotics if no improvement in 2-3 days of worsening symptoms is the treatment of choice for most children. For adults, it is recommended to start antibiotics rather than observe. Amoxicillin for 7 to 10 days.
- Referral for tympanostomy and pressure-equalizing tubes (PET) for severe chronic or recurrent infections.

> **Review Video:** Otitis Media
> *Visit **mometrix.com/academy** and enter **Code: 328778***

Mastoiditis

Mastoiditis usually results from extension of acute otitis media because the mucous membranes of the middle ear are continuous with the mastoid air cells in the temporal bone. All patients with otitis media should be considered at risk for mastoiditis. Patients with chronic otitis media also often develop chronic mastoiditis, which can result in formation of benign cholesteatoma. Signs and symptoms of mastoiditis include persistent fever, pain in or behind the ear (especially during the night), and hearing loss. Differential diagnoses may include Bell's palsy, otitis externa, and otitis media. Diagnosis is based on symptoms, CBC, audiometry, tympanocentesis or myringotomy with culture and sensitivities, and CT scan (definitive). Acute mastoiditis is treated with antibiotics, usually beginning with a 3rd generation cephalosporin or penicillin/aminoglycoside combination until culture and sensitivity results return. If spreading empyema or osteitis is present, then surgical mastoidectomy is required.

Ménière disease

Ménière disease occurs when a blockage in the endolymphatic duct of the inner ear causes dilation of the endolymphatic space and abnormal fluid balance, which causes pressure or rupture of the inner ear membrane. Symptoms include:

- Progressive fluctuating sensorineural hearing loss.
- Tinnitus.
- Pressure in the ear.
- Severe vertigo that lasts minutes to hours.

- Diaphoresis.
- Poor balance.
- Nausea and vomiting.

Diagnosis includes:
- Complete physical exam and evaluation of cranial nerves. Tuning fork sounds may lateralize to unaffected ear.
- Assessment of hearing loss.

Treatment:
- Low Na diet.Vestibular suppressant (antihistamine): Meclizine. Benzodiazepine or SSRI for anxiety. Antiemetics, such as promethazine suppositories. Diuretics, such as hydrochlorothiazide.
- Referral for surgical repair for persistent vertigo, but this will not correct other symptoms.

Labyrinthitis

Labyrinthitis is a viral or bacterial inflammation of the inner ear, and it may occur secondary to bacterial otitis media. Viral labyrinthitis may be associated with mumps, rubella, rubeola, influenza, or other viral infections, such as upper respiratory tract infections. Because the labyrinth includes the vestibular system that is responsible for sensing head movement, labyrinthitis causes balance disorders. The condition often persists for 1 to 6 weeks with acute symptoms the first week and then decreasing symptoms. Symptoms include:
- Sudden onset of severe vertigo.
- Hearing loss and sometimes tinnitus.
- Nausea and vomiting.
- Panic attacks from severe anxiety related to symptoms.

Treatment includes:
- Bacterial: IV antibiotics
- Volume replacement.
- Antiemetics, such as promethazine suppositories.
- Vestibular suppressant (antihistamine): Meclizine
- Benzodiazepine or SSRI for anxiety.
- Referral to surgeon for I&D if necessary.
- Viral: Symptomatic as for bacterial (except for antibiotics).

Nasal fracture

Nasal fracture can result from any type of blunt trauma to the face. Fracture may be overlooked because of edema, so careful examination of the nose with facial injuries is important. Common causes include altercations and sporting injuries. Septal cartilage is often fractured as well as nasal bones. Symptoms include:
- Edema.
- Pain.
- Crepitation.
- Ecchymosis.
- Deformity.
- Nasal bleeding.

Diagnosis is based on clinical examination and otoscope. Radiographic studies are not indicated unless other facial fractures are suspected. Clear nasal discharge following injury to the face may indicate leaking of cerebrospinal fluid from torn meninges resulting from fracture of cribriform plate. A drop of clear drainage should be placed on filter paper and examined for a clear area around a central stain of blood. If CSF drainage is suspected, the patient should be placed upright, and have a CT scan and neurological consult.

Treatment for fracture includes:
- Realignment if necessary.
- Analgesia
- Nasal decongestant.
- Protective covering.
- Packing only for persistent epistaxis.

Recurrent epistaxis

Recurrent epistaxis is common in young children (2 to 10 years), especially boys, and is often related to nose picking, dry climate, or central heating in the winter. Incidence also increases between 50 to 80 years of age, and may be caused by NSAIDs and anticoagulants. Kiesselbach plexus in the anterior nares has plentiful vessels and bleeds easily. Bleeding in the posterior nares is more dangerous and can result in considerable blood loss. Bleeding from the anterior nares is usually confined to one nostril, but from the posterior nares, blood may flow through both nostrils or backward into the throat and the person may be observed swallowing. People abusing cocaine may suffer nosebleeds because of damage to the mucosa. Hematocrit and hemoglobin should be done to determine if blood loss is significant. Bleeding should stop within 20 minutes.

Treatment:
- Upright position, leaning forward so blood does not flow down throat.
- Applying pressure below the nares or by pinching the nostrils firmly for 10 minutes.
- Severe bleeding: packing and/or topical vasoconstrictors.
- Humidifiers may decrease irritation.

Sinusitis

Sinusitis is inflammation of the nasal sinuses, of which there are 2 maxillary, 2 frontal, and 1 sphenoidal, as ethmoidal air cells. Inflammation causes obstruction of drainage with resultant discomfort. Symptoms include:
- Frontal and maxillary presents with pain over sinuses.
- Ethmoidal present with dull aching behind eye.
- Tenderness to palpation and percussion of sinuses.
- Mucosa of nasal cavity edematous and erythematous.
- Purulent exudate.

Diagnosis includes:
- Transillumination of sinus (diminished with inflammation).
- CT for those who are immunocompromised or if diagnosis is not clear.
- Careful examination to rule out spreading infection, especially with signs of fever, altered mental status, or unstable vital signs.

Treatment includes:
- Symptomatic relief with analgesia: topical decongestants, nasal irrigation.
- Antimicrobial therapy if symptoms persist at least 7 days or are severe (avoid routine use): amoxicillin or TMP/SMX.
- Steroid nasal spray twice daily.

Temporomandibular fracture and/or dislocation

Temporomandibular fracture and/or dislocation can occur as a result of trauma, such as a direct blow to the jaw, or chronic disorders. Dislocations may be anterior (most common and often after extreme mouth opening), posterior, lateral, or superior. Symptoms include:
- Acute pain. Dysphagia. Difficulty speaking.
- Edema and rigidity of surrounding muscles.
- Inability to open mouth.

Diagnosis includes:
- Complete head, neck, ear, and dental examination.
- Radiography, such as x-rays or CT, with significant trauma.
- Tongue blade test: patient bites hard on tongue blade while examiner twists blade, attempting to break it. If fracture, patient opens mouth to release blade.

Treatment (dislocation) includes:
- Short-acting muscle relaxant.
- Narcotic analgesia/conscious sedation.
- Reduction: Patient on chair with head against hard surface.
- Examiner in front of patient places gloved thumbs in patient's mouth, posteriorly over the surface of the mandibular molars.
- Examiner applies pressure posteriorly and inferiorly.
- Alternately, examiner stands behind recumbent patient and applies pressure posteriorly and inferiorly.

TMB

Temporomandibular disorder (TMB) is jaw pain caused by dysfunction of the temporomandibular joint (TMJ) and the supporting muscles and ligaments. It may be precipitated by injury, such as whiplash, or grinding or clenching of the teeth, stress, or arthritis. Symptoms include:
- Clicking or popping noises on jaw movement.
- Limited jaw movement or "locked" jaw.
- Acute pain on chewing or moving jaw.
- Headaches and dizziness.
- Toothaches

Diagnosis includes:
- Complete dental exam with x-rays to rule out other disorders.
- MRI or CT may be needed.

Treatment usually begins conservatively:
- Ice pack to jaw area for 10 minutes followed by jaw stretching exercises and warm compress for 5 minutes 3 to 4 times daily.
- Avoidance of heavy chewing by eating soft foods and avoiding hard foods, such as raw carrots and nuts.
- NSAIDs to relieve pain and inflammation.
- Night mouthguard.
- Referral for dental treatments to improve bite as necessary.

Maxillary fractures

Maxillary fractures of the face often are associated with significant other trauma because of the degree of force necessary to fracture the maxilla. Three primary types include:
- Le Fort I: horizontal (low downward force)
- Le Fort II: pyramidal (low or mid maxilla force)
- Le Fort II: transverse (force to bridge of nose or upper maxilla)

However, many injuries are a combination with more than one type of fracture. Symptoms may include:
- Malocclusion and open bite.
- Apparent lengthening of face.
- CSF rhinorrhea (clear nasal discharge).
- Periorbital ecchymosis.

Diagnosis:
Grasping and moving the hard palate back and forth may shift the facial bones. Complete head, neck, ear, oral, and nasal examination with slit headlamp, suction as needed, nasal speculum, and otoscope. CT scans of face and brain.

Treatment:
- Stabilize patient and ensure patent airway.
- Disimpaction of displaced fragments manually.
- Obtain pre-injury photograph to guide surgical fixation.
- Referral to surgeon for fixation.

Dental avulsions

Dental avulsions are complete displacement of a tooth from its socket. The tooth may be reimplanted if done within 1 to 2 hours after displacement, although only permanent teeth are reimplanted, not primary. Procedure:
- Tooth can be transported from accident site to the ED in Hank solution, saline, or milk.
- Cleanse tooth with sterile NS or Hank solution, handling only the crown and avoiding any disruption of fibers.
- If tooth has been dry for 20 to 60 minutes, soak tooth in Hank solution for 30 minutes before reimplantation.
- If tooth has been dry for more than 60 minutes, soak tooth in citric acid for 5 minutes, stannous fluoride 2% for 5 minutes, and doxycycline solution for 5 minutes prior to reimplantation.
- Remove clot in socket and gently irrigate with NS.

- Place tooth into socket firmly, cover with gauze, and have patient bite firmly on gauze until splinting can be applied.
- Apply splinting material and mold packing over implanted tooth and 2 adjacent teeth on both sides (encompasses 5 teeth).

Dental fractures

Dental fractures, most commonly of the maxillary teeth, may occur in association with other oral injuries and may be overlooked unless a careful dental examination is carried out. Fractures are classified according to severity of fracture with treatment to prevent further damage and necrosis:
- Ellis I: chipping of enamel. Tx: Smooth rough edges.
- Ellis II: fracture of enamel and dentin with pain on pressure and air sensitivity. Tx: Protect dentin with glass ionomer dental cement and refer to dentist within 24 hours.
- Ellis III: fracture of enamel, dentin, and pulp with pain on movement, air and temperature sensitivity. Blood may be evident. Tx: Protect dentin with ionomer dental cement or calcium hydroxide base and refer to dentist for prompt treatment. Oral analgesics.
- Alveolar/Root fracture: Loose tooth and malocclusion, sensitivity to percussion. Tx: Prompt referral to dentist for splinting and/or root canal.

> **Review Video:** Anotomical and Clinical Parts of Teeth
> *Visit **mometrix.com/academy** and enter **Code: 683627***

Corneal abrasions

Corneal abrasion results from direct scratching or scraping trauma to the eye, often involving contact lenses. This causes a defect in the epithelium of the cornea. Infection with corneal ulceration can occur with abrasions. Symptoms include:
- Pain.
- Intense photophobia.
- Tearing.

Determining the cause and source of the abrasion is important for treatment as organic sources pose the danger of fungal infection and soft contact lenses pose the danger of *Pseudomonas* infection. Diagnosis includes:
- Topical anesthetic prior to testing for visual acuity.
- Fluorescent staining and examination with cobalt blue light.
- Eversion of eyelid to check for foreign body.
- Examine cornea and assess anterior chamber with slit lamp.

Treatments include:
- Cycloplegic agent to relieve spasm and pain: cyclopentolate 1%.
- Erythromycin ophthalmic ointment 4 times daily with or without eye patch if not related to contact lens AND without eye patch if related to organic source.
- Tobramycin ophthalmic ointment 4 times daily without eye patch if related to contact lens.

Chemical eye burns

Chemical burns are caused by splashing of chemicals (solid, liquid, or fumes) into any part of the eye, often related to facial burns. Chemical burns may damage the cornea and conjunctiva, although other layers of the eye may also be damaged, depending upon the chemical and degree of saturation. Many injuries are work-related and involve alkali (greater than 7 pH), acid (less than 7 pH) (muriatic acid or sulfuric acid), or other irritants (neutral pH) such as pepper spray. Alkali chemicals (such as ammonia, lime, and lye) usually cause the most serious injuries.

Symptoms include:
- Pain.
- Blurring of vision.
- Tearing.
- Edema of eyelids.

Diagnosis includes:
- History of event.
- Eye exam showing corneal irritation.

Treatment includes:
- Irrigate eye and other areas of contact with copious amounts of water or normal saline.
- Litmus paper exam of eye to determine residual pH and continue irrigation until pH returns to neutral.
- Cycloplegic agent to relieve spasm and pain: cyclopentolate 1%.
- Antibiotic ointment to prevent infection.

Snow blindness and flash burns

Ultraviolet keratitis results from injury to the corneal epithelium from exposure to ultraviolet rays from the sun (as in snow blindness where the snow reflects UV rays into the eyes) or from artificial light sources, such as tanning beds, halogen lights, or welding torches (flash burn). Symptoms usually occur 6 to 12 hours after exposure:
- Pain.
- Tearing.
- Photophobia.
- Decreased visual acuity.
- Spasm of eyelids.
- Exam shows punctate irregularities of corneal surface and corneal haze.

An accurate history that details exposure to UV rays should be done. Diagnostic studies include:
- Examination of eye and lids.
- Slit lamp exam with fluorescein staining.

Treatment includes:
- Cycloplegic agent to relieve spasm and pain: cyclopentolate 1%.
- Antibiotic ophthalmic ointment, such as erythromycin.
- Analgesia: opiate (oxycodone) and NSAIDs (ibuprofen 600 mg 4 times daily).
- Topical NSAIDs are sometimes used.

Healing should be evident within 24 to 48 hours.

Infectious conjunctivitis

Infectious conjunctivitis is inflammation of the conjunctiva of the eye from bacteria or viruses. If it occurs less than 30 days after birth, it is referred to as *ophthalmia neonatorum* and is commonly acquired during delivery: Pathogenic agents include *Chlamydia trachomatis, Neisseria gonorrhea,* and herpes virus. Antibiotic drops are applied to the newborn's eyes to prevent conjunctivitis. IV acyclovir is given to infants exposed to herpes virus. Infectious conjunctivitis in older children (or adults) is usually caused by *Staphylococci, Streptococci, Pneumococci,* or viruses, and is extremely contagious, so good hand hygiene is essential. It is difficult to differentiate between bacterial and viral infections without cultures. The child should be kept from school and other children for 24 hours after starting treatment or until symptoms subside:

- Red, swollen, itchy conjunctiva.
- Eye pain.
- Purulent discharge.
- Scratchy feeling under eyelids.
- Mild photophobia.

Treatment is usually antibiotic drops or ointment and cool compresses, although many cases are caused by viruses and the condition often disappears without treatment in 3 to 5 days.

Acute angle-closure glaucoma

Acute angle-closure glaucoma is a medical emergency that involves increased intraocular pressure and impairment of vision in those without history of glaucoma because of occlusion of drainage, which forces the iris forward. This condition is most common in elderly patients. Symptoms include eye pain (periorbital) associated with headache, nausea and vomiting, decreased visual acuity with halos, intraocular pressure greater than 21 mm Hg (may be as high as 50), conjunctival injection, edema of epithelium of cornea, pupil nonreactive and mid-dilated, and shallower anterior chamber. Treatment aims to reduce pressure in the eye by reducing production of aqueous humor:

- Topical beta-blocker (timolol 0.5%, one drop).
- Topical alpha-adrenergic agonist (apraclonidine 0.1%, one drop).
- Topical steroid (prednisolone 1%, 1 drop every 15 minutes for 1 hour and then every hour).
- Acetazolamide 500 mg IV or by mouth.
- Mannitol 1 to 2 g/kg IV.
- Pilocarpine 1% to 2% after pressure reduced.
- Continued monitoring of intraocular pressure every hour.

Hyphema

Hyphema is the accumulation hemorrhaging blood in the anterior chamber of the eye after an injury. It is usually caused by a projectile hitting the eye and resulting in blunt or penetrating trauma. Hyphema are classified according to degree:

- Grade 1: Blood (layered) occupies less than one-third of chamber.
- Grade 2: Blood (filling) occupies one-third to one-half of chamber.
- Grade 3: Blood (layered) occupies more than one-half of chamber.
- Grade 4: Clotted blood occupies total chamber.

Symptoms in addition to bleeding include:
- Increased intraocular pressure greater than 22 mm Hg initially (in about one-third of patients) followed by reduction in 2 to 6 days for those with less than three-fourths filling of chamber. Those with more than three-fourths of complete filling of chamber may have continued increase in intraocular pressure.
- Secondary hemorrhage may occur, especially in children and African American patients.

Treatments include:
- Patch and shield for injured eye.
- Tylenol for analgesia. (NSAIDs should be avoided.)
- Topical steroids.
- Systemic aminocaproic acid to prevent secondary hemorrhage.
- Anti-glaucoma topical medications, such brimonidine, for increased IOP.

Penetrating or blunt ocular trauma with ruptured globe

Penetrating or blunt ocular trauma with resultant ruptured globe (full-thickness injury to cornea or sclera) can occur from many things, such as pellets, BBs, knife wounds, gunshot wounds, and other projectiles. Sports injuries are common. Blunt trauma usually has better outcomes than penetrating. If injury is suspected, get complete history of injury and examine eye carefully with slit lamp. Symptoms include:
- Laceration of eyelid.
- Shallow anterior chamber.
- Pain varies in intensity, but may be severe.
- Decreased visual acuity.
- Irregularity of pupil, especially teardrop shaped.
- Hyphema.
- Difficulty viewing optic nerve on exam.

Diagnostic studies include:
- Careful eye examination.
- Tetanus toxoid or tetanus immune globulin as needed.
- Waters view x-ray to confirm foreign body **OR**
- CT scan, MRI, or ultrasound to confirm rupture.

Treatment after ruptured globe is diagnosed or suspected:
- Do NOT check IOP.
- Place metal eye shield over eye for protection.
- Administer cephalosporin.
- Refer to ophthalmologist for surgical repair.

Anterior uveitis

Anterior uveitis (iritis) is inflammation of the iris. Iridocyclitis includes inflammation of the ciliary body. Uveitis is often related to autoimmune and other disorders, such as ankylosing spondylosis, multiple sclerosis, Reiter syndrome, juvenile idiopathic arthritis, and Crohn's disease. Symptoms include:

- Pain.
- Photophobia with increased pain.
- Reddening of eye.
- Irregularly shaped pupil.
- Decreased visual acuity
- Headache.

Diagnosis: The infection causes white blood cells to shed into the anterior chamber, and the numbers of these that are evident on slit lamp examination determine the degree of the disorder, graded 1 to 4 in increasing severity. Shining a bright light in the unaffected eye causes the pupil to constrict in the affected eye with an increase in pain. Applying topical anesthetic will not relieve pain.

Treatment includes:

- Topical steroid, such as prednisolone 1% (unless infection is also present), every 30 to 60 minutes during awake hours.
- Cycloplegic agent to relieve spasm and pain: cyclopentolate 1%.
- Dark glasses to reduce photophobia.
- Analgesia: acetaminophen or ibuprofen.

Eyelid laceration

The eyelids are thin and provide little protection of the ocular globe from blunt or penetrating trauma, so eyelid lacerations should prompt complete and careful eye examination for injuries or foreign bodies prior to repair. The eyelid comprises 5 layers:

1. Skin.
2. Subcutaneous tissue.
3. Muscle (orbicularis oculi) that controls closure of the lid and forms the medial and lateral canthus.
4. Tarsal plate.
5. Conjunctiva.

Usually only superficial horizontal lacerations are sutured in the ED. More serious injuries should be referred to ophthalmologists or ocular plastic surgeons.

Treatment includes:

- Local anesthesia (supra- or infraorbital).
- Wound irrigation with NS prior to suturing.
- Suturing with 6-0 or 7-0 coated or plain nylon suture (to be removed in 3 to 5 days), using care to avoid suturing into globe.
- Ophthalmic topical antibiotic in place of dressing.

Retinal artery occlusion

Central retinal artery occlusion (CRAO) and branch retinal artery occlusion (BRAO) usually results from an embolus lodging in the central retinal artery or a branch, most commonly the temporal vessels. It is most common in elderly patients (older than 60) and is associated with hypertension and occlusion of carotid arteries. Symptoms include:
- Sudden, painless vision loss on one side.
- History of episodes of temporary visual deficits.

Diagnosis includes:
- Examination with slit lamp shows whitening of retina in affected area and sometimes retinal edema. Embolus may be visible with BRAO.
- ESR to rule out temporal arteritis.
- CBC to evaluate for blood disorders and blood culture to rule out endocarditis or sepsis.
- Fluorescein angiography.

Treatment:
- Usually supportive without intervention.
- tPA may be used for CRAO (success limited).
- Transluminal nd: YAG laser embolysis to clear embolus may improve vision.

Keratitis

Keratitis is inflammation of the cornea, and it may be superficial or deep, which usually results in scarring. The multiple causes for keratitis include bacterial, fungal, viral, and parasitic infections, as well as allergic response to antigens and photokeratitis from exposure to ultraviolet rays. It can also arise from wearing contact lenses. Any corneal ulceration can allow pathogens to enter the eye and cause infection.

Symptoms include:
- Pain and tearing.
- Photophobia.
- Decreased visual acuity.
- Discharge.

Diagnosis includes:
- Careful examination with slit lamp.
- Culture of discharge.

Treatment includes:
- Antifungal or antibacterial drops as indicated.
- Trifluridine every 2 to 3 hours during awake hours to maximum of 9 drops daily for herpes simplex until healing and then 4 times daily for about 1 week.
- Artificial tears.
- Analgesia.

Retinal detachment

Retinal detachment occurs when the retinal pigment epithelial (RPE) layer separates from the underlying sensory layer. There are 4 types of detachment:
- Rhegmatogenous: a tear occurs in the sensory retina and liquid vitreous seeps through, detaching the RPE.
- Traction: bands of scar tissue provide traction that pulls on retina, usually related to diabetes, vitreous hemorrhage, or retinopathy of prematurity.
- Exudative: the choroid produces serous fluid under the retina, usually related to uveitis or macular degeneration.
- Combination of other types.

Symptoms include:
- Painless visual changes, such as floaters, "cobwebs," photopsia (flashes of light), shadow over vision, or loss of central vision.

Diagnosis includes:
- Check visual acuity.
- Dilated fundus exam with indirect ophthalmoscope and Goldman 3-mirror to create a detailed retinal diagram.

Treatment:
- Referral to retinal surgeon for surgical repair.

Orbital fractures

Orbital fractures most often occur with blunt force against the globe causing a rupture through the floor of the orbital bone or a direct blow to the orbital rim, often related to an assault. Injuries are most common in adolescents and young adults.

Symptoms include:
- Essentially asymptomatic.
- Ecchymosis and edema of eyelid.
- Infraorbital anesthesia from pressure or damage to infraorbital nerve.
- Decrease sensation of cheek and upper gum on injured side.
- Diplopia.
- Enophthalmos (sunken globe).

Diagnosis includes:
- Complete eye (slit lamp) and vision examination.
- IOP measurement.
- CT scan.

Treatment:
- Usually supportive.
- Topical steroids for severe edema.
- Patient advised not to blow nose for several weeks.

- Surgical repair about 2 weeks after injury when edema has subsided for extensive fracture (at least 33% of orbital floor) or enophthalmos greater than 2 mm remaining 10 to 14 days post-injury.

Zygomatic fractures

Zygomatic fracture involves the arch of bone that forms the lateral border of the eye orbit and the bony cheek prominence, most commonly associated with a blow to the lateral cheek from an altercation or accident. Fracture can result in a tilting of the eye and flattening of the cheek, which may be obscured by initial edema. Fracture may be only of the arch or may be a more extensive tripod fracture of the infraorbital rim, diastasis of the zygomaticofrontal suture, and disruption of the zygomaticotemporal arch junction. Diagnosis is by CT scan, which shows the extent of the fracture as well as the amount of displacement. Treatment for tripod fracture is referral to surgeon for open reduction with fixation and exploration and reconstruction of orbit as needed.

Traumatic amputation

Amputations may be partial or complete. The amputated limb should be treated initially as though it could be reattached or revascularized. Single digits, except the thumb, are not usually reattached. Initial treatment includes stabilizing patient and stopping bleeding by applying a BP cuff proximal to injury 30 mm Hg above systolic for less than 30 minutes. Instruments, such as clamps and hemostats, should be avoided. Other treatment includes:
- Tetanus prophylaxis.
- Analgesia.
- Prophylactic antibiotics may be needed.
- Irrigation of stump with NS (not antiseptics) if contaminated.
- Splint and elevate stump, with saline-moistened sterile dressing in place.
- Neurovascular examinations of stump.

The Allen test should be done to determine arterial injury if digits are amputated. In the Allen test, both the radial and ulnar artery are compressed and the patient is asked to clench the hand repeatedly until it blanches, and then one artery is released, and the tissue on that side should flush. Then the test is repeated again, releasing the other artery.

Care of amputated part prior to reattachment or revascularization

The amputated part should be cooled to 4°C to extend the time of viability and decrease damage from ischemia. (Single digits and lower limbs are not usually reattached, but the limbs should be treated as though they will until determination is made, especially for children.) The part should be reattached within 6 hours if possible but up to 24 hours if properly cooled. Initial care of amputated part includes:
- Removal of jewelry.
- Irrigation with NS to remove debris or contamination.
- Part stored wrapped in saline moistened dressing but NOT immersed in saline or hypotonic solution.
- Minimal handling to prevent tissue damage.
- Cool by placing wrapped part in sealed plastic bag and immersing the bag in ice water (1:1 ice to water). Avoid freezing part and do not allow part to directly be exposed to ice.

If the amputation is partial, treatment is similar but NS wrapped part is splinted and ice packs or commercial cold packs are applied over area that is devascularized.

Compartment syndrome

Compartment syndrome occurs when muscle perfusion is inadequate because of constriction caused by a cast or tight dressing or because of increase in contents of a muscle compartment because of edema or hemorrhage (often related to fractures or crush injuries). It most often affects the forearm and leg muscles. Symptoms include:
- Severe, throbbing pain unrelieved by opiates.
- Numbness and tingling as pressure on nerves increases.
- Cyanosis and decreased or lacking pulse.
- Edema.

Diagnosis includes:
- Clinical examination.
- Doppler ultrasonography to verify pulses.
- Tissue pressure measurement (normal is 8 mm Hg or less).

Treatment must be initiated immediately to prevent neurovascular damage and necrosis:
- Elevation of affected limb above the heart.
- Release of constricting cast or dressings.
- Tissue fasciotomy to relieve constriction if condition is advanced or there is no response to medical treatment. The wound is left open, allowing the muscle tissue to expand, and covered with moist sterile NS dressing. The limb is splinted and elevated until swelling decreases.

Costochondritis

Costochondritis is inflammation of the cartilage that connects the sternum and the ribs in the anterior chest wall without edema. Costochondritis may be precipitated by exercise (especially repetitive activities that cause micro-damage), blunt trauma, postsurgical infection, fibromyalgia, or referred pain. It is most common in women older than 40, but is also a common cause of chest pain in children. Symptoms may mimic those of a myocardial infarction and include:
- Costochondral pain, especially on the left, increasing with breathing or coughing and with associated dyspnea.

Diagnosis includes:
- Clinical examination and pain on palpation of the costochondral junctions.
- ECG and chest x-rays may be done to rule out other disorders.

Treatments include:
- NSAIDs, such as ibuprofen.
- Steroid injection if nonresponsive to other medications.
- Local application of heat.
- Intercostal nerve block if pain refractory.
- Tricyclic antidepressants may aid with sleep.

Foreign bodies in subcutaneous tissue

Foreign bodies (FB) imbedded in subcutaneous tissue can include metal, glass, plastic, and wood. Symptoms may include pain, infection, or inflammatory response, pseudotumor, sinus tracts, or osteomyelitis. Patients often sense presence of FB. Treatment includes careful history and examination to determine if the trauma of removing the foreign object is worse than leaving the object in place. Inert objects, such as metal and sometimes plastic or glass may be left in place, but wood always causes infection and must be removed. Diagnosis includes:
- Radiographs of soft tissue (metal and glass).
- Ultrasound (wood or thorns).
- CT for dangerous FB only.

MRIs are usually only done if the initial attempt to remove the FB was unsuccessful and infection has developed, but metal fragments may move during an MRI so it is contraindicated for intraorbital or intracranial FBs.

Removal
Treatment to remove a foreign body (FB) should not exceed 30 minutes in the ED. Open tissue should not be probed with a gloved finger to locate FB because of the danger of tearing a glove:
- Palpate tissue and use metal instrument to search for glass fragments rather than gloved finger.
- Local anesthetic: lidocaine with epinephrine.
- Use radiographs or ultrasound for guidance, using metal markers or inserting 2 needles to isolate location.
- BP cuff or tourniquet may be needed to slow arterial flow to extremity.
- Incise tissue adequately and use hemostat to remove FB.
- Irrigate wound with normal saline.
- Wound is usually left opened and bandaged; large wounds may be sutured closed in 3 to 5 days.
- Antibiotics as indicated.
- FBs under nails may require removing all or part of nail:
- Digital block.
- Sterile hypodermic needle (straight or bent) slid under nail to capture the FB.
- CO_2 laser vaporization may be used to vaporize nail above foreign object.

Inflammation resulting from tattoos and piercing

Tattoos and piercing have both been implicated in MRSA infections. Tattooing uses needles that inject dye, sometimes resulting in local infection with erythema, edema, and purulent discharge. Body piercing for insertion of jewelry carries similar risks. Piercings of concern include the upper ear cartilage, nipples, navel, tongue, lip, penis, and nose. Some people who do piercings use reusable piercing equipment that is difficult to adequately clean and sterilize. Infections resulting from piercing in cartilage are often resistant to antibiotics because of lack of blood supply.

- 136 -

Copyright © Mometrix Media. You have been licensed one copy of this document for personal use only. Any other reproduction or redistribution is strictly prohibited. All rights reserved.

Treatment includes:
- Cleansing wounds. Jewelry may need to be removed in some cases.
- Antibiotics: Culture should be obtained, but medications for community-acquired MRSA should be started immediately:
- Mupirocin may be used topically 3 times daily for 7 to 10 days with or without systemic antimicrobials.
- Trimethoprim-sulfamethoxazole DS (TMP 160 mg/SMX 800 mg), 1 to 2 tablets twice daily. Children, dose based on TMP: 8 to 12 mg/kg/day in 2 doses.

Infectious arthritis

Infectious arthritis may be bacterial, viral (rubella, parvovirus, and hepatitis B), parasitic, or fungal, with bacterial arthritis causing the most rapid destruction to the joint. *Neisseria gonorrhoeae* (most common), *Staphylococcus, Streptococcus, and Escherichia coli* are the most common bacterial agents. The infection may be bloodborne or spread from an infection near the joint or from direct implantation or postoperative contamination of the wound. Usually the infection involves just one joint. Symptoms include acute edema, erythema, and pain in a joint. Systemic reactions, such as fever and polyarthralgia, may occur, especially with gonorrhea. Diagnosis requires a complete history and physical examination, arthrocentesis and synovial fluid culture, and WBC.

Treatment includes:
- Antibiotics as indicated by organism.
- Arthrocentesis to drain fluid accumulation in joint (may need to be repeated).
- Analgesia.

Bursitis and tendinitis

Bursitis is inflammation of the bursa, fluid-filled spaces or sacs that form in tissues to reduce friction, causing thickening of the lining of the bursal walls. This can be the result of infection, trauma, crystal deposits, or chronic friction from trauma. Tendinitis is inflammation of the long, tubular tendons and tendon sheaths, adjacent to bursa. Causes of tendinitis are similar to bursitis but tendinitis may also be caused by quinolone antibiotics. Frequently, both bursa and tendons are inflamed. Common types of bursitis include shoulder, olecranon (elbow), trochanteric (hip), and prepatellar (front of knee). Common types of tendinitis include wrist, Achilles, patellar, and rotator cuff. Symptoms include pain with movement, edema, dysfunction, and decreased range of motion.

Diagnosis is by clinical examination, although x-rays may rule out fractures. The bursa may be aspirated diagnostically to aid in ruling out other diagnosis, like gout or infection. Treatment for bursitis and tendinitis includes:
- Rest and immobilization.
- NSAIDs.
- Application of cold packs to affected area.
- Steroid injections.

Carpal tunnel syndrome

Carpal tunnel syndrome is a type of entrapment neuropathy in which the median nerve is compressed by thickening of the flexor tendon sheath, skeletal encroachment, or mass in the soft tissue. Carpal tunnel syndrome is often associated with repetitive hand activities, arthritis, hypothyroidism, diabetes, and pregnancy. Patients complain of pain in wrist, radiating to forearm, and numbness and tingling in the first 2 to 3 fingers, especially during the night. Diagnosis is based on symptoms and tests:
- Positive Tinel test: Gentle percussion over medial nerve in inner aspect of wrist elicits numbness and pain.
- Positive Phalen test: The backs of the hands are pressed together and the wrists sharply flexed for 1 minute to elicit pain and numbness.

Treatment includes identifying and treating underlying cause:
- Steroid injection may relieve symptoms.
- Splint during the night or during repetitive activities.
- Modification of activities.
- Referral for decompression surgery in recalcitrant cases or those with severe loss of sensation.

Joint effusion and arthrocentesis

Joint effusion is the accumulation of fluid (clear, bloody, or purulent) within a joint capsule. Joint effusion can cause pressure on the joint and severe pain. Arthrocentesis relieves the pressure and the fluid aspirated can be examined to aid in diagnosis. Arthrocentesis is usually contraindicated in the presence of overlying infection, prosthetic joint, and coagulopathy without referral to an orthopedic specialist.

Procedure:
- Patient is positioned according to joint to be aspirated and encouraged to relax muscles.
- Overlying area is cleansed with povidone-iodine solution, air-dried a few minutes, and cleansed of iodine with alcohol wipe.
- Local anesthetic is given to area (but not into joint) with 25 to 30 gauge needle (lidocaine 1% to 2% lidocaine) or a regional nerve block for severe pain.
- Joint is aspirated with insertion in a straight line, using a 30 to 60 mL syringe (depending upon expected amount of fluid) and an 18 to 22 gauge needle or IV catheter.
- The joint is completely drained of fluid.
- Observe for complications: bleeding, infection, allergic reaction.

Gout

Gout (metabolic arthritis) is a group of conditions associated with a defect of purine metabolism that results in hyperuricemia with oversecretion of uric acid, decreased excretion of uric acid, or a combination. The increased uric acid levels can cause monosodium urate crystal depositions in the joints, resulting in severe articular and periarticular inflammation. With chronic gout, sodium urate crystals, called tophi, accumulate in peripheral body areas, such as the great toe (75%), hands, and ears, although other joints may be affected. Patients often present to the ED with acute gout, and these flares can be a recurrent part of the chronic condition. Symptoms include abrupt onset of pain with erythema and edema lasting 3 to 10 days. Attacks become more frequent over time and some may develop kidney stones. Diagnosis is based on clinical examination, history, and uric acid level greater than 7 mg/dL. The most specific and secure diagnosis is made when urate crystals are visualized in fluid aspirated from synovial joint under microscope. Treatment includes:

- NSAIDs (first line, such as naproxen 500 mg PO every 12 hours or indomethacin 50 mg PO three times a day), colchicine (tapering dose as symptoms resolve),
- Prophylactic for chronic gout: Probenecid (to prevent tophi formation), Allopurinol (to prevent formation of uric acid). Restriction of high-purine foods (organ meats) and alcohol.
- Weight control methods.

Lumbosacral pain

Lumbosacral (low back) pain may be related to strain, muscular weakness, osteoarthritis, spinal stenosis, herniated disks, vertebral fractures, bony metastasis, infection, or other musculoskeletal disorders. Disk herniation or other joint changes put pressure on nerves leaving the spinal cord, causing pain to radiate along the nerve. Pain may be acute or chronic (more than 3 months). Symptoms include local or pain radiating down the leg (radiculopathy), impaired gait and reflexes, difference in leg lengths, decreased motor strength, and alteration of sensation, including numbness. Diagnosis is by careful clinical examination and history as well as x-ray (fractures, scoliosis, dislocations), CT (identifies underlying problems), MRI (spinal pathology), and/or EMG and nerve conduction studies. Diagnostic studies may be deferred in many cases for 4 to 6 weeks as symptoms may resolve over time. Treatments for nonspecific back pain include:

- Analgesia: acetaminophen, NSAIDS, opiates.
- Encourage activity to tolerance but not bed rest.
- Muscle relaxants: diazepam 5 to 10 mg every 6 to 8 hours.
- Cold compresses and/or heart compresses.

Peripheral vascular trauma

Peripheral vascular trauma may be blunt (auto accident, bites) or penetrating (gunshot and stab wounds, iatrogenic injuries). Fractures and dislocations can compromise blood flow. Most injuries (80%) affect the lower extremities. Symptoms include hematoma, hemorrhage, pain on extension, thrill or bruit, lack of pulse, decreased sensation, delay in capillary refill, and temperature change and pallor in affected limb. Ischemia greater than 4 to 6 hours can result in necrosis of tissue so prompt identification is critical. Diagnosis includes CBC, radiographs to determine cause, angiography/CT angiography to determine arterial injury, ankle-brachial index, color-flow duplex ultrasound, and Doppler pressure measurements. Treatment varies according to underlying cause:

- Reduction of fractures or dislocations.
- Control of hemorrhage with pressure or BP cuff (avoid the use of hemostats and clamps, which can injure vessels).
- Referral for surgical consultation if indicated.

Osteomyelitis

Osteomyelitis is infection of the bone, usually from extension of soft tissue infection (infected ulcer), puncture wound (bone surgery or trauma), and bloodborne infection. Osteomyelitis is common in the foot with *Pseudomonas* most often in nondiabetic persons and *Staphylococcus aureus* in diabetic persons, who are 3 times more likely to develop osteomyelitis. Symptoms vary according to cause. Onset may be sudden if bloodborne with constant throbbing pain. The area may be erythematous and edematous if from adjacent infection, and chronic conditions may exhibit constant or intermittent drainage and pain. Diagnosis includes x-ray, radioisotope bones scans, MRI, and CBC, and wound and blood cultures. Treatment includes identifying and treating underlying cause:

- IV antibiotic therapy based on diagnosis is begun around the clock initially and modified with results of culture, usually continuing for 2 to 3 weeks.
- Supportive measures: Diet high in vitamins and protein, good hydration.
- Immobilization of affected area to reduce pain and prevent fractures.
- Warm wet soaks 20 minutes 4 times daily.
- Referral for surgical debridement as indicated.

Strains and sprains

A strain is a overstretching of a part of the musculature ("pulled muscle") that causes microscopic tears in the muscle, usually resulting from excess stress or overuse of the muscle. Onset of pain is usually sudden with local tenderness on use of the muscle. A sprain is damage to a joint, with a partial rupture of the supporting ligaments, usually caused by wrenching or twisting that may occur with a fall. The rupture can damage blood vessels, resulting in edema, tenderness at the joint, and pain on movement with pain increasing over 2 to 3 hours after injury. An avulsion fracture (bone fragment pulled away by a ligament) may occur with strain, so x-rays rule out fractures. Treatment for both strains and strains includes:

- RICE protocol: rest, ice, compression, and elevation.
- Ice compresses (wet or dry) should be applied 20 to 30 minutes intermittently for 48 hours and then intermittent heat 15 to 20 minutes 3 to 4 times daily.
- Monitor neurovascular status (especially for sprain).
- Immobilization as indicated for sprains for 1 to 3 weeks.

> **Review Video:** <u>R.I.C.E.</u>
> *Visit **mometrix.com/academy** and enter **Code: 654264***

Fractures and dislocations

Fractures and dislocations usually occur as the result of trauma, such as from falls and auto accidents, but pathologic fractures can result from minor force to diseased bones such as those with osteoporosis or metastatic lesions. Stress fractures are caused by repetitive trauma, such as from forced marching. Salter fractures involve the cartilaginous epiphyseal plate near the ends of long bones in children who are growing. Damage to this area can impair bone growth. Orthopedic injuries that are of special concern include:

- Open fractures with soft tissue injury overlying the fracture, including puncture wounds from external forces or bone fragments, can result in osteomyelitis.
- Subluxation, partial dislocation of a joint, and luxation (complete dislocation) can cause neurovascular compromise, which can be permanent if reduction is delayed. Dislocation of the hip can result in avascular necrosis of the femoral head.

Fractures and dislocations are commonly diagnosed by clinical examination, history, and radiographs. Careful inspection and observation of range of motion, palpation, and observation of abnormalities is important because pain may be referred. Neurovascular assessment should be done immediately to prevent vascular compromise. Radiographs should usually precede reduction of dislocations to ensure there are no fractures and follow reduction to ensure the dislocation is reduced.

Treatment includes:
- Analgesia and sedation as indicated.
- Application of cold compresses and elevation of fractured area to reduce edema.
- Reduction of fracture: steady and gradual longitudinal traction to realign bone.
- Immobilization with brace, cast, sling, or splint indicated.
- Reduction of dislocation: Varies according to area of dislocation.
- Open fracture:
- Wound irrigation with NS.
- Tetanus prophylaxis.
- Antibiotic prophylaxis.
- Referral to orthopedic specialist for open fractures, irreducible dislocations, and complications such as compartment syndrome or circulatory impairment.

Immobilization techniques for fractures and dislocations include:
- Cast: Plaster and fiberglass casts are applied after reduction to ensure that bone is correctly aligned. Cast should be placed over several layers of padding that extends slightly beyond the cast ends. Cast material, such as plaster, should NOT be immersed in hot water but water slightly above room temperature (70°F).
- Splint: Plaster splints use 12 or more layers of plaster measured to the correct length and then several layers of padding (longer and wider than splint should be measured and cut). The plastic splint is submerged in water to saturate, removed, laid on a flat surface, and massaged to fuse the layers. The padding is laid on top and the splint positioned and wrapped with gauze to hold in place. While setting the splint, position can be maintained by holding in place with the palm of the hand (not the fingers). After setting, the splint may be wrapped by elastic compression bandage.

> **Review Video:** Range of Motion Therapy
> *Visit mometrix.com/academy and enter Code:* **191142**

Crutches

Crutches should be properly fitted before patient attempts ambulation. Correct height is one hand-width below axillae. The handgrips should be adjusted so the patient supports the body weight comfortably with elbows slightly flexed rather than locked in place. The patient should be cautioned not to bear weight under the axillae as this can cause nerve damage but to hold the crutches tight against the side of the chest wall. The type of gait that the patient uses depends on the type of injury. Typical gaits include:
- Two-point in which both crutches are placed forward and then the well leg advances to the crutches.
- Three-point in which the injured extremity and both crutches are advanced together and then the well leg advances to the crutches.

The patient should be advised whether there is partial or no weightbearing and demonstration provided. Stair climbing should be practiced:
- Ascending: well foot goes first and then crutches and injured extremity.
- Descending: Crutches go first and then the well foot.

Abrasion, contusion, laceration, and avulsion

Abrasion is damage to superficial layers of skin, such as with road burn or ligature marks. Contusion occurs when friction or pressure causes damage to underlying vessels, resulting in bruising. Contusions that are bright red/purple with clear margins have occurred within 48 hours and those with receding edges or yellow-brown discoloration are older than 48 hours. Laceration is a tear in the skin resulting from blunt force, often from falls on protuberances, such as elbows, or other blunt trauma. Lacerations may be partial to full-thickness. Avulsion is tissue that is separated from its base and lost or without adequate base for attachment. Treatments include:

- Local anesthetic if needed.
- Low pressure, high volume irrigation with 35-50 ml syringe of open wound with normal saline, water, or non antiseptic nonionic surfactants, such as Shur-Clens®, and mechanical scrubbing of surrounding tissue with disinfectant.
- Topical antibiotics as indicated.
- Prophylactic antibiotics or antibiotic irrigation if wound contaminated.
- Suturing/debridement as needed.
- Hydrocolloids, Steri-Strips, and transparent dressings to stabilize flaps.

Skin stripping and lacerations

Mechanical trauma may result in stripping of the epidermis and sometimes the dermis of the skin or lacerations. Mechanical trauma may occur from tape removal or blunt trauma, such as colliding with furniture. Skin tears are categorized with the Payne-Martin Classification System:

- Skin tear leaves avulsed skin adequate to cover wound. Tears may be linear or flap-type.
- Skin tear with loss of partial thickness, involving either scant (less than 25% of epidermal flap over tear is lost) to moderate-large (more than 25% of dermis in tear is lost).
- Skin tear with complete loss of tissue, involving a partial-thickness wound with no epidermal flap.

Treatment includes:

- Recognizing fragile skin and treating carefully.
- Applying emollients, skin sealants, and skin barriers as indicated.
- Applying and removing tape appropriately.
- Avoiding adhesives when possible.
- Using hydrocolloids, Steri-Strips, and transparent dressings to stabilize flaps.

Missile injuries

Missile injuries include arrow, gunshot, paint gun, nail gun, and shrapnel wounds. These injuries are usually circular, oval, or triangular, and may have both an entry (with abrasion at periphery) and exit site. Other residue, such as gunpowder, may be evident at the entry. Careful documentation should be done and clothes retained for evidence in gunshot wounds. Puncture wounds are difficult to properly cleanse and become easily infected, even with treatment. Treatment varies according to the site, type, and degree of injury and may include:

- Tetanus prophylaxis.
- Irrigation of wound with NS if both entry and exit.
- Incision over puncture wound to create a linear incision that can be irrigated and cleansed adequately.

- Removal of foreign body if in place.
- Antibiotics as indicated.
- Follow-up care to check for infection.

High-Pressure Injection Injuries

High-pressure injection injuries involve injection of materials (such as nails) or substances (water, air, oil, paint) into the tissue under high pressure. The severity of the injury depends on the location of the injury, the material or substance, and the size or amount of the injection. High-pressure injection injuries may result in ischemia, tissue destruction, open wounds, and inflammatory response even though the external injury may appear small. Signs and symptoms include pain and swelling. Crepitus may be present with air injection. Ischemia may occur. These injuries may result in fractures, contractures, amputations, fibrosis, and fistulae. Common substances involved in high-pressure injection injuries include grease (over half of injuries) and diesel fuel. Injuries often occur on fingers of the non-dominant hand. Diagnosis includes clinical symptoms and may include CBC (as some substances may cause increase WBC count) and electrolytes (some substances cause imbalance). Treatment depends on the extent of injury and includes supportive care, tetanus prophylaxis, and broad-spectrum antibiotic. Surgical repair may be required.

Medical maggots

Medical Maggots are applied to the open wound; periwound tissue must be protected:
- A wound pattern is transferred onto a hydrocolloid pad, opening cut, and pad applied to the skin with the wound exposed. The pattern is used to cut an opening in a semi-permeable film for an outer dressing.
- Maggots are wiped from the container with a saline-dampened 2 X 2 gauze (about 5 to 10 maggots per cm^2 wound size). The gauze is loosely packed into the wound.
- A porous mesh (Creature Comfort) is placed over the wound and secured to the hydrocolloid with tape or glue, creating a maggot cage.
- Transparent film is placed over the hydrocolloid, making sure that the cutout area is over the cage so that the maggots have air and drainage can escape. Saline-dampened gauze is placed loosely over cage.
- Dry gauze is used for the outer dressing and changed every 4 to 8 hours as needed.
- Maggots are wiped from the wound after 48 hours and wound irrigated with normal saline.

Environment and Toxicology Emergencies, and Communicable Diseases

Tick bites

Ticks, blood-feeding parasites, are the primary vector of infectious diseases in the United States. Ticks transmit a wide variety of pathogens, including bacteria such as *Rickettsiae*, protozoan parasites, and viruses. Lyme disease is the most common tick-borne disease, but there are increasing reports of other diseases, such as babesiosis, human anaplasmosis, and ehrlichiosis. Many tick-borne diseases present with similar, nonspecific flu-like symptoms and can easily be misdiagnosed. Ticks should be carefully removed if still feeding:

- Using fine-tipped tweezers, tick is grasped close to the skin and pulled upward with even and steady pressure, avoiding jerks or twists that may break mouthparts.
- The tick must not be handled with bare hands.
- Disinfect skin site.
- Tick should be saved for identification: place tick in a plastic bag, date, and place in freezer in case illness occurs in 2 to 3 weeks.

People should be cautioned to immediately seek medical attention for flu-like or neurological symptoms or erythema migrans (bull's eye rash) typical of Lyme disease.

Bee stings

Bees and wasps sting by puncturing the skin with a hollow stinger and injecting venom. Wasps and bumblebees can sting more than once but honeybees have barbs on their stingers, and the barbs keep the stinger hooked into the skin. Local reactions to bee sting:

- Raised white wheal with central red spot of about 10 mm appearing within a few minutes and lasting 20 minutes (honeybees)
- Edema and erythema, which may last several days (vespid wasps).
- Pain, swelling, and redness confined to sting site.
- Swelling may extend beyond the sting site and may, for example, involve swelling of an entire limb.

Some people may develop an anaphylactic reaction, including a biphasic reaction, in which the symptoms recede and then return 2 to 3 hours later. About 50% of deaths occur within 30 minutes of the sting, and 75% within 4 hours. Symptoms of an allergic reaction/anaphylaxis may become increasingly severe with generalized urticaria, edema, hypotension, and respiratory distress.

Treatment of bee stings initially includes:

- Wash the site with soap and water.
- Remove stinger using 4 x 4–inch gauze wiped over the area or by scraping a sharp instrument over the area.
- NEVER squeeze the stinger or use tweezers, as this will cause more venom to go into the skin.
- Apply ice to reduce the swelling (10 to 20 minutes on/10 to 20 minutes off for 24 hours).
- Antihistamines may be prescribed.

- A paste of baking soda and water or meat tenderizer and water may reduce itching.
- Topical corticosteroids may relieve itching.
- Tetanus toxoid or tetanus immune globulin as needed.

Allergic responses/anaphylaxis requires immediate, aggressive medical intervention:
- Epinephrine.
- Antihistamines.
- Corticosteroids.
- IV fluids as needed.
- Oxygen and other supportive treatments.

People with extensive local or anaphylactic reactions should be advised to carry an epinephrine autoinjector for emergency use if stung.

Spider bites

Spider bites are frequently a misdiagnosis of a *Staphylococcus aureus* or MRSA infection, so unless the spider was observed, the wound should be cultured and antibiotics started. If the wound responds to the antibiotic, then it probably was not a spider bite. There are 2 main types of venomous spider bites:
- Producing neurological symptoms (black widow).
- Producing local necrosis (brown recluse, yellow sac, and hobo spiders).

Treatment includes:
- Cleanse wound and apply cool compress and elevate body part if possible.

Black widow bites:
- Narcotic analgesics.
- Nitroprusside to relieve hypertension.
- Calcium gluconate 10% solution IV for abdominal cramps.
- Latrodectus antivenin for those with severe reaction.

Necrotic/ulcerated bites (e.g., brown recluse):
- There is no consensus on the best treatment, as ulceration caused by the venom may be extensive and surgical repair with grafts may be needed.
- Treatment as for other necrotic ulcers, with moisture-retentive dressings as indicated.
- Hyperbaric oxygen therapy (HBOT) has been used in some cases.

Animal bites

There is no one topical therapy for traumatic wounds because they vary so widely in the type and degree of injury. A scrape on the knee is treated very differently from a car accident that involves massive tissue injury or tissue loss. Animal bites, including human, are frequent causes of traumatic injury. Treatment includes:
- Cleanse wound by flushing with 10 to 35 cc syringe with 18-gauge Angiocath to remove debris and bacteria using normal saline or dilute Betadine solution.
- Hand, puncture, and infected wounds or those more than 12 hours old may be closed by secondary intention.

- Moisture-retentive dressings as indicated by the size and extent of injury of wound left open. Dry dressings may be applied to injuries with closure by primary intention.
- Topical antibiotics may be indicated, although systemic antibiotics are commonly prescribed for animal bites.
- Tetanus toxoid or immune globulin is routinely administered.

Snake bites

Coral snakes
About 45,000 snakebites occur in the United States each year, about 8,000 of which are venomous. In the United States, about 25 species of snakes are venomous. There are 2 types of snakes that can cause serious injury, classified according to the type of fangs and venom. Coral snakes have short, fixed permanent fangs in the upper jaw and venom that is primarily neurotoxic, but may also have hemotoxic and cardiotoxic properties:
- Wounds show no fang marks but there may be scratches or semi-circular markings from teeth.
- There may be little local reaction, but neurological symptoms may range from mild to acute respiratory and cardiovascular failure.

Treatment includes:
- Cleanse wound thoroughly of dirt and debris and leave open or cover with dry dressing.
- Antibiotics not usually needed.
- Administer antivenin immediately even without symptoms, which may be delayed.
- Tetanus toxoid or immune globulin.

Pit vipers
The second type of snakes that can cause serious injury include the pit vipers. Rattlesnakes, copperheads, and cottonmouths have erectile fangs that fold until they are aroused, and venom is primarily hemotoxic and cytotoxic but may have neurotoxic properties.
- Wounds usually show 1 or 2 fang marks.
- Edema may begin immediately or may be delayed up to 6 hours.
- Pain may be severe.
- There may be a wide range of symptoms, including hypotension and coagulopathy with defibrination that can lead to excessive blood loss, depending upon the type and amount of venom.
- There may be local infection and necrosis.

Treatment includes:
- Cleansing wound thoroughly and dressings as indicated.
- Tetanus toxoid or immune globulin.
- Analgesics, such as morphine sulphate
- Avoiding NSAIDs and aspirin because of anticoagulation properties.
- Marking edema every 15 minutes.
- Antivenin therapy if indicated (observation for serum sickness if horse serum used).
- Prophylactic antibiotics for severe tissue necrosis.
- Platelets, plasma, or packed RBCs for coagulopathy.

Shark bites

Even small shark bites can crush bones. Hit and run attacks may cause small lacerations or minimal damage, but other types of attacks can result in loss of limbs or large chunks of flesh, with loss of muscle and bone. Internal organs may be exposed and damaged. Extensive soft tissue trauma and damage to arteries and veins may occur, as well as crushing internal injuries. The wounds are often contaminated with sand, algae, fragments of shark teeth, and other materials and pathogens, such as *Mycobacterium marinum* and *Vibrio spp.* Life-threatening injuries need to be addressed first, including control of hemorrhage:
- IV fluids and blood products.
- Tetanus toxoid or tetanus immune globulin.
- Wounds must be flushed with copious amounts of normal saline and debris removed.
- Treatment for hypothermia if needed.
- X-rays to identify fractures or debris in wound.
- Fixation of fractures.
- Prophylactic antibiotics:
- Ciprofloxacin
- Trimethoprim-sulfamethoxazole
- Doxycycline
- Surgical repair, debridement, and/or skin grafting.

Alligator bites

Alligators are found in 10 coastal states in the southeastern United States with the largest population in Florida, where most injuries are reported. Animals between 4 and 8 feet often bite once and release, but larger animals may bite repeatedly, engaging in typical biting and feeding activities, which result in severe injury, amputations, or death. Most wounds involve the limbs, with the hands and arms the most frequently bitten. Treatment includes:
- Treatment for shock and blood loss.
- Applying pressure to wound.
- Retrieving amputated limbs if possible.
- Flushing wound with copious amounts of normal saline to reduce contamination.
- Wound cultures.
- Prophylactic broad-spectrum antibiotics for gram-negative organisms, such as *Aeromonas hydrophila* and *Clostridium.*
- Observation for signs of infection, such as erythema, cellulitis, exudate, and necrosis.
- Tetanus toxoid or immune globulin.
- Repair fractures.
- Surgical repair and debridement as indicated with wounds usually healing by secondary intention or delayed primary closure.

Stingray stings

The tail of a stingray is thrust forward, driving serrated spines into the victim, causing a jagged laceration. The stinger injects a toxin that causes severe pain. Wounds often become infected. Symptoms include:
- Intense, excruciating pain with envenomation lasting 2 to 3 days.
- Bleeding.
- Systemic: dizziness, GI upset, seizures, hypotension.

Treatment includes:
- Rinse the wound with fresh water or saline and remove visible pieces of spine with forceps or tweezers.
- Heat immersion: Deactivate the venom and relieve pain by immersing the wound in hot water for 30 to 90 minutes at 113°F (45°C). May repeat up to 2 hours.
- Radiographs may be necessary to locate the spine or fragment.
- Tetanus toxoid or tetanus immune globulin.
- Infiltration of wound with a local anesthetic, such as lidocaine or bupivacaine, to relieve severe pain.
- Opiates for pain.
- Open wounds are usually allowed to heal without primary closure or with loose primary closure.
- Prophylactic antibiotics may be given for 5 days to prevent infections.

Diarrhea related to bacterial infections from contaminated food or water

A wide range of bacterial and viral pathogens can cause mild to severe life-threatening diarrhea:
- *Campylobacter jejuni* transmitted from pets to children younger than 7 years through contaminated food and water, usually in the summer. Diarrhea with fever, vomiting, and abdominal pain persists 7 to 12 days. Treatment: (in complicated cases) levofloxacin 500 mg orally for 3 days or until symptoms improve.
- *Clostridium difficile* occurs secondary to antibiotic use as normal flora of the gut is killed and c. difficile colonizes the GI tract. Some people are asymptomatic carriers, but severe illness is life-threatening with bloody diarrhea and abdominal pain leading to megacolon. Treatment: stop inciting antibiotic, contact precautions with soap and water instead of hand sanitizer to remove spores. Metronidazole (moderate) or vancomycin for 10-14 days (severe).
- *Yersinia enterocolitica* found in uncooked pork or unpasteurized milk causes secretory diarrhea with fever, foul, green, bloody stool, and pain in RLQ of abdomen. Usually resolves in 3-4 days.
- *Shigella* is transmitted fecal-oral route from contaminated food and water and occurs primarily in children from 6 to 36 months of age. Characterized by blood diarrhea, abdominal pain, and fever. Treatment: Tailored to cultures but use fluroquinolones once daily x 3 days while waiting for culture results or Trimethoprim-sulfamethoxazole (TMP-SMZ): TMP 8 mg/kg and SMZ 40 mg/kg per day given orally in 2 divided doses every 12 hours for 5 days.

Salmonella

Salmonella causes up to 4 million infections in the United States, resulting in 500 deaths, primarily of young children. There are two main types of salmonella, with nontyphoidal salmonella being the most common in the United States. Nontyphoidal *Salmonella* is spread by the fecal-oral route through ingestion of contaminated food or water, including all meats, milk, eggs, and vegetables. Raw or undercooked meat, unpasteurized milk, and unwashed produce are high risk. *Salmonella* may be found in the feces of pets, particularly reptiles such as snakes and turtles.

Symptoms appear 12 to 72 hours after infection and include bloody diarrhea with abdominal pain, fever, and vomiting. Most cases resolve within 7 to 10 days, and are often indistinguishable from any other gastroenteritis. The mainstay of treatment is keeping the patient from becoming hypovolemic and keeping electrolytes balanced. In some cases, life-threatening sepsis may occur, requiring treatment with antibiotics, and fluoroquinolones are the antibiotics of choice. Antibiotic prophylaxis is usually contraindicated except in children younger than 1 year of age who are at risk for bacteremia or those who are immunocompromised. Patients who handle food as an occupation and those who are healthcare workers should not return to work until symptoms abate.

Escherichia coli

E. coli strains are part of the normal flora of the intestines and serves to inhibit other bacteria, but some serotypes can cause intestinal disease and severe diarrhea. Onset of symptoms is generally about 4 days after being exposed. Some strains of E. coli are more common in developing countries and may occur in people who are traveling in areas where feces have contaminated food supplies and water. Severe outbreaks of *E. coli* infection have occurred in the United States with a toxic strain, O157:H7, known as an enterohemorrhagic E. coli. This strain produces a toxin that can cause damage to the intestinal lining, including blood vessels, resulting in hemorrhage and watery diarrhea that becomes bloody, especially in children and elderly persons. This hemorrhagic colitis usually clears with supportive treatment after 10 days. However, about 15% of children develop sepsis and hemolytic uremic syndrome with kidney failure, hemolytic anemia, and thrombocytopenia. Death rates are 3% to 5%, but residual renal and neurological damage may result. Treatment is supportive with IV therapy, blood transfusions, and kidney dialysis. Antibiotics and antidiarrheals are contraindicated because they may worsen *E. coli* infections.

Hemolytic uremic syndrome

Hemolytic uremic syndrome is a life-threatening disorder usually follows an *E. coli* infection. Mortality rates are 3% to 5%, but chronic renal problems develop in 50% and a few have lifelong complications, including blindness, paralysis, and kidney failure requiring dialysis. Symptoms include:
- Weakness, lethargy.
- Nausea and increased diarrhea, blood in stool
- Fever.
- Hematuria and decreased urinary output.
- Petechiae and ecchymosis, bleeding from the nose or mouth occurs as platelets decrease and clotting time increases.
- Jaundice.
- Alterations in consciousness, seizures (rare), paralysis (cerebral blood clot).
- Hypertension.
- Edema.

Treatment includes:
- Antibiotics are contraindicated unless sepsis is present because they may increase release of toxins associated with E. coli.
- IV fluids and nutritional supplements.
- Protein limitation and ACE inhibitors to prevent permanent kidney damage.
- Transfusions may be needed.
- Plasmapheresis is sometimes used to remove Blood antibodies from the blood.

Ingestion or exposure to pesticides

Insecticides, organophosphorus compounds, and carbamates can cause severe CNS toxicity, usually within 8 to 24 hours of exposure by ingestion, inhalation, or contact. History, clinical exam, cholinesterase assays, and tests for specific compounds. Staff must use protective measures caring for patients with external contamination. Symptoms include:

- Salivation, lacrimation
- Urinary incontinence and defecation.
- GI irritation with n/v.
- Bradycardia, heart block, ventricular dysrhythmias.
- Bronchorrhea and bronchospasm.
- Hydrocarbon/garlic odor. 1 to 4 days after ingestion: paralysis of neck flexor, proximal limb, and respiratory muscles may occur. 1 to 3 weeks after ingestion: irreversible neurological and neurobehavioral abnormalities and paralysis may occur.

Treatment includes:

- Supportive:
  - Gastric decontamination (if ingested orally).
  - Decontamination (varies according to type of contamination).
  - Oxygen (100%), oximetry, and cardiac monitoring.
- Antidotes: atropine 1 mg (adult) or 0.01 to 0.04 mg/kg (children) IV initially and may be repeated and pralidoxime 1 to 2 g (adults) or 20 to 40 mg/kg (children) in NS over 10 minutes or IM to resolve paralysis.

Intestinal parasites

Giardia lamblia
Giardia lamblia is a protozoan that infects water supplies and spreads through the fecal-oral route. It is the most common cause on nonbacterial diarrhea in the United States, causing about 20,000 cases of infection each year in all ages. Children often become infected by swallowing recreational waters (pools, lakes) while swimming or putting contaminated items into the mouth. *Giardia* lives and multiplies within the small intestine where cysts develop. Symptoms occur 7 to 14 days after ingestion of 1 or more cysts and include diarrhea with greasy, floating stools (rarely bloody), stomach cramps, nausea, and flatulence, lasting 2 to 6 weeks. A chronic infection may develop that can last for months or years. Treatment includes furazolidone 5 to 8 mg/kg/day in 4 doses for 7 to 10 days or metronidazole 40 mg/kg/day in 3 doses for 7 to 10 days. Chronic infections are often very resistant to treatment.

Pinworms
Enterobius vermicularis (pinworms) are tiny (3 to 13 mm) worms that hatch in the small intestine after ingestion of eggs. The mature worms crawl through the rectum to lay eggs in the perianal folds, causing intense itching, often resulting in repeat self-infection; the person scratches and touches the hand to the mouth or contaminates food. Infection may result from contact with contaminated surfaces as well. The larvae hatch in the small intestines, but the adults live in the colon. Pinworms are the most common helminthic infection in the United States, affecting about 40 million people, especially children. Many are asymptomatic except for intense perianal itching, although some may have abdominal discomfort and anorexia or develop secondary infections from scratching. Girls may develop vulvovaginitis from invasion of the genital tract. Diagnosis is made by the "scotch tape" test or anal swabs.

Treatment includes albendazole 400 mg for 1 dose repeated in 2 weeks or mebendazole 100 mg for 1 dose repeated in 2 weeks or pyrantel pamoate 11 mg/kg for 1 dose repeated in 2 weeks.

Roundworms

Worldwide, there are numerous helminthes (worms) that can cause intestinal infections. Studies estimate that 50 million children in the United States are infected with worms. Risk factors include:

- Young age.
- Going barefoot.
- Poor sanitation of food and water.
- Poor hygiene.
- Living in or traveling to an endemic area.
- Immigrant status, especially from Mexico.

Roundworms (Ascaris lumbricoides) can grow 6 to 13 inches in length, and a child may have up to 100 worms. After ingestion of eggs from contaminated raw foods or vegetables, the worms migrate to the intestines but can migrate to other organs, such as the lungs, and cause serious damage. They may also multiply in clumps and cause intestinal obstruction or may penetrate the intestinal wall causing peritonitis. Symptoms include malnutrition, abdominal discomfort, and passing worms in stool or emesis. Treatment includes albendazole 400 mg orally once **OR** mebendazole 100 mg times 3 days **OR** pyrantel pamoate 11 mg/kg in 1 dose. Piperazine citrate 75 mg/kg/day for 2 days for intestinal obstruction.

Hookworms

Necator americanus is the most common species of hookworm found in the southeastern United States. Hookworm larvae may be swallowed directly or penetrate the skin, often the feet of children going barefoot, and migrate to the lungs, where they are coughed up and swallowed, and then carried to the small intestines, where they attach themselves to the walls to suck blood and multiply. Severe infection can result in hypochromic, microcytic anemia along with hypoproteinemia and malnutrition. Infection with hookworms can result in dyspnea, cardiomegaly, and arrhythmias, and can be fatal in infants. Infected children may have restricted growth and mental development, which may be irreversible. Diagnosis is with serial stool specimens. Symptoms include itching and rash at the site of infection, followed by abdominal pain, diarrhea, anorexia, weight loss, and anemia. Treatment includes albendazole 400 mg once **OR** mebendazole 100 mg times 3 days. Iron supplements may be necessary. Stools must be rechecked 1 week after treatment so that repeat treatment can be done if needed.

Tapeworm

Cestodes, or tapeworms, are parasitic worms that live in the intestinal tracts of some animals/fish. There are several different species that can infect humans who eat raw or undercooked meat or fish that contains the immature form of the tapeworm. The worms mature and lay eggs that usually undergo maturation in the small bowel (autoinfection) or pass through the host feces. Many infections are asymptomatic, but heavy infections can cause nausea, vomiting, weight loss, diarrhea, and epigastric and abdominal pain. Pork tapeworms may invade the subcutaneous tissue and CNS, causing epilepsy and neurological compromise. Fish tapeworm may cause pernicious anemia. Diagnosis: stool ova and parasites.

Treatment includes:
- Praziquantel 5 to 10 mg/kg one time (drug of choice for all types) **OR**
- Nitazoxanide 500 mg for 3 days (dwarf tapeworm)
  - 1 to 3 years, 100 mg twice daily for 3 days
  - 4 to 11 years, 200 mg twice daily for 3 days **OR**
- Niclosamide 1 g one time (beef, pork, fish, and double-pored dog tapeworm)
  - 50 mg/kg one time pediatric dose.

Lice

Pediculosis is infestation with lice, transmitted by direct contact with someone who is infested:
- Head lice (most common in children).
- Body lice (most common in transient populations). They feed on the body but live in clothing or bedding and are spread by sharing bedding, clothes, or towels.
- Pubic lice spread by sexual contact or (rare) sharing clothes or bedding, and may infest the genital area, eyebrows, eyelids, lower abdomen, and beard.

Symptoms include persistent itch (usually worse at night), irritation, excoriation, and sometimes secondary infection. Diagnosis is by clinical exam and finding of lice or nits.

Treatment includes: Permethrin 1% (treatment of choice): This is a cream rinse applied after body or hair is shampooed with a non-conditioning shampoo and then towel dried. It is left on for 10 minutes and then rinsed off, leaving residue designed to kill nymphs emerging from eggs not killed with the first application. Treatment is often repeated in 7 to 10 days. Nits should be manually removed.

Scabies

Scabies is caused by a microscopic mite, *Sarcoptes scabiei hominis,* which tunnels under the outer layer of skin, raising small lines a few millimeters long. Mites prefer warm areas, such as between the fingers and in skin folds, but can infest any area of the body. As the mites burrow, they cause intense itching and subsequent scratching can result in excoriation and secondary infections. Some develop a generalized red rash. Scabies is spread very easily through person-to-person contact and has become a problem in nursing homes and extended-care facilities where staff spread the infection. Incubation time is 6 to 8 weeks and itching usually begins in about 30 days, so people may be unaware they are transmitting scabies. Most infestations involve only about a dozen mites, but a severe form of scabies infection, Norwegian or crusted scabies, can occur in elderly patients or those who are immunocompromised, and usually causes less itching. However, lesions can contain thousands of mites, making this type highly contagious. Diagnosis of scabies is through skin scrapings, but because so few adult females usually infest a person, a negative finding does not mean that the person does not have scabies. When examining a patient with suspected scabies, it is helpful when searching for burrows to use a magnifying glass and a small flashlight held at an oblique angle.

Treatment for scabies includes:
- Scabicide:
  - Permethrin 5% cream (drug of choice) applied from chin to toes and left on for 12 hours and then showered off with a repeat treatment in 1 week.
  - Sulfur in petrolatum 10% concentration applied to entire body below the head on 3 successive nights and then bathe 24 hours after each application (safe for small children and pregnant women).
- Oral medication: Ivermectin oral medication in 2 doses, 1 week apart, especially effective for crusted form.
- Itching: Antihistamines.
- Secondary infections: Antibiotics.

Hantavirus pulmonary syndrome

Hantavirus pulmonary syndrome is a deadly disease that is contracted through contact with infected rodents, their urine, or feces, primarily in the Southeast or Northeast. Incubation time is unclear but probably about 1 to 5 weeks after contact. Early symptoms are flu-like with headache, fever (more than 101.3° F), chills, myalgia, GI upset such as diarrhea, nausea, and vomiting, and dizziness. About 4 to 10 days after onset, patients develop severe cough, dyspnea (respiratory rate 26 to 30), and tachycardia associated with interstitial pulmonary infiltrates and compromise similar to ARDS. Condition deteriorates quickly after cough begins. Diagnosis is based on history, clinical exam, serologic assays, and radiographs. Treatment is supportive, but prognosis is poor as there is no specific treatment for the virus.
- Oxygen therapy.
- Broad-spectrum antibiotics initially until diagnosis confirmed.
- Endotracheal intubation and ventilation may be necessary.
- Monitoring and control of fluid and electrolyte balances.
- Ribavirin is NOT recommended.

Fungal infections

Tinea capitis and tinea corporis
Tinea capitis is a fungal infection of the scalp, usually affecting children between 1 and 10. It is spread through the sharing of combs, brushes, or caps. Symptoms include:
- Circumscribed areas of hair loss with fine scaling and superficial pustules with mild itching.

Treatment:
- Griseofulvin orally 8 to 12 weeks.
- Selenium sulfide shampoo 2 to 3 times weekly, leaving shampoo on scalp for 10 minutes before rinsing.

Tinea corporis is a fungal infection of the skin of the trunk, although it can occur on the face or other parts of the body. It is spread by direct contact. Symptoms include:
- One or multiple circular patches that may be scaly and erythematous with slightly raised borders.

Treatment:

- Selenium sulfide shampoo wash of area before applying medication.
- Topical antifungal (clotrimazole, miconazole, tolnaftate, naftifine, terbinafine) 2 times daily for 4 weeks.
- Systemic agents: terbinafine, fluconazole, and itraconazole.

Tinea cruris and tinea pedis

Tinea cruris (jock itch) is a fungal infection of the perineal area, penis, inner thighs, and inguinal creases, but may also occur under breasts in women and beneath abdominal folds where skin is warm and moist. It rarely occurs before adolescence. Symptoms include: Scaly, itching, erythematous rash that may contain papules or vesicle and is usually bilateral and symmetrical.

Treatment:

- Selenium sulfide shampoo wash of area before applying medication.
- Topical antifungal (clotrimazole, miconazole, tolnaftate, naftifine, terbinafine) 2 times daily for 4 weeks.

Tinea pedis (athlete's foot) is a fungal infection of the feet and toes. It is rare before adolescence and is more common in males. Symptoms include:

- Severe itching with vesicles or erosion of instep and with peeling maceration and fissures between toes.
- Dry, scaly, mildly erythematous patches on plantar and lateral foot surfaces.

Treatment:

- Same as tinea cruris.
- Keep feet dry with absorbant talc.
- Allow feet to air dry and use 100% cotton socks, changed twice daily.

Fungal diaper rash

Candidiasis, infection of the epidermis with *Candida* spp. (commonly referred to as "yeast" or "thrush"), causes a pustular erythematous papular rash that is commonly scaly, crusty, and macerated with a white cheese-like exudate. It may burn and is usually extremely pruritic and grows in warm, moist areas of the skin, such the perineal area, and is aggravated by the use of disposable diapers. Candidiasis must be differentiated from bacterial infections because antibiotic treatment will worsen the condition.

Treatment includes:

- Preventing humid, moist conditions of skin.
- Controlling hyperglycemia.
- Careful cleansing and exposing area to air as much as possible.
- Topical antifungal creams (nystatin) with each diaper change or 4 times daily.
- Zinc chloride ointment over antifungal to provide barrier protection.
- Topical antifungal powders for mild cases.
- Oral antifungal (fluconazole) for severe cases.

> **Review Video:** Diaper Rash
> *Visit **mometrix.com/academy** and enter Code:* **937853**

Burn injuries

Burn injuries may be chemical, electrical, or thermal, and are assessed by the area, percentage of the body burned, and depth:
- First-degree burns are superficial and affect the epidermis, causing erythema and pain.
- Second-degree burns extend through the dermis (partial thickness), resulting in blistering and sloughing of epidermis.
- Third degree burns affect underlying tissue, including vasculature, muscles, and nerves (full thickness).

Burns are classified according to the American Burn Association's criteria:
- Minor: Less than 10% body surface area (BSA). 2% BSA with third degree without serious risk to face, hands, feet, or perineum.
- Moderate: 10% to 20% combined second- to third-degree burns (children younger than 10 years or adults older than 40 years). 10% or less full thickness without serious risk to face, hands, feet, or perineum.
- Major: 20% BSA; at least 10% third-degree burns. All burns to face, hands, feet, or perineum that will result in functional/cosmetic defect. Burns with inhalation or other major trauma.

Systemic complications
Burn injuries begin with the skin but can affect all organs and body systems, especially with a major burn:
- Cardiovascular: Cardiac output may fall by 50% as capillary permeability increases with vasodilation and fluid leaks from the tissues.
- Urinary: Decreased blood flow causes kidneys to increase ADH, which increases oliguria. BUN and creatinine levels increase. Cell destruction may block tubules, and hematuria may result from hemolysis.
- Pulmonary: Injury may result from smoke inhalation or (rarely) aspiration of hot liquid. Pulmonary injury is a leading cause of death from burns and is classified according to degree of damage:
  - First: Singed eyebrows and nasal hairs with possible soot in airways and slight edema.
  - Second: (At 24 hours) Stridor, dyspnea, and tachypnea with edema and erythema of upper airway, including area of vocal chords and epiglottis.
  - Third: (At 72 hours) worsening symptoms if not intubated and if intubated, bronchorrhea and tachypnea with edematous, secreting tissue.

Multisystem complications of burn injuries include:
- Neurological: Encephalopathy may develop from lack of oxygen, decreased blood volume and sepsis. Hallucinations, alterations in consciousness, seizures and coma may result for recovery is usual.
- Gastrointestinal: Ileus and ulcerations of mucosa often result from poor circulation. Ileus usually clears within 48-72 hours, but if it returns it is often indicative of sepsis.

- 155 -

- Endocrine/Metabolic: The sympathetic nervous system stimulates the adrenals to release epinephrine and norepinephrine to increase cardiac output and cortisol for wound healing. The metabolic rate increases markedly. Electrolyte loss occurs with fluid loss from exposed tissue, especially phosphorus, calcium and sodium, with an increase in potassium levels. Electrolyte imbalance can be life-threatening if burns cover >20% of BSA. Glycogen depletion occurs within 12-24 hours and protein breakdown and muscle wasting occurs without sufficient intake of protein.

<u>Management</u>
Management of burn injuries must include both wound care and systemic care to avoid complications that can be life threatening. Treatment includes:
- Establishment of airway and treatment for inhalation injury as indicated:
  o Supplemental oxygen, incentive spirometry, nasotracheal suctioning.
  o Humidification.
  o Bronchoscopy as needed to evaluate bronchospasm and edema.
  o β-Agonists for bronchospasm, followed by aminophylline if ineffective.
  o Intubation and ventilation if there are indications of respiratory failure. This should be done prior to failure. Tracheostomy may be done if ventilation >14 days.
- Intravenous fluids and electrolytes, based on weight and extent of burn. Parkland formula: 4 ml/kg/wt x BSA per 24 hours.
- Enteral feedings, usually with small lumen feeding tube into the duodenum.
- NG tube for gastric decompression to prevent aspiration.
- Indwelling catheter to monitor urinary output. Urinary output should be 0.5-2 ml/kg/hr.
- Analgesia for reduction of pain and anxiety.
- Topical and systemic antibiotics.
- Wound care with removal of eschar and dressings as indicated.

Electrical Injuries

Electrical injuries are most commonly work-related injuries or mouth injuries to young children (from sucking on an electrical cord or plug). The tissue damage depends on the amperage and the tissue resistance because the more resistant the tissue, the greater the heat damage. Tissue resistance from greatest to least is bone—fat—tendons—skin—muscles—blood vessels—nerves. High voltage injury, however, tends to damage all tissues regardless of resistance. AC injuries are usually more severe than DC.

<u>Low voltage</u> (<1000 volts)
Effects: Cardiac dysrhythmia (usually VF), tetanic skeletal muscle contractions, fractures, burns
Treatment: Telemetry, supportive care, wound management, analgesia, tetanus prophylaxis

<u>High voltage</u> (>1000 volts)
Effects: Cutaneous burn (flash-flame) of various degree, myonecrosis, vessel thrombosis, nerve entrapment, compartment syndrome, myoglobinuria
Treatment: Fluid replacement at >4 mL/kg/% TBSA; mannitol for myoglobinuria; wound management with excision, debridement, topical antimicrobials, pain management; fasciotomy, if needed; tetanus prophylaxis

SSSS

Staphylococcal scalded skin syndrome (SSSS) is a superficial partial-thickness infection of the skin caused by toxins produced by a localized *Staphylococcus aureus* infection, resulting in generalized erythema followed in 24 to 48 hours with blisters that rupture and peel off, leaving large areas of superficial necrosis and denuded skin, giving the skin a burned or "scalded" appearance. It is most common in neonates and children younger than 5, and can be confused with noninfectious diaper rash or candidiasis. It can affect adults who are immunocompromised or in renal failure. Pain is usually mild unless the infection is very widespread.

Treatment includes:
- IV antibiotics (such as flucloxacillin) are usually needed initially, followed by a course of oral antibiotics.
- Maintenance of fluids and electrolytes.
- Debridement of skin.
- Moisture-retentive dressings, such as foam dressings, sheet hydrogels, and alginates; avoid adhesives.
- Excessive tissue loss may be treated the same as partial-thickness burns.

CSD

Cat scratch disease (CSD) is a bacterial disease caused by *Bartonella henselae*. Cats can carry the bacteria in their saliva and transfer it to their paws when they clean themselves. CSD can result from bites or scratches by a cat. CSD is one of the most common causes of prolonged fever and painful lymph node swelling in children. Symptoms include:
- Blister or sore with or without pus at site where bacteria entered the body.
- Swollen lymph nodes, especially in head, neck, or upper limbs (2 weeks or less)
- Flu-like symptoms (fever, headache, anorexia)
- Rare: bacillary angiomatosis and Parinaud oculoglandular syndrome

Diagnosis is often made on the basis of exposure to a cat and typical clinical signs as well as failure to find another cause. Indirect fluorescent antibody (IFA) for Bartonella is 84% to 88% sensitive and 94% to 96% specific.

Treatment includes:
- Antipyretics and analgesics.
- Local heat to affected lymph nodes.
- Aspiration of nodes may relieve pain if suppurative.
- Antibiotics not usually recommended except for immunocompromised patients.

Rabies

Rabies is caused by a lyssavirus that causes acute encephalitis in animals and humans. Rabies is found in most species of warm-blooded animals, so bites from both wild and domesticated animals, including bats, pose danger. Most dogs in the United States are vaccinated, but many cats and all wildlife are not. Rabies is almost always fatal once symptoms develop. Incubation varies 2 weeks to 2 years. Early symptoms include fever, headache and malaise progressing to severe neurological symptoms (insomnia, anxiety, paralysis, hallucination, agitation, hypersalivation, hydrophobia, dysphagia, and death) within 2 to 20 days of onset. Diagnosis by postmortem direct fluorescent

- 157 -

antibody on the animal is easiest. Human testing requires RT-PCR of saliva, finding serum and spinal fluid antibodies, and skin biopsy to examine for rabies antigen in cutaneous nerves at hair follicle bases. Treatment is preventative or supportive. Supportive: Two people survived rabies with induced coma, ventilator support, and IV ribavirin. Preventitive treatment is pre- or postexposure prophylaxis (PEP) and appropriate wound care after reported bite. Post exposure prophylaxis is a 4-step 14-day immune globulin and rabies vaccine protocol as per CDC guidelines. One of the most important steps to prevent rabies after being bitten by an animal is wound care. Good cleaning with a virucidal agent can reduce the chance of getting rabies by 90%.

Lyme disease

Lyme disease, first identified in 1975, is contracted through the bite of a tick infected with the bacterium *Borrelia burgdorferi.* There is a wide range of symptoms:
- Early localized: erythema migrans (EM) bull's-eye rash occurs 3 to 30 days after bite in 70% to 80%, flu-like symptoms.
- Early disseminated: migratory pain in joints, additional EMs, flu-like symptoms, fever, fatigue, headache, stiff neck, vision changes.
- Late (weeks, months): arthritis of 1 to 2 large joints, neurological problems (confusion, memory loss, disorientation, peripheral numbness), cardiovascular disorders.

Diagnosis requires 2 steps: ELISA or IFA with positive results confirmed by Western blot test.

Treatment:
- Exact amount and route of antibiotics will be decided by the stage of the disease which is indicated by the presenting symptoms.
- Oral antibiotics: doxycycline or amoxicillin, 21 to 28 days.
- IV antibiotics (for more serious symptoms): ceftriaxone or penicillin G 4 to 6 weeks.
- No vaccine is currently available as it was withdrawn from the market.
- Prophylaxis after tick bite in highly endemic area where an engorged tick is found and removed: doxycycline, single 200 mg dose.

> **Review Video:** Lyme Disease
> *Visit* ***mometrix.com/academy*** *and enter* ***Code: 505529***

Rocky Mountain spotted fever

Rocky Mountain spotted fever is a tick-borne disease caused by the bacterium *Rickettsia rickettsii* resulting in vascular injury. It can occur throughout the United States with highest incident in the South Atlantic area between April and September. Early symptoms include flu-like syndrome with fever, headache, myalgia, anorexia, severe headache, nausea, and vomiting. Most patients develop a rash 2 to 5 days after onset, usually macular lesions on arms, wrists, and ankles. By day 6, the typical rash is red, spotted, and petechial, and may spread to palms and soles. Later symptoms include abdominal pain, arthralgia, and diarrhea with damage to internal organs resulting in pulmonary edema, respiratory distress, myocarditis and heart failure, CNS abnormalities, such as meningocephalitis and paralysis, renal failure, hepatomegaly, splenomegaly, and death (within 5 days). Diagnosis is by serologic assay, such as IFA. Treatment includes: Doxycycline 100 mg every 12 hour or 4 mg/kg per day in 2 doses for children for 5 to 10 days (3 days after fever), begun immediately before laboratory confirmation.

Plague

Yersinia pestis causes plague, usually from fleas of infected rats, and can be aerosolized to use as a biologic weapon. There are 3 forms of plague, which sometimes occur together. Bubonic and septicemic plague can develop into pneumonic, a concern of bioterrorism:
- Bubonic occurs when a person is bitten by an infected flea with flu-like symptoms, nausea, vomiting (sometimes with blood), constipation/diarrhea with tarry stools, headache, purpuric macules, and formation of buboes (usually 5 cm or less) in inguinal, axillary, cervical, or epitrochlear areas.
- Pneumonic occurs with inhalation and results in pneumonia with fever, headache, cough, and progressive respiratory failure.
- Septicemic occurs when *Y. pestis* invades the bloodstream, often after initial bubonic or pneumonic plague, with severe generalized symptoms.

Diagnosis is by clinical exam, CBC, gram stain of secretions, blood culture, serologic testing, and chest radiograph. Pneumonic plague can spread easily from person to person.

Treatment:
- Antibiotics: Gentamicin 5 mg/kg IV/IM daily (2.5 mg/kg IV IM for children) for infection and prophylaxis for those exposed.
- Droplet precautions.

Botulism

Clostridium botulinum produces a neurotoxin that causes botulism. There are 4 primary forms of botulisms:
- Foodborne botulism from contamination of food through improper canning or handling. Symptoms usually appear 12 to 36 hours after ingestion but may be delayed for 2 weeks and include nausea, vomiting, dyspnea, dysphagia, slurred speech, blurred vision, diplopia, progressive weakness, and paralysis.
- Infant botulism (younger than 1 year) results from C. botulinum spores ingested into the intestinal tract. Constipation, poor feeding, impaired feeding, and progressive weakness are presenting symptoms.
- Injection from overdose of Botox.
- Wound botulism results from contamination of open skin, but symptoms are similar to foodborne botulism.

Diagnosis is by history and clinical exam and mouse inoculation test to identify antitoxin in blood serum or stool.

Treatment includes:
- Gastric emptying of food remaining in stomach.
- Antitoxin: trivalent antitoxin as per CDC.
- Supportive care, including mechanical ventilation if necessary.
- Infant botulism: *BabyBIG* (botulism immune globulin) is now available.

Carbon monoxide poisoning

Carbon monoxide (CO) poisoning occurs with inhalation of fossil fuel exhausts from engines, emission of gas or coal heaters, indoor use of charcoal, and smoke and fumes. The CO binds with hemoglobin, preventing oxygen carriage and impairing oxygen delivery to tissue. Diagnosis includes history, on-site oximetry reports, neurological examination, and CO neuropsychological screening battery (CONSB) done with patient breathing room air, CBC, electrolytes, ABGs, ECG, chest radiograph (for dyspnea). Symptoms include:
- Cardiac: chest pain, palpitations, decreased capillary refill, hypotension, cardiac arrest.
- CNS: malaise, nausea, vomiting, lethargy, stroke, coma, seizure.

Secondary injuries:
- Rhabdomyolysis with renal failure
- Non-cardiogenic pulmonary edema
- Multiple organ failure (MOF).
- DIC.
- Encephalopathy.

Treatment includes:
- Immediate support of airway, breathing, and circulation.
- Non-barometric oxygen (100%) by non-breathing mask with reservoir or ETT if necessary.
- Mild: Continue oxygen for 4 hours with reassessment.
- Severe: hyperbaric oxygen therapy (usually 3 treatments) to improve oxygen delivery.

Tissue damage related to chemical trauma

Chemical trauma may be caused by leakage or incontinence of body fluids, such as urine, feces, and exudate, or chemicals applied to the skin, such as lotions, iodine, soap, organic solvents, acids, and adhesives. Reactions to irritant contact dermatitis may vary widely from an itching rash similar to allergic contact dermatitis to cracks and fissures in the skin, especially on the hands, or denouement of skin, often in the perineal area. The skin reaction may be rapid and extremely painful. Treatment includes:
- Identifying irritant and eliminating contact with skin.
- Gentle cleansing of skin to remove irritant but avoid further skin irritation.
- Use of skin sealants or skin barriers as indicated to protect the skin and allow healing.
- Use of appropriate skin care products and containment devices.
- Monitoring of dressings and periwound condition daily.

Allergic contact dermatitis

Contact dermatitis is a localized response to contact with an allergen, resulting in a rash that may blister and itch. Common allergens include poison oak, poison ivy, latex, benzocaine, nickel, and preservatives, but there is a wide range of items, preparations, and products to which people may react. Treatment includes:
- Identifying the causative agent through evaluating the area of the body affected, careful history, or skin patch testing to determine allergic responses.
- Corticosteroids to control inflammation and itching.
- Soothing oatmeal baths.
- Pramoxine lotion to relieve itching.

- Antihistamines to reduce allergic response.
- Lesions should be gently cleansed and observed for signs of secondary infection.
- Antibiotics are used only for secondary infections as indicated.
- Rash is usually left open to dry.
- Avoidance of allergen will prevent recurrence.

Radiation injuries

Radiation injuries may be caused by direct radiation in which waves pass through the body (locally or to the entire body), which can result in acute radiation illness and genetic damage. Contamination usually occurs from radioactive dust or liquid contacting the skin. It can be absorbed into the tissues (eventually causing chronic illnesses, such as cancer) or contaminate others who contact it. Contaminated material may also be ingested. The lethal dose of 50% of those exposed within 60 days (LD50/60) is 4.5 Gy with immediate intensive treatment. Diagnosis for direct radiation is symptomatic as there is no specific test; however, contamination can be measured by Geiger counter. Syndromes of acute radiation sickness vary according to exposure:
- Hematopoietic: (at least 2 Gy exposure) affects blood cell production.
  - 2 to 12 hours after exposure: anorexia, nausea, vomiting, lethargy.
  - Symptom-free week during which blood cell production decreases causing decreased WBC and platelet count, resulting in infection and hemorrhage with weakness and dyspnea.
  - Recovery begins in 4 to 5 weeks if patient survives.
- GI: (at least 4 Gy exposure).
  - 2 to 12 hours after exposure: nausea, vomiting, diarrhea, dehydration.
  - 4 to 5 days, fewer symptoms but lining of GI tract sheds, leaving ulcerated tissue.
  - Severe diarrhea (bloody) and dehydration and systemic infections.
- Cerebrovascular: (20 to 30 Gy exposure) always fatal.
  - Alterations in mental status, nausea, vomiting, and diarrhea (bloody), progressing to shock, seizures, coma, and death.
  - Treatment includes:
    - Decontamination if contamination irradiation or if source of irradiation not clear.
    - Complete history of event, including source of radiation.
    - Protocol for decontamination and securing of area should be followed, including use of individual dosimeters and protective coverings.
- Localized: burn care and analgesia.
- Internal: gastric decontamination, collection of urine and feces for 4 days to monitor rate of radioisotopes excretion, and collection of body fluids for bioassay.
- Whole body irradiation: Supportive treatment and prophylactic measures to combat opportunistic infections, hematopoietic growth factor for bone marrow depression.

Drowning accidents

Drowning is the leading cause of death in children younger than 5 and the second in children younger than 15:
- Infants: Bathtub injuries usually associated with intentional injury or lack of supervision.
- Toddler: Injuries in pools, bathtub, spa, toilet, or places where children have access with lack of supervision.

- 161 -

- Children: Injuries in swimming pool or spa.
- Adolescents/Adults: Injuries in lakes, rivers, or oceans related to risk-taking and/or altered level of awareness of drugs or alcohol.

Submersion usually causes aspiration (wet drowning) but may trigger severe laryngospasm (dry drowning):
- Laryngospasm leads to this sequence:
  1. Cardiac arrest with hypoxic/acidosis to brain.
  2. Decreased oxygen, glucose, and adenosine triphosphate.
  3. Decreased sodium, potassium pump.
  4. Increased Na and water in intracellular fluid (ICF).
  5. Cerebral intracellular edema leading to neuronal death.
- Aspiration leads to this sequence:
  1. Cardiac arrest with hypoxic/acidosis to other organs (heart, kidneys).
  2. Decreased oxygen, glucose, adenosine triphosphate.
  3. Decreased sodium, potassium pump.
  4. Increased Na and water in ICF.
  5. Hypovolemia with shock and death.

Near-drowning asphyxia

Submersion asphyxiation can cause profound damage to the central nervous system, pulmonary dysfunction related to aspiration, cardiac hypoxia with life-threatening arrhythmias, fluid and electrolyte imbalances, and multi-organ damage, so treatment can be complex. Hypothermia related to near drowning has some protective affect because blood is shunted to the brain and heart. Treatment includes:
- Immediate establishment of airway, breathing and circulation (ABCs).
- NG tube and decompression to reduce risk of aspiration.
- Neurological evaluation.
- Pulmonary management includes monitoring for $\geq$72 hours for respiratory deterioration. Ventilation may need positive-end expiratory pressure (PEEP), but this poses danger to cardiac output and can cause barotrauma, so use should be limited.
- In patients that are symptomatic but do not yet need intubation, use supplemental oxygen to keep SpO_2 > 94%.
- Monitoring of cardiac output and function.
- Neurological care to reduce cerebral edema and increased intracranial pressure, and prevent secondary injury.
- Rewarming if necessary (0.5 to 1°C/hr).

Heat-related illness

Children and the elderly are particularly vulnerable to heat-related illness, especially when heat is combined with humidity. Heat-related illnesses occur when heat accumulation in the body outpaces dissipation, resulting in increased temperature and dehydration, which can then lead to thermoregulatory failure and multiple organ dysfunction syndromes. Each year in the United States, about 29 children die from heat stroke after being left in automobiles. At temperatures of 72° to 96°F, the temperature in a car rises 3.2° every 5 minutes, with 80% of rise within 30 minutes. Temperatures can reach 117°F even on cool days. There are 3 types of heat-related illness:

- Heat stress: Increased temperature causes dehydration. Patient may develop swelling of hands and feet, itching of skin, sunburn, heat syncope (pale moist skin, hypotension), heat cramps, and heat tetany (respiratory alkalosis). Treatment includes removing from heat, cooling, and hydrating, and replacing sodium is usually sufficient.
- Heat exhaustion: Involves water or sodium depletion, with sodium depletion common in patients who are not acclimated to heat. Heat exhaustion can result in flu-like aching, nausea and vomiting, headaches, dizziness, and hypotension with cold, clammy skin and diaphoresis. Temperature may be normal or elevated to less than 106°F. Treatment to cool the body and replace sodium and fluids must be prompt in order to prevent heat stroke. Careful monitoring is important and reactions may be delayed.
- Heat stroke: Involves failure of the thermoregulatory system with temperatures that may be more than 106°F and can result in seizures, neurological damage, multiple organ failures, and death. Exertional heat stroke often occurs in young athletes who engage in strenuous activities in high heat. Young children are susceptible to nonexertional heat stroke from exposure to high heat. Treatment includes evaporative cooling, rehydration, and supportive treatment according to organ involvement.

Hypothermia

Hypothermia occurs with exposure to low temperatures that cause the core body temperature to fall below 95°F (35°C). Hypothermia may be associated with immersion in cold water, exposure to cold temperature, metabolic disorders (hypothyroidism, hypoglycemia, hypoadrenalism), or CNS abnormalities (head trauma, Wernicke disease). Many patients with hypothermia are intoxicated with alcohol or drugs. Symptoms of hypothermia include pallor, cold skin, drowsiness, alterations in mental status, confusion, and severe shivering. The patient can progress to shock, coma, dysrhythmias (T-wave inversion and prolongation of PR, QRS, and QT), including atrial fibrillation and AV block, and cardiac arrest. Diagnosis requires low-reading thermometers to verify temperature. Treatment includes:

- Passive rewarming if cardiac status stable.
- Active rewarming (external) with immersion in warm water or heating blankets at 40°C, radiant heat.
- Active rewarming (internal) with warm humidified oxygen or air inhalation, heated IV fluids, and internal (bladder, peritoneal pleural, GI) lavage. Warming with extracorporeal circuit, such as arteriovenous or venovenous shunt that warms the blood.
- Supportive treatment as indicated.

Frostnip and frostbite

Frostnip is superficial freeze injury that is reversible. Frostbite is damage to tissue caused by exposure to freezing temperatures, most often affecting the nose, ears, and distal extremities. As frostbite develops, the affected part feels numb and aches or throbs, becoming hard and insensate as the tissue freezes, resulting in circulatory impairment, necrosis of tissue, and gangrene. There are 3 zones of injury:
- Coagulation (usually distal) is severe, irreversible cellular damage.
- Hyperemia (usually proximal) is minimal cellular damage.
- Stasis (between other 2 zones) is severe but sometimes reversible damage.

Symptoms vary according to the degree of freezing:
- Partial freezing with erythema and mild edema, stinging, burning, throbbing pain.
- Full-thickness freezing with increased edema in 3 to 4 hours, edema and clear blisters in 6 to 24 hours, desquamation with eschar formation, numbness and then aching and throbbing pain.
- Prognosis is very good for first-degree and good for second-degree frostbite.
- Full-thickness and into subdermal tissue freezing with cyanosis, hemorrhagic blisters, skin necrosis, and "wooden" feeling, severe burning, throbbing, and shooting pains.
- Freezing extends into subcutaneous tissue, including muscles, tendons, and bones with mottled appearance, nonblanching cyanosis and eventual deep black eschar.

Prognosis is poor for third-degree and fourth-degree freeze injuries. Determining the degree of injury can be difficult because some degree of thawing may have occurred prior to admission to the hospital. Treatment includes:
- Rapid rewarming with warm water bath (40° to 42°C [104° to 107.6°F]) 10 to 30 minutes or until the frostbitten area is erythematous and pliable.
- Treatment for generalized hypothermia.

Treatment after warming:
- Debridement of clear blisters but not hemorrhagic blisters.
- Aloe vera cream every 6 hours to blistered areas.
- Dressings, separating digits.
- Tetanus prophylaxis.
- Ibuprofen 12 mg/kg daily in divided doses.
- Antibiotic prophylaxis if indicated (penicillin G 500,000 units IV every 6 hours for 24 to 72 hours).

Pediatric poisoning

Pediatric poisoning is one of the most common medical problems with young children, accounting for about 5% of childhood mortality. Over 90% of poisonings occur within the home environment and over half of toxic poisonings occur to children younger than 6. Most poisonings of young children are accidental and involve small amounts of one substance, generally a household product, such as cosmetics or medications. Adolescent poisoning is more often intentional, as a suicide attempt or substance abuse, often with multiple substances ingested and a delay in treatment. Recreational drugs, such as ecstasy, have been implicated in increased poisonings. Assessment of children with suspected ingestion of toxic substances includes: Airway. Breathing. Circulation. Disability, drugs/decontamination. ECG, exposure. Thorough examination to determine the toxidrome (characteristic patterns of symptoms related to specific toxins) must include assessment of the following:
- Vital sign changes.
- Alterations in mental status.
- Specific symptoms.
- Clinical findings.
- Results of laboratory testing, including serum and urine toxicology screens.

Toxic ingestions

Treatment for toxic ingestions is related to the type of toxin and whether or not it is identified:
- Administration of reversal agent if substance is known and an antidote exists. Antidotes for common toxins include:
  - Opiates: Naloxone (Narcan®).
  - Toxic alcohols: Ethanol infusion and/or dialysis.
  - Acetaminophen: N-acetylcysteine.
  - Calcium channel blockers, beta-blockers: Calcium chloride, Glucagon.
  - Tricyclic antidepressants: Sodium bicarbonate.
  - Ethylene glycol: fomepizole.
  - Iron: deferoxamine
- GI decontamination at one time was standard procedures (Ipecac® and gastric lavage followed by activated charcoal). It is no longer advised for routine use although selective gastric lavage may be appropriate if done within 1 hour of ingestion.
- Activated charcoal (1 g/kg/wt) orally or per NG tube binds to many toxins if given within one hour of ingestion. It may also be used in multiple doses (q 4-6 hrs) to enhance elimination
- Forced diuresis with alkalinization of urine (>7.5) may prevent absorption of drugs that are weak bases or acids.

Cyanide poisoning

Cyanide poisoning, from hydrogen cyanide (HCN) or cyanide salts, can result from inhalation of burning plastics, intentional or accidental ingestion or dermal exposure, occupation exposure, ingestion of some plant products, manufacture of PCP, and sodium nitroprusside infusions. Inhalation of HCN causes immediate symptoms; and ingestion of cyanide salts, within minutes. Diagnosis is by history, assessment, and normal PaO_2 and metabolic acidosis. Symptoms increase in severity and alter with the amount of exposure:

- Cardiovascular: Tachycardia, hypertension, bradycardia, hypotension, and cardiac arrest.
- Skin: May appear pink or cherry-colored because of oxygen remaining in the blood.
- CNS: Headaches, lethargy, seizures, coma.
- Respiratory: Dyspnea, tachypnea, and respiratory arrest.

Treatment includes:
- Supportive care as indicated.
- Removal of contaminated clothes.
- Gastric decontamination.
- Copious irrigation for topical exposure.
- Antidotes:
  - Amyl nitrate ampule cracked/inhaled 30 secs.
  - Sodium nitrite (3%) 10 mL IV.
  - Sodium thiosulfate (25%) 50 mL IV.
  - Childrens doses adjusted according to Hgb level.

> ➢ **Review Video:** Cyanide
> *Visit **mometrix.com/academy** and enter **Code: 975006***

Caustic ingestions

Caustic ingestions of acids (pH <7) such as sulfuric, acetic, hydrochloric, and hydrofluoric found in many cleaning agents and alkalis (pH >7) such as sodium hydroxide, potassium hydroxide, sodium tripolyphosphate (in detergents) and sodium hypochlorite (bleach) can result in severe injury and death. Acids cause coagulation necrosis in the esophagus and stomach and may result in metabolic acidosis, hemolysis, and renal failure if systemically absorbed. Alkali injuries cause liquefaction necrosis, resulting in deeper ulcerations, often of the esophagus, but may involve perforation and abdominal necrosis with multi-organ damage. Diagnosis is by detailed history, airway examination (oral intubation if possible), arterial blood gas, electrolytes, CBC, hepatic and coagulation tests, radiograph, and CT for perforations. Symptoms may vary but can include:

- Pain.
- Dyspnea.
- Oral burns.
- Dysphonia.
- Vomiting.

Treatment includes:
- Supportive and symptomatic therapy.
- NO ipecac, charcoal, neutralization, or dilution.
- NG tube for acids only to aspirate residual.
- Endoscopy in first few hours to evaluate injury/perforations.
- Sodium bicarbonate for pH <7.10.
- Prednisolone (alkali injuries).

Acetaminophen toxicity

Acetaminophen toxicity from accidental or intentional overdose has high rates of morbidity and mortality unless promptly treated. Diagnosis is by history and acetaminophen level, which should be completed within 8 hours of ingestion if possible. Toxicity occurs with dosage >140 mg/kg in one dose or >7.5g in 24 hours. Symptoms occur in stages:
1. (Initial) Minor gastrointestinal upset.
2. (Days 2-3) Hepatotoxicity with RUQ pain and increased AST, ALT, and bilirubin.
3. (Days 3-4) Hepatic failure with metabolic acidosis, coagulopathy, renal failure, encephalopathy, nausea, vomiting, and possible death.
4. (Days 5-12) Recovery period for survivors.

Treatment includes:
- GI decontamination with activated charcoal (orally or NG) <24 hours.
- Toxicity is plotted on the Rumack-Matthew nomogram with serum levels >150 requiring antidote. The antidote is most effective ≤8 hours of ingestion but decreases hepatotoxicity even >24 hours.
- Antidote: 72-hour N-acetylcysteine (NAC) protocol includes 140 mg/kg initially and 70 mg/kg every 4 hours for 17 more doses (orally or IV).
- Supportive therapy.

Gastric emptying for toxic substance ingestion

Gastric emptying for toxic substance ingestion should be done ≤60 minutes of ingestion for large life-threatening amounts of poison. The patient requires IV access, oximetry, and cardiac monitoring. Sedation (1-2 mg IV midazolam) or RSI and endotracheal intubation may be necessary. Patients should be positioned in left lateral decubitus position with head down at 20° to prevent passage of stomach contents into duodenum although intubated patients may be lavaged in the supine position. With a bite block in place, an orogastric Y-tube (36-40 Fr. for adults) should be inserted after estimating length. Placement should be confirmed with injection of 50 mL of air confirmed under auscultation and aspiration of gastric contents. Irrigation is done by gravity instillation of about 200-300 mL warmed (45° C) tap water or NS. The instillation side is clamped and drainage side opened. This is repeated until fluid returns clear. A slurry of charcoal is then instilled, and tube clamped and removed when procedures completed.

Amphetamine and cocaine toxicity

Amphetamine toxicity may be caused by IV, inhalation, or insufflation of various substances that include methamphetamine (MDA or "ecstasy"), methylphenidate (Ritalin®), methylenedioxymethamphetamine (MDMA), and ephedrine and phenylpropanolamine. Cocaine may be ingested orally, IV or by insufflation while crack cocaine may be smoked. Amphetamines and cocaine are CNS stimulants that can cause multi-system abnormalities.

Symptoms may include chest pain, dysrhythmias, myocardial ischemia, MI, seizures, intracranial infarctions, hypertension, dystonia, repetitive movements, unilateral blindness, lethargy, rhabdomyolysis with acute kidney failure, perforated nasal septum (cocaine) and paranoid psychosis (amphetamines). Crack cocaine may cause pulmonary hemorrhage, asthma, pulmonary edema, barotrauma, and pneumothorax. Swallowing packs of cocaine can cause intestinal ischemia, colitis, necrosis, and perforation. Diagnosis includes clinical findings, CBC, chemistry panel, toxicology screening, ECG, and radiography. Treatment includes:

- Gastric emptying (≤1 hour).
- Charcoal administration.
- IV access.
- Supplemental oxygen.
- Sedation for seizures: Lorazepam 2 mg or diazepam 5 mg IV titrated in repeated doses.
- Agitation: Haloperidol.
- Hypertension: Nitroprusside or phentolamine IV.
- Cocaine quinidine-like effects: Sodium bicarbonate.

> **Review Video:** Addiction to Crack Cocaine
> *Visit mometrix.com/academy and enter Code:* **460412**

Withdrawal syndromes

Opioids (morphine, oxycodone, heroin, fentanyl)
Symptoms: *6 to 12 hours:* Anxiety, diaphoresis, piloerection, pupil dilation, anorexia, tremor, rhinorrhea, tearing. *48 to 72 hours:* Diarrhea, agitation/excitation, fever, abdominal cramping, hypertension, tachycardia, insomnia, restlessness.
Treatment: Naloxone may be given for overdose but may trigger withdrawal. Methadone or buprenorphine reduce withdrawal symptoms. Clonidine or lofexidine are also used but are less effective.

> **Review Video:** Opiod Use Guidelines
> *Visit mometrix.com/academy and enter Code:* **677051**

Stimulants (cocaine, amphetamines)
Symptoms: Withdrawal is relatively mild with fatigue, anxiety, depression, and prolonged sleeping; however severe craving for the drugs may persist for weeks.
Treatment is primarily supportive.

Sedative-hypnotics (benzodiazepines)
Symptoms: Severe drug craving by 24 hours, seizures, delirium, and cardiac and respiratory arrest may occur.
Treatment: Patients must be closely monitored for the above symptoms which can be life threatening. Flumazenil may be used for overdose but is controversial in patients who abuse benzodiazepines due to the possibility of withdrawal seizures. Long-acting drugs, such as diazepam, chlordiazepoxide, or phenobarbital may be given to substitute for abused drug and dosage tapered.

Rohypnol ingestion

Rohypnol (flunitrazepam) is a type of benzodiazepine, commonly referred to as the "date rape drug" or "roofie" because it causes anterograde amnesia. Rohypnol is popular with teens and young adults and is often taken with alcohol, which potentiates its effects. Rohypnol is a CNS depressant that causes muscle relaxation, slurs speech, and reduces inhibitions. The effects occur within 20 to 30 minutes of ingestion but may persist 8 to 12 hours. Repeated use can result in aggressiveness, and withdrawal may cause hallucinations and seizures. Overdoses cause hypotension, altered mental status, vomiting, hallucinations, dyspnea, and coma. Diagnosis is by history and clinical examination. Treatment includes:

- Assessment for rape and rape kit if indicated with tests for STDs.
- Gastric emptying (less than 1 hour).
- Charcoal.
- Monitoring for CNS/respiratory depression.
- Supportive care.
- Flumazenil (antagonist) 0.2 mg each minute to total 3 mg may be used in some cases but not routinely advised because of complications related to benzodiazepine dependency or coingestion of cyclic antidepressants.
- Counseling referral for rape.

GHB and related drug toxicity

Gamma-hydroxybutyrate GHB is commonly known as "fantasy" or "blue nitro" (when blue dye is added) and is used as a hallucinogen and date-rape drug as it causes deep sedation and loss of memory. Similar drugs include butanediol (BD) and gamma butyrolactone (GBL). GHB may produce states of euphoria and hallucinations and is often taken with steroids to increase growth hormones affecting muscles. Symptoms of ingestion are dose-dependent:

- Less than 1 g: relaxation, reduced inhibitions.
- 1 to 2 g: increased relaxation, bradycardia, bradypnea, hypotension, impairment of motor ability.
- 2 to 4 g: severe lethargy, motor impairment, coma.
- Other symptoms include nausea, vomiting, amnesia, delusions, seizures, and depression.

Diagnosis is by history and clinical examination.

Treatment includes:

- Assessment for rape and rape kit if indicated and tests for STDs.
- Gastric emptying (less than 1 hour).
- Charcoal administration.
- Careful monitoring for CNS/respiratory depression.
- Supportive care.
- Referral for counseling in instances of rape.

Overdose of TCAs

Tricyclic antidepressants (TCAs), such as amitriptyline and imipramine, cause the most prescription-related deaths. They are prescribed for depression and other psychiatric and medical conditions. Toxicity may result from intentional overdose, excessive therapeutic dose, poly-drug combinations, serotonin syndrome (increased serotonin in CNS), and medical conditions. Symptoms of toxicity vary widely and can include:
- Alterations of consciousness, slurred speech, seizures, coma.
- Dilated or constricted pupils, blurred vision
- Pulmonary edema.
- Ataxia, tremor, myoclonus, hyperreflexia.
- Tachycardia, hypertension or hypotension, heart block, depressed cardiac contractility. ECG: sinus tachycardia with right-axis deviation (terminal 40 ms), prolonged PR, QRS, and QT (develop in <6 hrs).
- Urinary retention and overflow incontinence.

Diagnosis includes positive serum TCA and clinical findings, urine drug screening, ECG, serum electrolyte, creatinine, glucose levels, ABGs. Treatment may includes IV access, cardiac monitoring, urinary catheter if necessary, gastric decontamination with gastric lavage (1 hour or less) and charcoal, sodium bicarbonate (dysrhythmias, hypotension), IV dextrose, thiamine, naloxone, barbiturates (seizures), and isotonic crystalloid fluids and/or vasopressor, such as norepinephrine (hypotension).

Salicylate toxicity

Salicylate toxicity may be acute or chronic and is caused by ingestion of OTC drugs containing salicylates, such as ASA, Pepto-Bismol, and products used in hot inhalers. Symptoms vary according to age and amount of ingestion. Co-ingestion of sedatives may alter symptoms: Less than 150 mg/kg: nausea and vomiting. 150 to 300 mg/kg: Vomiting, hyperpnea, diaphoresis, tinnitus, alterations in acid-base balance. More than 300 mg/kg: Pediatrics: Metabolic acidosis in children younger than 4 but respiratory alkalosis and metabolic acidosis with alkalemia (pH greater than 7.5) in older children. Chronic toxicity is more serious and includes hyperventilation, volume depletion, acidosis, hypokalemia, and CNS abnormalities. Adults (usually intentional): Nausea, vomiting, diaphoresis, tinnitus, hyperventilation, respiratory alkalosis and metabolic acidosis. Chronic toxicity results in hyperventilation, tremor, papilledema, alterations in mental status, pulmonary edema, seizures, and coma. Diagnosis is by ferris chloride or Ames Phenistix tests. Treatment includes: Gastric decontamination with lavage (1 hour or less) and charcoal. Volume replacement (D5W). Sodium bicarbonate 1 to 2mEq/kg. Monitoring of salicylate concentration, acid-base, and electrolytes every hour. Whole-bowel irrigation (sustained-release tablets).

Benzodiazepine toxicity

Benzodiazepine toxicity may result from accidental or intentional overdose with such drugs as alprazolam, chlordiazepoxide, diazepam, lorazepam, oxazepam, midazolam, and temazepam. Mortality is usually the result of co-ingestion of other drugs. Symptoms are often nonspecific neurological changes: lethargy, dizziness, alterations in consciousness, ataxia. Respiratory depression and hypotension are rare complications. Coma and severe central nervous depression is usually is caused by co-ingestions. Diagnosis is based on history and clinical exam, as benzodiazepine level does not correlate well with toxicity.

Treatment includes:
- Gastric emptying (less than 1 hour).
- Charcoal.
- Concentrated dextrose, thiamine, and naloxone if co-ingestion suspected, especially with altered mental status.
- Monitoring for CNS/respiratory depression.
- Supportive care.
- Flumazenil (antagonist) 0.2 mg each minute to total 3 mg may be used in some cases but not routinely advised because of complications related to benzodiazepine dependency or co-ingestion of cyclic antidepressants. Flumazenil is contraindicated in the presence of increased intracranial pressure.

Ethanol overdose

Ethanol is the form of alcohol found in alcoholic beverages, flavorings, and some medications. It is a multisystem toxin and CNS depressant. Teenagers and young adults and those older than 60 frequently use ethanol as the drug of choice, but binge drinking can lead to serious morbidity or death. Ethanol has direct effects of the CNS, myocardium, thyroid, and hepatic tissue. Ethanol is absorbed through the mucosa of the mouth, stomach, and intestines, with concentrations peaking about 30 to 60 minutes after ingestion. About 90% of ethanol is metabolized in the liver and the rest excreted through the pulmonary and renal systems. Chronic abuse of ethanol (alcoholism) is also associated with alcohol withdrawal syndrome (delirium tremens) with abrupt cessation of alcohol intake, resulting in hallucinations, tachycardia, diaphoresis, and sometimes psychotic behavior. It may be precipitated by trauma or infection and has a high mortality rate: 5% to 15% with treatment and 35% without treatment.

Ethanol overdose affects the central nervous system as well as other organs in the body. Ethanol is absorbed through the mucosa of the mouth, stomach, and intestines, with concentrations peaking about 30-60 minutes after ingestion. If people are easily aroused, they can usually safely sleep off the effects of ingesting too much alcohol, but if the person is semi-conscious or unconscious, emergency medical treatment should be initiated. Symptoms include:
- Altered mental status with slurred speech and stupor.
- Nausea and vomiting.
- Hypotension.
- Bradycardia with arrhythmias
- Respiratory depression and hypoxia.
- Cold, clammy skin or flushed skin (from vasodilation).
- Acute pancreatitis with abdominal pain.
- Lack of consciousness
- Circulatory collapse leading to death.

Treatment includes:
- Careful monitoring of arterial blood gases and oxygen saturation.
- Ensure patent airway with intubation and ventilation if necessary.
- Intravenous fluids.
- Dextrose to correct hypoglycemia if indicated.
- Maintain body temperature (warming blanket).
- Dialysis may be necessary in severe cases.

Ethanol overdose affects young children differently than teenagers or adults. Additionally, young children often ingest alcohol in products such as perfumes and cleaning solutions, which are often more toxic than beer or alcoholic beverages.

Infants and young children:
- Seizures and coma. Respiratory depression and hypoxia.
- Hypoglycemia (especially infants and toddlers).
- Hypothermia.

Teenagers:
- Altered mental status.
- Hypotension.
- Bradycardia with arrhythmias.
- Respiratory depression and hypoxia.
- Cold, clammy skin or flushed skin (from vasodilation).
- Acute pancreatitis with abdominal pain.
- Lack of consciousness.
- Circulatory collapse leading to death.

Treatment includes:
- Careful monitoring of ABGs and oxygen saturation.
- Ensure patent airway with intubation and ventilation if necessary.
- IV fluids.
- Dextrose to correct hypoglycemia if indicated.
- Maintain body temperature (warming blanket).
- Dialysis may be necessary in severe cases.

Wernicke-Korsakoff syndrome

Wernicke-Korsakoff syndrome (alcoholic encephalopathy) results from long-term abuse of alcohol that causes malnutrition and thiamine (B1) deficiency, which causes damage to both the central and peripheral nervous systems. Diagnosis includes: Serum thiamine, increased pyruvate, decreased transketolase, increased blood alcohol level, increased liver enzyme levels. Symptoms include:
- Mild to severe alcohol withdrawal psychological and physical symptoms: shakiness, depression, anxiety, headache, diaphoresis, anorexia, nausea and vomiting, tachycardia, dilated pupils, tremor progressing to severe agitation, seizures, blackouts, delirium tremens, coma.
- Visual disturbances: diplopia, nystagmus, eyelid ptosis.
- Ataxia.
- Poor memory and severe memory loss, hallucinations.
- Malnourished appearance.

Treatment stops progression but does not reverse mental deterioration.
- Thiamine IM, IV, or orally;
- abstinence from alcohol;
- Dietary supplementation and nutritional counseling.

Patients are usually hospitalized until condition stable.

Mumps

Mumps is a viral disease that causes fever and swollen parotid glands but can cause deafness, meningitis, and swelling of the testicles. Mumps is spread through contact with saliva or aerosolized droplets from someone infected. The incubation period is 2 to 3 weeks. Incidence has decreased since vaccinations have become routine. Diagnosis is by clinical exam and virus culture if necessary.

Symptoms include:
- Painful swelling of glands on one or both sides of the face.
- Fever.
- Weakness, fatigue.
- Complications (rare) include orchitis, encephalitis, meningitis, ovarian inflammation, pancreatitis, and permanent hearing loss.

Treatment is supportive. There is no effective prophylaxis after exposure, although vaccination is not harmful and may protect against future infections if exposure does not cause disease. There is no effective treatment for mumps except for supportive care:
- Acetaminophen or ibuprofen.
- Standard barrier precautions.

Measles

Rubeola (measles) is a viral disease characterized by fever and rash but can cause serious morbidity and death. It is highly infectious by droplets 4 days before and 4 days after onset of rash and has an incubation period of 7 to 18 days. Symptoms include:
- Flu-like symptoms: cough, fever, running nose
- Red maculopapular rash.
- Koplik spots on mucous membranes.
- Complications include: pneumonia, seizures, severe neurological damage from encephalitis.

Vaccination (MMR) or previous infection provides immunity. The vaccine may be used as a prophylaxis for 72 hours after exposure while immunoglobulin may provide protection if given within 6 days.

Treatment for measles is supportive because nothing eradicates the virus:
- Acetaminophen or ibuprofen.
- Vitamin A (small children).
- Standard barrier precautions.

Chickenpox

Varicella (chickenpox) is a common infectious childhood disease caused by the varicella zoster virus, resulting in fever, rash, and itching, but it can cause skin infections, pneumonia, and neurological damage. After infection, the virus retreats to the nerves by the spinal cord and can reactivate years later, causing herpes zoster (shingles), a significant cause of morbidity in adults. Infection with varicella conveys immunity, but because of associated problems, it is recommended that all children receive varicella vaccine. Two doses are needed:
- 12 to 15 months.
- 4 to 6 years (or at least 3 months after first dose).

Children at least 13 years and adults who have never had chickenpox or previously received the vaccine should receive 2 doses at least 28 days apart. Children should not receive the vaccine if they have had a serious allergic reaction to gelatin or neomycin. Most reactions are mild and include soreness, fever, and blistering, itchy rash. Complications (rare) include febrile seizures, encephalitis, and pneumonia.

Treatment is supportive:
- Acetaminophen or ibuprofen.
- Barrier precautions.

Reye syndrome

Reye syndrome is a serious, sometimes fatal, systemic disorder that follows a viral infection, such as chickenpox, upper respiratory tract infections, and influenza, usually in children. The primary problems include fatty accumulation in the liver and other organs and encephalopathy. Early diagnosis is critical for prevention of permanent brain damage or death. There is an association between the use of salicylates (aspirin, aspirin compounds) for viral infections, so children younger than 19 should not receive salicylates. Symptoms usually appear as a viral infection recedes:
- Infants: diarrhea with or without vomiting, hyperventilation or periods of apnea, seizures.
- Others: Sudden onset of vomiting, usually without diarrhea, alterations in mental status with lethargy, agitation, stupor, extensor spasms, decerebrate rigidity, and coma. Symptoms common to salicylate poisoning may occur.

Diagnosis is based on increased AST and ALT (at least 200 units) but no jaundice, increased blood NH_3. Hypoglycemia is common in infants.

Treatment includes:
- Hypertonic glucose 10% IV.
- Supplemental oxygen and ventilation as necessary.
- Supportive care to reduce cerebral edema and as indicated by symptoms.

Rubella

Rubella, also known as German measles, is a viral disease that can cause rash, fever, and arthritis, but the big danger is that it can cause a woman who is pregnant to miscarry or deliver a child with serious birth defects. Transmission is through airborne droplets. The incubation period is 2 to 3 weeks after exposure. Symptoms persist 2 to 3 days and include:
- Fever 102°F or lower.
- Rhinitis.
- Conjunctivitis.
- Poor appetite, nausea.
- Rash, red or pink and sometimes itchy, starts on the face and moves down the body with the face clearing of rash as it progresses.
- Inflamed lymph nodes behind ears and at back of neck.

Children born with congenital rubella may shed the virus in stool and urine, which can infect caregivers. There is no effective prophylaxis after exposure.

Treatment is supportive:
- Acetaminophen or ibuprofen.
- Referral to obstetrician/gynecologist (pregnant women).
- Barrier precautions.

Whooping cough

Pertussis (whooping cough) is a very infectious respiratory tract infection characterized by a persistent cough lasting at least 2 weeks, caused by *Bordetella pertussis.* It is spread by droplets and is contagious as long as infection continues. Whooping cough usually clears without a problem in teenagers and adults but can be a serious illness in children, especially younger than 6 months.

Symptoms include:
- Initial: fever, rhinitis, sneezing, watery eyes, dry cough.
- 1 to 2 weeks later: severe repeated paroxysmal coughing with inspiratory "whoop," productive of thick phlegm and post-tussive emesis.
- Petechiae may occur on the upper body or sclera of eyes from exertion related to coughing.

Complications vary by age:
- Infants: ear infections, pneumonia, bradypnea or apnea, dehydration, CNS damage.
- Children: hernia, muscle damage (from coughing).
- Adults: hernia, fractured rib.

Treatment includes:
- Bed rest and fluids. Infants may require hospitalization and IV fluids.
- Mist vaporizer.
- Antibiotics: azithromycin or erythromycin may shorten course of disease. Supportive care and barrier precautions.

Mononucleosis

Mononucleosis is an infectious disorder caused by the Epstein-Barr virus. It is spread through saliva and airborne droplets and occurs most common in teenagers and young adults. Incubation period is 4 to 6 weeks. Symptoms are usually similar to an upper respiratory tract infection or flu, with adults affected more than children, and may persist for weeks:

- Weakness.
- Headaches.
- Fever.
- Persistent sore throat.
- Enlarged lymph nodes in neck and axillae.
- Enlarged tonsils.
- Generalized red macular rash.
- Enlarged spleen, rupture may occur in rare cases.

Diagnosis may include clinical examination, antibody tests (such as Monospot), and CBC. Treatment is primarily supportive as there is no treatment for the virus:

- Rest and restricted activity to avoid spleen rupture.
- Acetaminophen or ibuprofen.
- Adequate fluid intake.

TB

Tuberculosis (TB), caused by *Mycobacterium tuberculosis,* is not a new disease, but an increase in resistant strains has brought control and prevention of tuberculosis to the forefront of infectious disease control. TB is a particular danger to those who are immunocompromised, with 8% to 10% of those with HIV developing TB. Patients with TB may develop weight loss, general debility, night sweats, and fever. With pulmonary involvement, a progressive cough resulting in dyspnea and bloody sputum is common. Diagnosis is based on skin and sputum testing as well as x-ray. Transmission is from airborne particles small enough to suspend in the air, so anyone in contact to someone with active TB is at risk of inhaling particles.

Precautions:

- Prompt diagnosis and anti-tuberculosis drugs per protocol.
- Airborne infection isolation.
- Skin testing/x-rays of those in contact.
- Preventive isoniazid therapy for those with latent infection or newly converted to positive on TB testing.

<u>Exposure of healthcare workers</u>
Exposure to TB in a health care facility is almost always the result of inadequate or delayed diagnosis of active TB in a patient. Upon diagnosis, immediate contact investigation must be done to determine all those who might be at risk of infection, including nursing, laboratory, and housekeeping staff. A 2-step PPD skin testing or the *QuantiFERON*-TB Gold test should be done to determine if those exposed have become infected. Those who test positive must be evaluated to ensure that they do not have active TB. Treatment protocols for latent or active TB must be initiated as soon as possible. There are a number of different protocols, but for latent TB, isoniazid (INH) for 9 months is the treatment of choice. Health care workers with active pulmonary or laryngeal TB or

who stopped treatment must be excluded from work until symptoms subside and 3 sputum tests are negative or treatment is completed.

MDR-TB and XDR-TB

Multi-drug resistant tuberculosis (MDR-TB) is resistant to at least 2 commonly used first-line drugs, isoniazid (INH) and rifampin, while extensively drug resistant tuberculosis (XDR-TB) is also resistant to all fluoroquinolones and at least 1 of the 3 second-line drugs: amikacin, kanamycin, or capreomycin. XDR-TB emerged as a worldwide concern in 2005. In the United States, it is at present most commonly found in foreign born patients but also occurs in immunocompromised patients. Active TB requires treatment for extended periods of time, usually 18 to 24 months, with multiple drugs. Since the 1980s there has been increased need to use second-line drugs to combat infection. There are 2 primary causes for the increased resistance:
- Failure to complete a course of treatment
- Mismanaged treatment, including incorrect medication, dosage, or duration of therapy.

People who have had previous TB are at increased risk and should be monitored carefully. Drug-resistant TB increasingly poses a risk for patients and staff in health care facilities.

DOT: The ED infection control plans should include provisions for referring patients and/or staff with TB for directly observed therapy (DOT) when indicated. DOT requires that a health care worker monitor every dose of an individual's anti-tuberculosis medication, ensuring that all medications are taken and the entire course of treatment is completed. Drug protocol may be changed to 2 to 3 times weekly rather than daily to facilitate DOT. Regulations about DOT vary from state to state.

DOT is frequently used in these circumstances:
- Sputum cultures are positive for acid-fast bacilli.
- There is concurrent treatment with antiretroviral drugs (for HIV) or methadone (for addiction).
- Infection is MDR-TB or XDR-TB.
- Comorbidity with psychiatric disease or cognitive impairment exists.
- Patient is homeless and lacks adequate facilities.
- Patient has demonstrated lack of reliability in treatment.

When patients are discharged from the hospital, plans must include continuation of DOT through the use of home health agencies or having the patient return to a clinic for administration of drugs.

Identifying those with communicable diseases

Identifying those with communicable diseases involves 4 different types of surveillance:
- Admitting history/admission physical can help to identify high-risk behaviors or symptoms that may not be current but can indicate a communicable disease. Questioning answers to elicit more information is also helpful.
- Admitting diagnosis serves as a key element to determine if further evaluation should be done, especially if the diagnosis is a common opportunistic infection involving particular infectious diseases. For example, cytomegalovirus is often related to HIV infection.
- Symptoms, such as chronic or severe cough or diarrhea, should trigger further investigation to determine if there is a contagious cause.

- Laboratory review should be ongoing after threshold rates are established for different lab tests. Any abnormality that is suggestive of an infectious disease process should be evaluated to determine if further follow-up or isolation is needed.

Responsibility of ED staff in reporting diseases

The CDC issues a list of reportable diseases, also called notifiable diseases, which are important to public health. Each state also has a list, which may include additional diseases, such as cancer or hospital-acquired infections. The ED staff is required to report those diseases in which mandatory reporting is required and should also report diseases of interest that do not require reporting but are a public health concern. Tracking these diseases allows for identifying disease outbreaks and can help the states make better decisions regarding public health, such as food handling laws and immunization needs. Reporting to the CDC is not name-based, so no personal information is maintained at the federal level; however, some state reporting, such as for HIV, is name-based, so the staff must be familiar with reporting statutes for the state of practice. In some cases (chickenpox), just the total number of cases is reported. Different types of reports are required, depending upon the disease:
- Written reports are required for those diseases that require follow-up to identify source of disease or contacts, such as syphilis and salmonella infection.
- Telephone reports are required for those diseases in which statistics are maintained, such as measles and pertussis.

CDC isolation guidelines

Through the years, the CDC has issued a number of different guidelines for isolation precautions. The 1996 CDC isolation guidelines were an update from the "Universal Precautions" guidelines that dealt with blood and some body fluids but did not directly address other types of transmission. There are now 2 tiers of isolation precautions.

Tier I, standard precautions
Tier I deals with standard precautions that should be in place for all patients:
- Standard precautions include protection from all blood and body fluids and the use of gloves, face barriers, and gowns as needed to avoid being splashed with fluids. Hand washing remains central to infection control and should be with plain (not antimicrobial) soap or instant antiseptic. Soiled linens should be placed in waterproof bags and sharps should be placed in appropriate containers. Private rooms are used for those who contaminate the environment (e.g., uncontrolled diarrhea, cough) or are unhygienic. If no private room is available, patients with the same type of infection, same colonizing organism, may share a room.
- In 2007, the standards were updated to add safe injection practices, using a mask when engaging in procedures that involve puncturing the spinal column, and respiratory hygiene/cough etiquette.

Tier II, transmission-based precautions
Tier II of the CDC isolation guidelines protects from 3 types of transmission.
- Airborne precautions include placing patient in a private room with monitored negative airflow and the door closed. People who are susceptible to the disease, such as those not immune against measles, should not enter the room. Respiratory precautions (a mask) should be worn if the patient has suspected or confirmed TB. Patient should wear mask

outside of room. This type of isolation provides protection from diseases spread by small airborne droplets (less than 5 mm), including measles, tuberculosis, SARS, and varicella, which can remain suspended in the air for some time.

- Droplet precautions include private room. Staff and visitors who are within 6-10 feet of the patient must wear masks, and the patient must wear a mask outside of room. Patient door may remain open. This type of isolation provides protection from diseases spread by large airborne droplets (greater than 5 mm), easily spread by talking, coughing, or sneezing, but do not travel more than 6-10 feet (the previous distance of 3 feet was changed in 2003). Diseases include viral influenza, pertussis, streptococcal pharyngitis or pneumonia, *Neisseria* meningitides, and mumps.
- Contact precautions include placing the patient in a private room or room with someone with the same infection. Gloves should be used as for standard precautions but should immediately be removed and hands sanitized after contact with infective material. A clean protective gown should be worn inside the room for close contact with patient, including caring for a patient who is incontinent or has uncontained drainage. The patient should not leave the room if possible and equipment should be dedicated for patient use or disinfected before use by other patients.

Some diseases may require some combination of airborne, droplet, and contact precautions: Lassa fever, Marburg virus, and smallpox.

Airborne infection isolation

Airborne infection isolation should be initiated with suspicion or confirmation of a diagnosis of disease that has airborne transmission, such as SARS, varicella, measles, variola (smallpox), and tuberculosis, with droplet size less than 5 mcm, or patients with multiple drug-resistant strains of organisms. Isolation should be continued until confirmation that patient is not infective. Isolation procedures include:

- Placing patient in a private room with at least 12 air exchanges per hour (ACH) under negative pressure with air from the outside in and exhaust, preferably, to the outdoors, or recirculation provided through high-efficiency particulate air (HEPA) filters.
- Door to the room should remain closed and sign or color/coding should be used at door to alert medical staff to isolation.
- Respirator use for personnel entering room when indicated because of disease transmission (TB and smallpox) or lack of immunity (measles).
- Patient transported in clean linens and wearing a face mask.
- Procedures done in the room whenever possible.

Professional Issues

Environment for ethical decision-making

An environment for ethical decision-making and patient advocacy does not appear when it is needed; it requires planning and preparation. The expectation for the institution should clearly communicate that nurses are legally and morally responsible for ensuring competent care and respecting the rights of patients, including allowing informed consent and protecting confidentiality. Decisions regarding ethical issues often must be made quickly with little time for contemplation; therefore, ethical issues that may arise should be identified and discussed. Clearly defined procedures and policies for dealing with conflicts, including an active ethics committee, inservice training, and staff meetings, must be established. Patients and families need to be part of the ethical environment, and that means empowering them by providing patient/family information (print form, video, audio) that outlines patient's rights and procedures for expressing their wishes and dealing with ethical conflicts. Respect for privacy and confidentiality and a nonpunitive atmosphere are essential.

Cultural diversity and assessment

Issues of cultural diversity must be considered during assessment. Individuals vary considerably in their attitudes, so assuming that all members of an ethnic or cultural group share the same values is never valid. The individual must be assessed as well as the group. It is important to take time to observe family dynamics and language barriers, arranging for translators if necessary to ensure that there is adequate communication. In patriarchal cultures, such as the Mexican culture, the eldest male may speak for the patient. In some Muslim cultures, females will resist care by males. Acknowledging biological differences, such as skin color, is important for assessing skin because wounds and bruising may have a different appearance. The attitudes and beliefs of the patient in relation to wound care must be understood, accepted, and treated with respect. In some cases, the use of healers or cultural traditions must be incorporated into a plan of care.

African American
- Drug response
  - Fast response to tricyclic antidepressants, more adverse effects
  - Less response to beta blockers and ACE inhibitors
- May avoid eye contact out of respect
- May be distrustful

Asian
- Drug response
  - Require lower dosages of tricyclic antidepressants and antipsychotics and have more adverse effects
  - Less able to metabolize codeine
  - Require lower dosage of propranolol
  - More sensitive to alcohol
- Generally express psychological problems somatically
- May not openly express feelings or pain
- Chinese – *Shenjing shuairuo* (neurasthenia): a mental health related condition with symptoms of headache, fatigue, anxiety, high blood pressure, and depressed mood

- Koreans – *Hwa-byung*: a mental illness brought about by long term suppression of anger and built up resentment; symptoms include burning sensation, chest pain, anorexia, insomnia, and feeling of suffocation.

Hispanic
- *Colera* – anger-related condition with trembling, headache, screaming, GI problems, and fainting
- *Ataque de nervios* – stress related condition with uncontrolled yelling, aggression, trembling, crying
- May want to use folk medicine and healers

Middle Eastern
- Expect male family spokesman to be addressed first and to make decisions
- Often want same-sex caregiver
- May misinterpret direct eye contact with opposite gender

Native American
- Ghost sickness – symptoms of weakness, anorexia, terror, and nightmares
- Drug response
  o Faster metabolism of alcohol and lower tolerance
- May avoid eye contact
- May tolerate prolonged silence in communication

Evaluating and implementing research findings

The nurse must be taught and understand the process of critical analysis and know how to conduct a survey of the literature. Basic concepts related to research include:
- Survey of valid sources: Information from a juried journal and personal website are very different sources, and evaluating what constitutes a valid source of data is critical.
- Evaluation of internal and external validity: Internal validity shows a cause-and-effect relationship between 2 variables, with the cause occurring before the effect and no intervening variable. External validity occurs when results hold true in different environments and circumstances with different populations.
- Sample selection and sample size: Selection and size can have a huge impact on the results, but a sample that is too small may lack both internal and external validity. Selection may be so narrowly focused that the results cannot be generalized to other groups.

Communicating and incorporating research results

Research results about procedures, products, or technology can be communicated in a number of ways:
- Presentations to administration and those in positions of leadership, such as team leaders or managers, to garner support for incorporating findings into practice.
- Inservice training/education that focuses on results of research and explains applicability.
- Print distribution in the form of flyers or newsletters that outline the research findings.
- Electronic newsletters or training modules that present the research findings.
- Discussions with intra- and interdisciplinary team members about the research and ways in which to apply the data to the practice of care.

Communicating is only one part of the process. Procedures must be in place in each organization that outlines the steps to incorporating research findings into practice. An interdisciplinary team should evaluate the research findings and together create a system-wide approach to application, with the goal of improving outcomes for patients.

Pain assessment

Pain is subjective and may be influenced by the individual's pain threshold (the smallest stimulus that produces the sensation of pain) and pain tolerance (the maximum degree of pain that a person can tolerate). The most common current pain assessment tool for adults and pre-teens/adolescents is the 1-10 scale:
- 0 = no pain.
- 1-2 = mild pain.
- 3-5 = moderate pain.
- 6-7 = severe pain.
- 8-9 = very severe pain.
- 10 = excruciating pain.

However, there is more to pain assessment than a number on a scale. Assessment includes information about onset, duration, and intensity. Identifying what triggers pain and what relieves it can be very useful when developing a plan for pain management. Patients may show very different behavior when they are in pain: Some may cry and moan with minor pain, and others may exhibit little difference in behavior when truly suffering. Thus, judging pain by behavior can lead to the wrong conclusions.

Patients with cognitive impairment or inability to verbalize pain may not be able to indicate the degree of pain, even by using a face scale with pictures of smiling to crying faces. The Pain Assessment in Advanced Dementia (PAINAD) scale may be helpful, especially for those with Alzheimer's disease. Careful observation of non-verbal behavior can indicate that the patient is in pain:
- Respirations: Patients often have more rapid and labored breathing as pain increases with short periods of hyperventilation or Cheyne-Stokes respirations.
- Vocalization: Patients may remain negative in speech or speak quietly and reluctantly. They may moan or groan. As pain increases, they may call out, moan or groan loudly, or cry.
- Facial expression: Patients may appear sad or frightened, may frown or grimace, especially on activities that increase pain.
- Body language: Patients may be tense, fidgeting, pacing and as pain increases may become rigid, clench fists, or lie in fetal position. They may become increasingly combative.
- Consolability: Patients are less distractible or consolable with increased pain.

> **Review Video:** ABCDE Pain Assessment
> *Visit **mometrix.com/academy** and enter Code:* **760328**

Assessing activities in relation to pain
Assessment of pain must include determining those factors or activities that increase pain.
- Site of pain: While pain is often focused on the wound site, it may extend to the surrounding tissues, especially in chronic wounds, making application and removal of dressings especially painful.

- Movement: Pressure and touch caused by changes of position can increase pain, limiting mobility.
- Time: Pain often increases at night, making sleep difficult.
- Dressings: Dressings that are too tight or the wrong choice for a wound may cause intense site pain. Allowing a wound to become dry can also increase pain.
- Personal/Cultural: Some people have difficulty expressing the degree of pain. Others react to the expectation of the medical personnel or family. Some believe that they should remain stoic or are afraid of becoming "addicted," so they resist taking pain medications until pain is severe.

> **Review Video:** Assessing Pain
Visit mometrix.com/academy and enter Code: **693250**

> **Review Video:** Assessment Tools for Pain
Visit mometrix.com/academy and enter Code: **634001**

> **Review Video:** Barriers to Pain Assessment
Visit mometrix.com/academy and enter Code: **187514**

Pain management

Acute pain is a biologic response to illness or injury and usually responds to opiates. Chronic pain, lasting at least 3 months or 1 month longer than usual for a condition, is a common cause for ED visits, but chronic pain can usually not be completely relieved. However, the patient can be taught to manage pain. Pain may be dull, sharp, cramping, shooting, burning, constant, or recurrent.

The 3 primary types of chronic pain include:
- Nociceptive: Usually responds well to centrally acting analgesics.
- Neuropathic: Often responds poorly to analgesia.
- Psychogenic: May be difficult to treat because of patient resistance.

Identifying the type of pain and triggers or aggravating conditions is important to help the patient to avoid inducing pain.

Management programs may include:
- Diet and exercise.
- Psychological counseling.
- Acupuncture.
- Analgesia: NSAIDs, opiates (cancer), corticosteroids (back pain), acetaminophen.
- Antidepressants: Amitriptyline 10 to 20 mg 2 hours before bedtime.
- Anticonvulsants: Carbamazepine 100 to 200 mg 2 times daily or valproic acid 1 mg/kg daily in 2 doses (neuropathic pain).

Discharge planning from the ED

Both federal and state regulations govern discharge planning and prevent patient "dumping" from an ED. All patients admitted to a hospital (including the ED) receiving federal funds, such as Medicare, must be provided discharge planning.

The Social Security Act and Conditions of Participation outline steps to the discharge planning process:

- Case finding/screening.
- Evaluation of continuity of care needs includes evaluating the ability of the patient to provide self-care or the possibility of others providing care in the patient's environment.
- Resource assessment.
- Identification of problem.
- Planning.
- Implementation.

Discharge planning should include patient education, assistance in coordinating medical appointments, follow-up (telephone, e-mail), and information about access to care. High-risk patients, such as patients who are elderly, homeless, or drug or alcohol abusers, or those with repeated ED visits, are especially in need of adequate discharge planning and follow-up.

Organ donation

Organ donation procedures must be in place in the ED so that organ procurement can take place. The United Network for Organ Sharing (UNOS) facilitates organ sharing, provides the Critical Pathway (guideline to effective management of donors so that organs remain viable) and provides protocols for organ procurement for the following:

- Donations after brain death.
- Donations after cardiac death.
- Donations after pediatric death.

Organ procurement specialists should be trained and available to EDs so they can meet with family when the opportunity for organ donation arises. In some cases, patients may carry a donor card or indicate on their driver's licenses that they agree to donate their organs. In other cases, the decision about organ donation will be made by the family at a very stressful time, so a sensitive and supportive approach is critical. Once a donor is identified, UNOS is notified of the available organs so that they can be assigned. Hospitals that receive payment from CMS must have an Organ Procurement Organization (OPO), and that OPO must be notified in a timely manner of patients whose death is imminent or who have died.

Advance directives

In accordance with federal and state laws, individuals have the right to self-determination in health care, including decisions about end-of-life care through advance directives such as living wills and the right to assign a surrogate person to make decisions through a durable power of attorney. Patients should routinely be questioned about an advance directive as they may present at the ED without the document. Patients who have indicated they desire a DNR order should not receive resuscitative treatments for terminal illness or conditions in which meaningful recovery cannot occur. Patients and families of those with terminal illnesses should be questioned as to whether the patients are hospice patients. For those with DNR requests or withdrawing life support, staff should provide the patient palliative rather than curative measures, such as pain control and/or oxygen, and emotional support to the patient and family. Religious traditions and beliefs about death should be treated with respect.

Evidence for legal/forensic situations and reportable situations

Preservation of evidence for legal/forensic situations requires preparation and protocols established in cooperation with local law enforcement. The documentation of a chain of custody of any evidence collected helps ensure the integrity of that evidence. The less people that can handle a piece of evidence, the stronger the chain of custody will be. In most states, the chain of custody is originally started by the RN that finds the evidence. That nurse should place each item in a sealed container with the patient's name, the describtion of the item, the name of the RN who sealed the evidence (along with the date/time sealed), and the source of the item sealed (such as the anatomical location). The sealed evidence should not leave the nurse, unless it can be placed in a locked safe until law enforcement arrives, and at that time a note of final transfer is made in the patient's record. The nurse should write down factual information and use direct quotes from the patient using quotation marks when possible.

Documentation must be made using accurate terminology and wounds should be labeled using numbers, not "entry" or "exit". In some cases, photographic documentation of injuries should be made.The ED should establish clear protocols that include what to report (communicable diseases, assaults, gunshot wounds, child abuse, elder abuse, spousal abuse), how to report (e-mail, internet, telephone, mail), who to report to (city, county, state, federal), when to report (minimum time frame), and how to document (forms to be filled out, record keeping).

Emergency Department-Based Surveillance Systems and Symptoms Clusters

Emergency department-based surveillance systems are used to collect data that can be utilized to track incidence and spread of disease through analysis of symptom clusters. Data can be collected for local, state, or national use. For example, emergency department-based surveillance systems may track firearm or weapon related deaths. The CDC partners with other agencies with a surveillance system called Distribute, which tracks influenza-like illness. Syndromic surveillance systems collect data regarding non-specific symptoms to determine if symptom clusters indicating a possible bioterrorism attack are evident.

Symptom clusters are comprised or two or more symptoms that occur together at the same time, such as nausea—vomiting, anxiety—depression, and fatigue—pain—insomnia. Symptoms clusters vary by the type of illness but can help to diagnose an illness or help to identify clusters of patients that indicate an outbreak. In some cases, symptoms clusters can be used to predict outcomes.

Safety

Medications
Yearly, about 7,000 deaths in the United States are attributed to medication errors. Studies indicate that there are errors in 1 in 5 doses of medication given to patients in hospitals. A caring environment is one in which patient safety is ensured with proper handling and administering of medications:
- Avoiding error-prone abbreviations or symbols. In many cases, abbreviations and symbols should be avoided altogether or restricted to a limited approved list.
- Preventing errors from illegible handwriting. Handwritten orders should be block printed to reduce erroneous changes.
- Instituting bar-coding and scanners that allow the patient's wristband and medications to be scanned for verification.
- Providing lists of similarly named medications to educate staff.

- Establishing an institutional/departmental policy for administration of medications that includes protocols for verification of drug, dosage, and patient, as well as education of the patient about the medications.
- Routine evaluation of patient's response to medication.

Staffing and infection control

Between 48,000 and 98,000 patients each year die in hospitals because of errors in patient safety. A caring environment must be a safe environment for patients and their families. Patient safety is impacted by a number of factors:

- Staffing practices: Patient-staff ratios are of primary importance as studies have indicated that fewer staff and long hours result in more errors. This is especially true in critical areas. The expertise of the staff is another important factor. Studies indicate that increased proportion of care (in hours) by registered nurses decrease both hospital stay and complications.
- Infection control: The rates of hospital infections have steadily increased with pathogens (such as Staphylococcus aureus and MRSA) endemic in some institutions. Patients with invasive devices, such as central lines or ventilators, are at increased risk. Much infection is related to poor handwashing and infection control practices on the part of staff.

Transfers and stabilization

Transfers from the ED may be intrahospital or to another facility. Stabilization of the patient with emergency conditions or active labor must be done in the ED prior to transfer. Stabilization requires treatment for emergency conditions and reasonable belief that, although the emergency condition may not be completely resolved, the patient's condition will not deteriorate during transfer. Women in the ED in active labor should deliver both the child and placenta before transfer. The receiving department or facility should be capable of treating the patient and dealing with complications that might occur. The ED staff should advise patient and family of transfer policies, and patient records regarding the emergency condition and treatment in the ED must accompany the transfer patient to ensure continuity of care. The patient must be accompanied by staff able to effectively monitor and treat patient during transfer. Transfer to another facility is indicated if the patient requires specialized services not available intrahospital, such as to burn centers or NICUs.

Triage

Triage is a method of prioritizing patient care based on severity of illness or injury and the availability of medical care. In disasters, triage may take place on site, usually through the guidance of an emergency physician or nurse trained in triage. Traditionally, patients are placed into color-coded categories for easy identification:

- Red: Urgent systemic life-threatening conditions.
- Yellow: Urgent systemic conditions but able to wait 45 to 60 minutes for treatment.
- Green: Localized and able to wait hours for treatment.
- Black: Death (sometimes includes those whose death is inevitable).

While triage may have taken place prior to arrival, all patients received in the ED should be triaged to determine the appropriate treatment area to which the patient is referred and to institute immediate life support as indicated. During the triage procedure, protocols should be followed in relation to identifying and tagging the patient, securing belongings, and informing family members.

Revised trauma scoring system

The revised trauma scoring system is used to rapidly assess and triage patients involved in trauma. It is often used at the scene of an accident by first responders, but scores should be verified on arrival at the ED. The revised trauma scoring system comprises 3 elements, with the 3 scores added together.

1. Respiratory rate per minute:
   - 4 points: 10 to 29   3 points: more than 29
   - 2 points: more than 6 to 9
   - 1 point: 1 to 5
   - 0 point: not breathing.

2. Systolic BP (mm Hg):
   - 4 points: more than 89. 3 points: 76 to 89
   - 2 points: 40 to 75
   - 1 point: 1 to 49
   - 0 point: no BP found.

3. Glasgow Coma Score (GCS):
   - 4 points: GCS 13 to 15.
   - 3 points: GCS 9 to 12
   - 2 points: GCS 6 to 8
   - 1 point: GCS 4 to 5
   - 0 point: GCS 2

Scores range from 12 (best) to 0 (most severe). Patients with scores 11 or less may require treatment in a trauma center. Scores are often used to predict patient outcomes.

Transitions of care

The nurse is usually the primary staff member responsible for external and internal hand off transitions of care, and should ensure that communication is thorough and covers all essential information. The best method is to use a standardized format:
- DRAW: Diagnosis, recent changes, anticipated changes, and what to watch for.
- I PASS the BATON: Introduction, patient, assessment, situation, safety concerns, background, actions, timing, ownership, and next.
- ANTICipate: Administrative data, new clinical information, tasks, illness severity, contingency plans.
- 5 Rs: Record, review, round together, relay to team, and receive feedback.

A reporting form or checklist may be utilized to ensure that no aspect is overlooked.
For external transitions, the nurse must ensure that the type of transport team and monitoring is appropriate for patient needs and that the mode of transportation is adequate: ground transfer for short distance, helicopter for medium to long distance, and fixed-wing aircraft for long distances.

Patient boarding

Patient boarding is maintaining a patient in the ED, sometimes for more than 24 hours, after the patient is admitted as an inpatient, usually because staffing is inadequate on the destination unit or no bed is available. Boarding results in over-crowding in the ED and impacts the quality of care because boarded patients often have intensive needs. Psychiatric patients are often boarded because of a lack of mental-health beds. According to the Joint Commission, patient boarding is a safety risk and indicates a problem in patient flow. Boarding should not exceed 4 hours. If a patient cannot be transferred promptly then added staff should be provided to care for the boarded patients. The hospital should have plans in place to facilitate rapid transfer. If the hospital is over capacity, then contingency plans may need to be implemented, such as diverting patients to other EDs or transferring patients to other hospitals.

Shift reporting

Shift reporting should include bedside handoff when possible with oncoming staff members. The nurse handing off the patient should follow a specific format for handoff (such as I PASS the BATON) so that handoff is done in the same manner every time, as this reduces the chance of omitting important information. The shift report should include introduction of the oncoming staff to the patient, the triage category or acuity level of the patient, diagnosis (potential or confirmed), current status, laboratory and imaging (completed or pending) and results if available, and medications or treatments administered and pending. Any monitoring equipment (pulse oximetry, telemetry) should be examined. Any invasive treatments (Foley catheter, IV) should be discussed and equipment examined. The nurse should report any plans for admission, transfer, or discharge. It is essential that all staff be trained in shift reporting and the importance of consistency.

Delegation of tasks to unlicensed assistive personnel

The scope of nursing practice includes delegation of tasks to unlicensed assistive personnel, providing those personnel have adequate training and knowledge to carry out the tasks. Delegation should be used to manage the workload and to provide adequate and safe care. The nurse who delegates remains accountable for patient outcomes and for supervision of the person to whom the task was delegated, so the nurse must consider the following:
- Whether knowledge, skills, and training of the unlicensed assistive personnel provides the ability to perform the delegated task.
- Whether the patient's condition and needs have been properly evaluated and assessed.
- Whether the nurse is able to provide ongoing supervision.

Delegation should be done in a manner that reduces liability by providing adequate communication. This includes specific directions about the task, including what needs to be done, when, and for how long. Expectations related to consultation, reporting, and completion of tasks should be clearly defined. The nurse should be available to assist if necessary. Activities that may not be delegated to UAP: performing nursing assessments, performing interventions that require nursing judgment, administering medications, formulating the plan of care or nursing diagnosis, providing education for the patient, documenting assessment or patient response to interventions, and evaluating progress toward outcomes.

Disaster preparedness and planning

Disaster plans should be in place for the facility and the ED based on the Hospital Emergency Incident Command System (HEICS), which provides a model for management, responsibilities, and communication. Disasters can include a multiple casualty influx of patients from a community emergency, such as a train accident; an epidemic; fire or other internal hospital problem requiring evacuation; or inadequate staffing to safely treat ED patients. Plans should include/address:
- Readily available information and disaster preparedness drills.
- Activation of the plan, including the individual(s) responsible.
- Chain of command.
- Facility damage assessment, usually conducted by plant safety officer.
- Hospital/ED capacity to receive patients.
- Triage, including in community and in the ED.
- Transfer protocols for distributing patients to other facilities.
- Staffing, including telephone tree to notify staff to report to facility.
- Intra- and interfacility communication and communication with prehospital EMS personnel.
- Supplies on hand and methods to obtain added supplies.
- Delineation of receiving and treatment areas.

Critical incident stress management

Critical incident stress management helps people cope with overwhelming experiences, such as mass casualties or unexpected deaths. Each person's threshold for tolerance is different, but people working in emergency care are exposed to high stress situations on an almost daily basis. An effective critical incident stress management program may include:
- A focus on prevention with intervention before incidents takes place, using peer leaders.
- Education may include workshops, handouts, reprints, newsletters.
- Ongoing peer support strategies.
- Availability of mental health professional for individual counseling.
- Demobilizing: Assembling group to provide information and support in the event of serious incidents, allowing time for them to manage stress.
- Defusing: Small group meeting 8 to 12 hours after event for short debriefing.
- Debriefing: Group meeting 12 to 48 hours after event for more in depth debriefing, and discussion of the event, feelings, and coping.
- Recognition that despite efforts, delayed posttraumatic stress reactions may occur and that support may need to be ongoing.

CQI related to improvement exercises for infection control

Continuous Quality Improvement (CQI) emphasizes the organization and systems and processes within that organization rather than individuals. It recognizes internal customers (staff) and external customers (patients) and utilizes data to improve processes. CQI represents the concept that most processes can be improved. CQI uses the scientific method of experimentation to meet needs and improve services, and various tools, such as brainstorming, multivoting, various charts and diagrams, story boarding, and meetings. Core concepts include:
- Quality and success is meeting or exceeding internal and external customer's needs and expectations.
- Problems relate to processes, and variations in process lead to variations in results.
- Change can be in small steps.

Steps to CQI include:
1. Forming a knowledgeable team.
2. Identifying and defining measures used to determine success.
3. Brainstorming strategies for change.
4. Plan, collect, and utilize data as part of making decisions.
5. Test changes and revise or refine as needed.

Practice Test

Practice Questions

1. A forty-year-old female presents to the emergency department (ED) complaining of chest pain. After triaging the client, obtaining vital signs including a blood pressure of 90/46, and establishing an adequate airway, what is the next most important intervention for this client?
   a. registering the patient into the system
   b. ordering serum blood laboratory tests
   c. placing the client on a cardiac monitor, administering oxygen, and obtaining an electrocardiogram (EKG)
   d. giving a sublingual nitroglycerin tablet for the immediate relief of pain

2. The purpose of the primary assessment in any emergency is to
   a. perform a quick look-see to determine the illness or injury
   b. assess for life-threatening problems that require an immediate intervention
   c. make the client comfortable and remove wet clothing for the assessment
   d. gain a medical and surgical history, including allergies and medication

3. The emergency medical services (EMS) team transports an adult male with chest pain to the ED. They have initiated a large-bore intravenous (IV) line, administered oxygen, and placed the client on the cardiac monitor. Upon arrival to the ED, the initial EKG shows ST deviation in two leads, and the client is pale, clammy, and restless. What is the next intervention the ED nurse should anticipate?
   a. The nurse will give a report to the intensive care unit (ICU).
   b. The nurse will give a large dose of heparin.
   c. The nurse will prepare the client for the cardiac catheterization laboratory (cath lab).
   d. The nurse will order a repeat EKG for 8 hours in the future.

4. Which factors about troponin levels are important to consider when caring for a client being evaluated for an acute myocardial infarction (MI)?
   a. The troponin level is not the most important factor when caring for a client with an acute MI.
   b. Troponin levels elevate 3 to 12 hours after MI onset.
   c. Troponin levels are specific to MI clients only.
   d. Troponin levels will elevate in unstable angina as well as in an MI. troponin levels ↑
   help determine both angina + MI.

5. Which factor is NOT a risk for heart disease but also should not be excluded when considering the diagnosis of MI when a client presents with chest pain?
   a. age greater than 65
   b. nonsmoking female
   c. smoking any gender
   d. obesity

6. An elderly female client presents to the ED with complaints of chest pain and a history of angina. After the initial triage, what would be the next appropriate interventions?
    a. cardiac monitor, oxygen, and sublingual nitroglycerin
    b. cardiac monitor, sublingual nitroglycerin, and Foley catheter
    c. cardiac monitor, IV, oxygen, and sublingual nitroglycerin
    d. oxygen, sublingual nitroglycerin, and Foley catheter

IV before nitro r/t hypotension esp elderly

7. Which condition in the pediatric population may lead to congestive heart failure and should be considered when gaining a medical history on a pediatric patient in the ED?
    a. history of prematurity
    b. low weight for age
    c. history of asthma
    d. congenital heart defect

8. Which intervention is the most immediate when caring for a pediatric client who appears to be in heart failure?
    a. maintain airway and breathing
    b. monitor for distress
    c. limit fluid intake
    d. get a complete medical history

ABC

9. Which diagnosis may describe a client with a long history of cardiac disease and heart failure who presents to the ED with fatigue, orthopnea, edema, and hypertension but without chest pain?
    a. obesity
    b. asthma
    c. cardiomyopathy   *Dx effects myocardium*
    d. MI

diff. breathing lying flat

10. What is the physical consequence of any cardiac dysrhythmia that causes the need for an intervention?
    a. There is no physical consequence unless pain is involved.
    b. There is a decrease in cardiac output that directly relates to the hemodynamic status of the client.
    c. It can increase blood pressure.
    d. It does not affect the airway.

11. A 64-year-old client presents to the ED complaining of shortness of breath and fatigue for two days. An initial EKG shows a non-q-wave myocardial infarction (previously called a non-transmural MI). Which of the following would not be true about this type of MI?
    a. ST depression is visible on the ECG
    b. Peak CK levels are usually reached in about 12-13 hours
    c. The coronary occlusion is usually complete.   *incomplete*
    d. Reinfarction is common.

incomplete

12. Which task would NOT be performed initially by the ED nurse when a client presents with chest pain?
    a. initiate monitoring and interpret EKG rhythm strips
    b. assess defibrillator for proper functioning
    c. auscultate heart sounds
    d. order a low-salt diet for the client

13. A patient presents to the ER with pain that he describes as sharp and ripping on the posterior chest. There is widening on the mediastinum on the chest x-ray, and a blood pressure differential is noted. What diagnosis does the nurse suspect?
    a. Myocardial infarction
    b. Cardiac tamponade
    c. Dissecting aortic aneurysm
    d. Tension pneumothorax

14. The ED nurse understands that the ongoing evaluation and monitoring of a client with chest pain includes which of the following?
    a. evaluating response to a low-sodium meal
    b. managing airway patency, blood pressure, and oximetry
    c. being prepared to insert an IV line as needed
    d. documenting the client's insurance information

15. Which symptom/s would be apparent with left-sided heart failure?
    a. pulmonary edema
    b. venous congestion
    c. absence of pain
    d. absence of any notable symptoms

16. Inspection when triaging a client with chest pain includes which of the following?
    a. observing the patient's interactions with the assistive personnel
    b. looking for family interactions
    c. observing skin color, signs of edema
    d. asking about medical history

17. Which statement explains abnormal liver function tests in the client with heart failure?
    a. The client may be an alcoholic.
    b. The abnormal results may be the result of hepatic vascular congestion.
    c. The client has hepatitis.
    d. The results are altered from the cardiac drugs the client may have taken.

18. Which statement(s) are true about dopamine? **Select all that apply**
    a. it is a vesicant
    b. it produces more instances of unwanted tachycardias than norepinephrine
    c. it increases contractility of the myocardium and increases cardiac output
    d. it increases myocardial workload

19. All of the following extracardiac sounds may be heard on auscultation of the heart EXCEPT
    a. pericardial friction rub
    b. venous hum
    c. clicks of valves
    d. clucks of valves

20. Which nursing diagnosis would be appropriate for a client with a cardiac history and shortness of breath?
    a. ineffective tissue perfusion
    b. low fluid volume
    c. ineffective breathing pattern
    d. none of the above

21. Which client with a possible cardiac dysrhythmia would require an immediate intervention because of a decrease in cardiac output?
    a. a 22-year-old athlete with a heart rate of 46 at rest who is pink and in no distress
    b. an 42-year-old male with a heart rate of 42 who is pale and clammy
    c. a 82-year-old febrile female with a heart rate of 90
    d. a 15-month-old with a heart rate of 110 who is laughing and playing

22. Which rate may indicate possible paroxysmal supraventricular tachycardia from what is understood about normal vital signs?
    a. one hundred thirty beats per minute in a three year old
    b. one hundred beats per minute in an adult with anxiety
    c. one hundred and fifty beats per minute in a newborn
    d. one hundred and thirty beats per minute in an adult

23. Which rhythm would be identified on an ECG/EKG six-second strip by a heart rate of 76 and a PR interval of 0.24, the P:QRS ratio is 1:1, the P and the QRS are normal and regular?
    a. sinus arrhythmia
    b. first-degree atrioventricular block
    c. sinus rhythm
    d. second-degree type I Block

24. What *constitutes the description or definition* of ventricular tachycardia?
    a. one or two premature ventricular contractions (PVCs) in a one-minute span
    b. any heart rate over 100
    c. a run of three or more PVCs with or without symptoms
    d. two PVCs together as a couplet

25. The initial intervention when a client develops ventricular fibrillation (VF) is which of the following?
    a. perform cardiopulmonary resuscitation (CPR)
    b. defibrillation
    c. doses of epinephrine
    d. doses of atropine

26. The term for the abdominal emergency best described as a part of the bowel telescoping into or within itself causing a bowel obstruction is which of the following?
    a. large bowel obstruction
    b. small bowel obstruction
    c. intussusception
    d. acute abdomen

27. Which one of the following is NOT a cause of acute gastritis?
    a. the use of NSAIDs
    b. excess alcohol consumption
    c. caustic ingestion of foods with excessive seasoning
    d. H. Pylori infection

28. Which bacteria may be a leading cause of chronic gastritis?
    a. streptococcus
    b. staphylococcus
    c. Helicobacter pylori
    d. gram-negative bacteria

29. Which fact is important to remember when dealing with pediatric abdominal trauma patients?
    a. Abdominal trauma in the pediatric population is rare.
    b. Low blood pressure is a late sign of shock in the pediatric population and doesn't appear until a child has lost greater than 25% of their circulating blood.
    c. Low blood pressure is an early sign of shock in the pediatric population and needs to be addressed immediately upon arrival to the ED.
    d. Children have a lower percentage of water than body weight and a lower metabolic rate making the acid-base balance difficult to maintain.

30. Which is the most common cause of intestinal obstruction requiring an intervention during infancy?
    a. intussusception
    b. pyloric stenosis
    c. obstructive colic
    d. reflux

31. The most important initial intervention for abdominal trauma is which of the following?
    a. assessing the airway, breathing, and circulation (ABCs)
    b. initiating a large-bore IV for fluid replacement
    c. preparing for a computed tomography (CT) scan of the abdomen
    d. inserting a Foley catheter to assess for urinary output and bladder or kidney injury

32. Hypocalcemia may result from which acute or chronic abdominal condition?
    a. appendicitis
    b. pancreatitis → releases lipase or binds to the Ca or is excreted.
    c. hepatitis
    d. gastritis

33. A patient presents to the ED with acute abdominal pain, nausea, and vomiting. Which of the following tests would cause the nurse to suspect pancreatitis?
    a. WBC count of 5.0
    b. hematocrit (HCT) of 40%
    c. WBC count of 28.0
    d. Lipase 500 U/L

34. Which medical intervention is appropriate for a client with a possible bowel obstruction after the ABCs have been established and an IV has been initiated?
    a. Place the patient on bedrest.
    b. Insert a nasogastric (NG) tube and attach to suction.
    c. Order a clear liquid tray.
    d. Massage the abdomen.

35. Which pharmacologic agent would be appropriate for an adult client with pancreatitis who is in severe pain?
    a. Compazine nausea
    b. aspirin
    c. narcotics, avoiding morphine if possible
    d. gentamicin anbio

36. The pain of acute diverticulitis can be described as dull or cramping. Where is the pain most likely to be located with an acute episode?
    a. right lower quadrant (RLQ)
    b. right upper quadrant (RUQ)
    c. left lower quadrant (LLQ)
    d. left upper quadrant (LUQ)

37. A client with bleeding esophageal varices is at risk for severe hemorrhage and even death. What specific emergency procedure should the nurse be prepared to assist with in the case of uncontrolled esophageal bleeding?
    a. insertion of a nasogastric tube for suction
    b. intubation and a Sengstaken-Blakemore tube
    c. administering an IV
    d. doing a type and cross match for blood

38. An 8 year old presents to the ED with blood diarrhea, abdominal pain, fever, and vomiting. On history, the mother mentions the child cleaned out his pet turtle's cage yesterday before lunch time. What is the nurse beginning to suspect?
    a. campylobacter jejuni
    b. clostridium difficile
    c. yersinia enterocolitica
    d. nontyphoidal salmonella

39. A 45-year-old man is admitted to the emergency department after a bout of bloody vomiting. He is noted to be mildly hypotensive with slight scleral icterus, palmar erythema, and hepatomegaly. There is no history of aspirin or NSAID use but he does admit to long-term alcohol abuse. The most likely source of the bleeding is:
    a. gastric ulcer
    b. esophageal varices
    c. gastric cancer
    d. angiodysplasia

40. A 45-year-old woman is brought to the emergency department complaining of acute, severe midabdominal pain, radiating from the epigastrium to the mid-back. There is marked guarding of the abdomen and mild abdominal distention is present. She denies alcohol abuse or prior abdominal surgery. There has been no recent change in her bowel habits. Bowel sounds are markedly diminished. What is the most likely diagnosis and the laboratory or imaging test to establish the diagnosis?
    a. acute pancreatitis and serum amylase *pain radiates to the back*
    b. small bowel obstruction and plain films of the abdomen *— fever, n/v, abpain*
    c. acute cholecystitis and ultrasound of the gall bladder
    d. acute appendicitis and CT of the abdomen

41. A 30-year-old man comes to the emergency department with the acute onset of left flank pain radiating to the groin. Microscopic hematuria is present on urinalysis. What is the most likely diagnosis?
    a. ureteral calcium oxalate calculus
    b. ureteral cystine calculus
    c. testicular torsion
    d. cystitis

42. A young woman with a history of lupus and recent aminoglycoside treatment of an infection develops nausea, extreme fatigue, and poor urinary output. Her serum creatinine is 4.5 mg/dL and urine output is severely diminished. An ECG shows peaked T waves, prolonged PR interval, and a slightly widened QRS complex. Which of the following would be appropriate emergency therapy?
    a. intravenous calcium
    b. intravenous glucose and insulin
    c. both A and B
    d. neither A nor B

43. While assessing a trauma patient, the nurse finds the client complaining of flank pain where there is also bruising noted. What intervention should the nurse be ready to perform because of these signs of injury?
    a. a CT scan of the client's head
    b. a urinalysis and a complete blood count (CBC)
    c. offer oral fluids to promote hydration
    d. administer oxygen

44. An important concept when evaluating for traumatic genitourinary injuries for both children and adults would be which of the following?
    a. Keep the client dressed to protect privacy and avoid direct observation.
    b. Assess the genitourinary system last, as it is the least important.
    c. Undress the client while protecting his or her privacy and directly observe the genitals for injury.
    d. Never insert a Foley catheter unless absolutely needed because of the risk for infection.

45. A client presenting to the ED complaining of flank pain, diaphoresis, and nausea may be experiencing which genitourinary emergency?
    a. MI
    b. kidney stones
    c. testicular torsion
    d. ovulation

46. Acute renal failure developing over a short period of time is the result of which of the following?
    a. calcium buildup
    b. fluid overload
    c. increase in nitrogenous waste products circulating
    d. decrease in potassium circulating

47. Which prerenal sign will the ED nurse recognize as the first indication of acute renal failure needing an immediate intervention?
    a. an increase in renal blood flow
    b. a prolonged period of hyperperfusion
    c. a prolonged period of overhydration
    d. a decrease in renal blood flow and ischemia

48. At what age are boys at the most risk for testicular torsion?
    a. the first year of life
    b. the ages of five to seven years
    c. the risk for testicular torsion is minimal at any age
    d. the ages of seven to nine years

49. Children are at a higher risk for kidney injury than adults. Which statement best explains this fact?
    a. Children are more active than adults.
    b. Children do not hydrate appropriately.
    c. The incomplete ossification of the 10th and 11th ribs during childhood.
    d. Children have kidneys that are three times the normal size of adult kidneys.

50. What is the most common symptom of a UTI?
    a. fever
    b. dysuria
    c. cloudy urine
    d. fruity odor of urine

51. Pyelonephritis is a serious infection that can lead to what complications during pregnancy?
    a. cystitis
    b. fever
    c. bleeding
    d. preterm labor and preeclampsia

52. The immediate nursing interventions for a client presenting to the ED with urinary complaints including flank pain would include which of the following?
    a. obtain a urine specimen and initiate IV fluids
    b. urinalysis, IV, and pain control
    c. observe for fever
    d. encourage oral fluid intake

53. Which condition would be considered a true urologic emergency requiring surgical intervention?
    a. renal calculi
    b. UTI
    c. bladder tumor
    d. testicular torsion

54. An adult male presenting to the ED with complaints of pain in the scrotum, a "duck waddle" gait, and fever may have what genitourinary emergency?
    a. priapism
    b. epididymitis
    c. inguinal hernia
    d. UTI

55. Which condition is the most emergent for a mother and fetus during the second and third trimesters of pregnancy?
    a. multiple fetuses by ultrasound
    b. placenta previa
    c. UTI
    d. abruptio placenta

56. What are the classic symptoms of abruptio placenta to note when assessing a pregnant client presenting to the ED with bleeding?
    a. hyperglycemia
    b. hypertension
    c. vaginal bleeding and uterine tenderness
    d. emesis

57. What is the most important element of neonatal resuscitation?
    a. keeping the infant warm
    b. maintaining a glucose level of greater than 45
    c. maintaining cardiac compressions of greater than 90
    d. establishing an adequate airway and administering oxygen

58. Which obstetric emergency is the leading cause of maternal death due to hemorrhagic shock?
    a. multiple births with retained placenta
    b. ruptured ectopic pregnancy implanted in the fallopian tube
    c. pelvic inflammatory disease (PID)
    d. placenta previa

59. Which symptoms are recognized as a positive indication of preeclampsia-eclampsia?
    a. low liver enzymes, abdominal pain, edema
    b. low blood pressure, proteinuria, edema
    c. high blood pressure, proteinuria, edema
    d. high platelet count, abdominal pain, edema

60. What symptoms may occur in late eclampsia that can be life threatening?
   a. proteinuria
   b. seizures
   c. hemolysis
   d. headache

61. The seriousness of hyperemesis gravidarum is related to which side effect/s?
   a. weight loss, dehydration, low thiamine
   b. obesity, low thiamine, high potassium
   c. overhydration, hyponatremia, edema
   d. high potassium, low magnesium, edema

62. The initial steps for neonatal resuscitation include which of the following?
   a. drying and doing chest compressions
   b. drying under a heat source and establishing an airway
   c. suctioning the stomach
   d. weighing and measuring the infant

63. Discharge instructions to a female client experiencing dysfunctional uterine bleeding (DUB) who has required an emergent dilation and curettage (D&C) should include which of the following?
   a. Stop taking pain medication 24 hours from procedure.
   b. Avoid eating red meat.
   c. Return to the ED for fever greater than 100.6°F.
   d. Stay on bed rest for 48 hours.

64. A female client presents to the ED with complaints of white thin vaginal discharge and a foul fishy odor. What would most likely be the cause of these symptoms?
   a. nothing–this is normal
   b. vaginitis
   c. trichomonas vaginitis
   d. bacterial vaginitis

65. The most common pharmacologic therapies ordered for a female in the ED diagnosed with pelvic inflammatory disease (PID) would include which of the following?
   a. antifungal
   b. sedation
   c. analgesics and antibiotics
   d. none of the above

66. A client presenting to the ED with an eating disorder is most likely to have what other emergent medical condition, requiring an immediate intervention?
   a. dysrhythmias due to electrolyte imbalances
   b. low potassium
   c. dehydration
   d. depression

67. All of the following are examples of organic psychoses EXCEPT
    a. dementia
    b. schizophrenia
    c. delirium
    d. toxic drug-induced psychosis

68. Suicidal behavior is best described as
    a. attempts to cause death by self-inflicted injury
    b. impulsive but not harmful
    c. never planned
    d. attempts by someone other than one's self to cause injury

69. During a pediatric resuscitation, family members should:
    a. be allowed to watch the procedure
    b. have a nursing team member assigned to explain and comfort
    c. have a specific space and be permitted to touch their child if possible
    d. all of the above

70. Clinical depression:
    a. results in suicide risk higher in men than women
    b. can be rapidly treated with antidepressant drugs
    c. alcohol and substance abuse may contribute
    d. does not require brain imaging or blood tests

71. A 40-year-old man comes to the emergency department complaining of chest pain and shortness of breath for about an hour. The onset occurred rapidly while he was riding on a crowded subway. He has no history of heart or other significant medical problem. His pulse and respiratory rate are increased but blood pressure and temperature are normal. His skin is damp and cool. His electrocardiogram, cardiac enzymes, chest x-ray, and other routine laboratory tests are all normal. What is the most likely diagnosis?
    a. panic attack
    b. depression
    c. acute coronary syndrome
    d. esophageal spasm

72. A 1-year-old child is brought to the emergency department in a comatose state. His parents state that he fell from a swing and hit his head. There is bruising of the scalp as well as retinal hemorrhages. There are additional bruised areas of the arms and legs and what appears to be a healed rib fracture on chest x-ray. An MRI indicates a subdural hematoma in the parietal portion of the brain. A pediatric neurosurgeon is asked to consult. What is the appropriate course of action for the emergency department nurse now?
    a. report possible child abuse to the appropriate agency per state law
    b. detailed questioning of the parents regarding the circumstances of the injury
    c. check medical records for prior emergency department visits for trauma
    d. all of the above

73. Which of the following is NOT appropriate for screening for domestic violence by the emergency department nurse?
   a. asking if the person has been hit, kicked, or otherwise hurt by someone in the past year; if so, by whom
   b. asking, "Do you feel safe in your present relationship?"
   c. avoid asking about intimate person violence if the patient is in the emergency department for a medical ailment, not trauma
   d. asking if there is a partner from a previous relationship that makes the individual feel unsafe

74. An elevated ventilation/perfusion (V/Q) ratio is most likely seen in:
   a. pneumonia
   b. pulmonary embolus
   c. acute respiratory distress syndrome
   d. atelectasis

75. A patient is intubated and on mechanical ventilation. The ventilator alarm rings and the airway pressure is found to be elevated. Possible causes include the following EXCEPT:
   a. endotracheal tube obstruction with sputum
   b. pneumothorax
   c. bronchospasm
   d. cuff leak

76. The initial assessment of any adult, infant, or child with any emergency diagnosis should include which of the following?
   a. Do a complete head-to-toe assessment.
   b. Establish the chief complaint or injury.
   c. Administer oxygen per mask.
   d. Establish an adequate airway.

77. Which statement best describes acute respiratory distress syndrome (ARDS)?
   a. ARDS is caused by trauma only.
   b. ARDS is sudden, progressive, and severe.
   c. ARDS is caused by an illness only.
   d. ARDS never results in lung scarring.

78. An elevated blood alcohol level may lead to what respiratory complication?
   a. increase in respirations
   b. no effect on the respiratory system
   c. decrease in respiratory effort and aspiration
   d. decrease in depression

79. A 30-week-gestation premature infant may need pharmacological interventions to improve respiratory status of the lungs. Which drug would most likely be administered in the first few hours after birth?
   a. epinephrine
   b. caffeine
   c. Survanta
   d. vitamin K

80. All of the following are appropriate ways to establish an initial airway on a nonresponsive client EXCEPT?

    a. nasal trumpet

    b. endotracheal tube

    c. esophageal-tracheal Combitube

    d. a Replogle tube

81. The nurse in the ED is caring for a patient who was brought over from dialysis with a suspected acute pulmonary embolism. Which of the following tests could provide the most definitive diagnosis?

    a. D-dimer

    b. ABG

    c. Chest x-ray

    d. Spiral CT

82. Which airway emergency would need to be treated first with an immediate intervention in the ED?

    a. an adult with mild wheezing who denies distress

    b. a child carried in by his dad who has a fever but is alert

    c. a teen in a wheelchair because of a possible long bone fracture

    d. a child arriving by EMS in status asthmaticus

83. Which respiratory illness affects children under the age of two and causes inflammatory obstruction of the airway?

    a. asthma

    b. bronchitis

    c. pneumonia

    d. bronchiolitis

84. Which of the following are patient care management tasks?

    a. providing community education

    b. identifying clients who are potential organ donors

    c. cooling a client following a cardiac arrest

    d. all of the above

85. Croup is an acute respiratory illness presenting with which of the following?

    a. fever greater than 103°F

    b. barking cough

    c. rash over extremities

    d. total airway obstruction

86. Anxiety may be a precipitating factor in which respiratory syndrome?

    a. chronic obstructive pulmonary disease

    b. emphysema

    c. hyperventilation

    d. asthma

87. Clients seen in the ED for transporting illegal drugs by swallowing packages and subsequently overdosing are called which of the following?
    a. condoms
    b. body packers
    c. rockets
    d. ice

88. The street drug phencyclidine (PCP) can cause which acute complication, requiring intervention?
    a. dissociation anesthesia
    b. delusions and tachycardia
    c. rhabdomyolysis and renal failure
    d. tachypnea and urethral calculi

89. The nurse assessing an adolescent for complaints of headache and nausea suspects the teen has been "huffing" an inhalant. Which objective data would support that suspicion?
    a. the odor of solvent on the client's face and hands
    b. a normal blood urea nitrogen (BUN) and creatinine
    c. a positive pregnancy test for the female teen
    d. increased reflexes

90. All of the below are present in all three types of shock EXCEPT:
    a. Systolic blood pressure below 110 mm Hg
    b. Decreased cardiac output
    c. Urine output less than 0.5 mL/kg/hr
    d. Peripheral vasoconstriction and vasodilation

91. Hypovolemia leads to all of the following EXCEPT?
    a. decreased venous return
    b. increased cardiac output
    c. diminished stroke volume
    d. decreased central venous pressure

92. Professional issues regarding emergency nursing include all of the following EXCEPT?
    a. participating in ethical decision making
    b. evaluating the client's capacity to make decisions
    c. protecting patient confidentiality
    d. keeping abuse ED cases confidential therefore not reporting them to the authorities

93. Which of the following is true regarding management of acute respiratory distress syndrome (ARDS)?
    a. Antibiotics have proved effective in the clinical management of ARDS.
    b. Patients with ARDS are usually hypovolemic, and giving volume of IVF is a cornerstone of treatment.
    c. Most of the care for ARDS is supportive and preventive of other injury.
    d. Higher than normal tidal volumes must be used in patients with ARDS.

94. You are caring for a patient that has been in the ED for 2 hours. The patient was brought in by ambulance already intubated and still sedated from drugs used for RSI on arrival. At the scene the paramedics were told the patient had been using cocaine immediately before collapsing and the ambulance being called. The patient just woke up, eyes wide, grabbing at anything she can get her hands on, biting the ETT. The patient's respiratory rate is 40 and the heart rate is 120. The patient's ABG shows pH 7.48, $PaCO_2$ 50 mm Hg, and a decreased H_2CO_3. The nurse attempts to calm the patient verbally and by decreasing the stimuli, with no result. What intervention should the nurse expect to perform?
    a. Immediately extubate the patient
    b. Increase the patient's tidal volume
    c. Give Benzodiazepines as ordered
    d. Decrease the patient's tidal volume

95. A young African American man presents with a painful, persistent erection lasting 12 hours after sexual intercourse. He denies use of sildenafil (*Viagra*) or other drugs for erectile dysfunction. Which of the following diagnostic studies would be most appropriate initially?
    a. ultrasound of the penis
    b. CT of the abdomen
    c. sickle cell test
    d. urinary catheterization for residual urine

96. A 24-year-old woman complains of a mucopurulent vaginal discharge and painful urination for about 5 days. Her last sexual encounter was 10 days ago. Her menstrual periods are regular. She takes birth control pills and has never been pregnant. Which of the following tests are indicated?
    a. urine for culture and sensitivity and analysis
    b. quick test of vaginal discharge for Chlamydia
    c. vaginal swab on modified Thayer-Martin agar
    d. all of the above

97. In differentiating the HELLP syndrome from ordinary preeclampsia, which of following is true?
    a. HELLP occurs more commonly in primigravidas
    b. hemolysis and thrombocytopenia are present in HELLP
    c. blood pressure is normal in HELLP
    d. proteinuria is absent in HELLP

98. A 27-year-old woman presents with left-sided pelvic pain and vaginal spotting of several days duration. She has a history of pelvic inflammatory disease in her early 20s. She is now married and trying to have a child. She has not had menses for 8 weeks and a home pregnancy test is positive. Bimanual pelvic exam reveals a normal size uterus and tenderness and fullness in the left adnexal region. Her β-hCG level is markedly elevated. Which diagnosis and treatment are most likely?
    a. ectopic pregnancy and intramuscular methotrexate
    b. ovarian cyst with surgical excision
    c. normal 10- to 12-week pregnancy; no treatment
    d. abruptio placenta; packed cell transfusion

99. Which of the following may be associated with rhabdomyolysis?
    a. use of statin drugs
    b. elevated creatine kinase (CK)
    c. both A and B
    d. hypokalemia

100. Which of the following is NOT true in the management of a sexual assault victim?
   a. many victims do not wish to report a rape to law enforcement
   b. many victims blame themselves or their actions for inviting sexual assault
   c. the hospital has discretion not to report the incident if the patient does not wish to do so
   d. chain of custody must be maintained by written record and time for all transfers of evidence

101. Which of the following is effective in the management of posterior epistaxis?
   a. pinching the nose to stop the blood flow
   b. topical vasoconstrictors such as phenylephrine
   c. silver nitrate or electric cautery
   d. insert a Merocel nasal sponge or Nasostat epistaxis nasal balloon

102. A 2-year-old is brought to the emergency department with mild fever, persistent restlessness, crying, and pulling his left ear. He has had a cold for about a week. Examination of the ear reveals a distorted light reflex and slight bulging of the tympanic membrane. What is the proper diagnosis and treatment?
   a. otitis externa and antibiotics
   b. otitis media and antibiotics
   c. otitis media and myringotomy
   d. acute labyrinthitis and antivertigo drug

103. A 45-year-old man presents with severe pain after being struck in the face during an auto accident while he was driving. He also reports some numbness of the upper lip. His face is bruised and somewhat distorted and edematous with nasal and periorbital swelling and subconjunctival hemorrhages. A CT scan of the facial structures is obtained. What is the likely diagnosis?
   a. orbital blowout fracture
   b. zygomatic fracture
   c. mandibular fracture
   d. middle third maxillary fracture (Le Fort II)

104. A 65-year-old Asian man comes to the emergency department complaining of headache, severe pain in his right eye, and nausea of several hours' duration. The pupil is slightly dilated and fixed to light and the globe is very hard. He also notes halos of light and a diminished peripheral vision. Left eye exam is normal. What is the likely diagnosis?
   a. open-angle glaucoma
   b. acute angle-closure glaucoma
   c. occlusion of the central retinal artery
   d. retinal detachment

105. A 12 year old presents with a Grade 3 hyphema, after being hit with a baseball at a game. Which of the following are true?
   a. Patch and shield will not be necessary.
   b. Motrin should be given for pain.
   c. Aminocaproic acid should be given to prevent secondary hemorrhage.
   d. System or topical antibiotics are a cornerstone of treatment for hyphema.

106. Your patient has been diagnosed with temporomandibular disorder. You should include all the following in the patient's discharge instructions except:
    a. Use NSAIDS to relieve pain and inflammation.
    b. Use ice and warm compresses several times a day.
    c. Use a night mouthguard when able.
    d. Do not stretch or use jaw until pain subsides.

107. Your patient presents with a dental avulsion. The tooth came out 1 hour ago. All of the following correctly relate to reimplanting a tooth EXCEPT:
    a. soak the tooth in Hank solution for 30 minutes
    b. only permanent teeth are reimplanted
    c. after reimplantation, apply splinting material over implanted teeth and 2 adjacent teeth on both sides.
    d. you cannot reimplant a tooth that has been out for more than 30 minutes

108. A 45-year-old man presents an eyelid laceration that is vertical and through the orbicularis oculi muscle. The patient is stable. The nurse should be prepared to:
    a. Do wound irrigation with NS prior to suturing
    b. Assist the physician with suturing with a 6-0 or 7-0 coated nylon suture
    c. Apply ophthalmic topical antibiotic in place of a dressing
    d. Transfer the patient to a facility that has an ocular plastic surgeon.

109. Which of the following is/are associated with a vascular migraine headache?
    a. family history of migraine
    b. prodromal aura
    c. unilateral, throbbing headache
    d. all of the above

110. A 75-year-old man has a history of several episodes of transient right-sided arm and hand weakness lasting an hour or two but with full recovery. He is diabetic and hypertensive and is taking medication for both conditions. This time the episode does not resolve and he is taken to the emergency department some 2 hours after the onset of symptoms. He is awake and able to answer questions and give a medical history. His chest is clear and no bruits are heard over the carotids. There is drift of the right arm on examination and his speech is slightly garbled. His blood pressure is 160/95 mm Hg and his pulse is irregular at 80 beats per minute. A CT of the brain reveals a small left-sided occlusion in a branch of the middle cerebral arterial circulation without hemorrhage. What should be the next step in his management?
    a. start nitroprusside to reduce his blood pressure to normal
    b. begin fibrinolytic therapy with alteplase (Activase)
    c. begin warfarin
    d. neurosurgical consultation for carotid endarterectomy

111. Which of the following best describes status epilepticus?
    a. a seizure that starts in one part of the body but there is no loss of consciousness
    b. a seizure that starts in one part of the body and spreads to others with loss of consciousness
    c. consecutive seizures without regaining consciousness
    d. seizure associated with automatism such as lip smacking or facial grimacing

112. Which of the following cranial nerves controls facial movements, lacrimation, taste, and salivation?
    a. III (oculomotor)
    b. IV (trochlear)
    c. VI (abducens)
    d. VII (facial)

113. A 24-year-old woman is brought to the emergency department, after an ATV accident. The patient's neurologic status, including the Glasgow Coma Scale, is quickly evaluated. Eye response is opening eyes in response to pain. Verbal response is incomprehensible sounds. Her motor response is withdrawal in response to pain. What is her score on the Glasgow Coma Scale?
    a. 7
    b. 8
    c. 9
    d. 10

114. A knowledge of the circulation to the brain is important in evaluating a patient with neurologic symptoms or signs. The anterior circulation to the brain is supplied by:
    a. internal carotid arteries
    b. vertebral artery
    c. basilar artery
    d. external carotid arteries

115. A 28-year-old HIV-positive man arrives at the emergency department with a history of intermittent fevers, headache of several weeks, and increasing confusion. Which procedure is likely to give the most accurate diagnosis?
    a. CT of the brain
    b. lumbar puncture (LP)
    c. blood cultures
    d. magnetic resonance angiography (MRA)

116. A 25-year-old woman presents with tingling of the extremities for several weeks and weakness in both lower extremities so that walking is difficult. These symptoms started soon after a flu-like illness and have progressed to date. On exam there is bilateral weakness in the lower extremities with decreased deep tendon reflexes. What is the most likely diagnosis?
    a. cerebrovascular accident (CVA)
    b. viral meningitis
    c. Guillain-Barré syndrome
    d. myasthenia gravis

117. Early signs of increased intracranial pressure (ICP) include the following EXCEPT:
    a. abnormal reflexes
    b. headache
    c. slurred speech
    d. sluggish pupillary light reflex

118. Which of the following is the most accepted method of reducing elevated ICP?
   a. hyperventilation
   b. mannitol intravenous bolus
   c. mannitol continuous intravenous drip
   d. hypotonic saline

119. A young man is hit on the head with a blunt object in a street mugging. He was briefly unconscious and has now arrived at the emergency department complaining of a severe headache and a dilated pupil on the side of the injury. As he is being examined he becomes more comatose. He is stabilized and taken for a CT exam of the head and neck. What is the most likely finding?
   a. epidural hematoma
   b. subdural hematoma
   c. intraventricular hemorrhage
   d. cervical spine injury

120. A 17-year-old high school football player was knocked unconscious for about a minute after a vigorous tackle during a game. On recovering consciousness, he was somewhat confused and complained of mild nausea and headache. Both of these resolved within a few minutes. He was examined by the trainer and team doctor. They did not find any neurologic deficits. He wants to go back into the game. How should this player be managed?
   a. send him back into the game after a brief rest
   b. bench him for the game but allow him to practice the following week
   c. hospitalize him for observation and CT scanning
   d. no athletics with continued observation for neurologic signs and gradual return to school and the team

121. All of the following are appropriate measures in stabilizing a patient with a suspected cervical spine injury EXCEPT:
   a. a four-person team is optimal
   b. strap the patient to the backboard at the shoulders, hips, and proximal to the knees
   c. do not attempt to remove a helmet
   d. a rigid cervical collar is applied by one person while the leader maintains in-line head position

122. A Hare traction splint is appropriate for which of the following fractures?
   a. mid-shaft fracture of the femur
   b. distal fracture of the tibia
   c. fracture of the fibula
   d. fracture of the hip

123. A farmer's arm is severed by a threshing machine at the mid-humerus. Which of the following would best preserve the amputated arm for possible reimplantation?
   a. no action; such arm injuries cannot be reimplanted
   b. irrigate the arm with normal saline and pack directly in ice water
   c. pack the arm directly in warm saline
   d. moisten with saline, wrap in a plastic bag, and preserve on crushed ice and water

124. In training a patient with a foot injury to use axillary crutches, which of the following is NOT true?
    a. tips of the crutches should be 6 inches to the side and 6 inches in front
    b. move crutches and injured leg forward at the same time
    c. each handpiece should be situated at the fingertips with the arms in full extension
    d. each crutch should be 2 inches below the axilla with no weight-bearing

125. A basketball player landed awkwardly after a rebound attempt and twisted his ankle. He is seen in the emergency department complaining of pain and tenderness of the ankle and there is swelling and discoloration around the joint. He claims he heard a snapping noise when landing and a small avulsion fracture is seen on x-ray. What is the most likely diagnosis?
    a. First-degree strain
    b. Second-degree strain
    c. Third-degree strain
    d. First-degree sprain

126. After an auto accident, x-rays of the patient's leg show a transverse fracture of the mid-femur with several bone fragments surrounding the fracture site. The skin of the leg is intact. This type fracture is called:
    a. compression fracture
    b. comminuted fracture
    c. avulsion fracture
    d. open fracture

127. A professional soccer player hears a loud snap in his leg while dodging an opposition player during a game. This is followed by severe pain in the heel and posterior leg. He is unable to walk or use the injured foot. Thompson sign done in the emergency department is positive in the affected foot. What is the most likely diagnosis?
    a. tibial fracture
    b. fibular fracture
    c. ruptured Achilles tendon
    d. calcaneus fracture

128. Which of the following is true about shoulder dislocations?
    a. most are posterior dislocations
    b. most are anterior dislocations
    c. they are uncommon in children
    d. they rarely recur

129. Which of the following injuries is LEAST likely to occur from the initial blast or airwave from an explosion?
    a. spinal fracture
    b. ruptured tympanic membrane
    c. pneumothorax
    d. perforated viscus

130. Which of the following is NOT true of the compartment syndrome?
  a. occurs most often in the arm or leg
  b. deep throbbing pain out of proportion to the original injury
  c. pressure of 30 to 60 mm Hg requires fasciotomy
  d. irreversible tissue damage does not occur until 24 to 48 hours of the injury

131. A 12-year-old is brought to the emergency department with a history of a dog bite the previous day. The dog was the household pet and her family treated it with 70% alcohol and bandage. Today the laceration continues to hurt and appears somewhat swollen and red with a dark exudate. Which of the following would be inappropriate in the treatment of this wound?
  a. irrigation followed by suturing
  b. debridement of nonviable tissue
  c. amoxicillin/clavulanate (Augmentin) orally for 5 days
  d. irrigation with povidone-iodine solution (Betadine)

132. Which of the following dressings would be most appropriate for an exudative, probably infected wound?
  a. gauze
  b. transparent film
  c. absorption dressing
  d. hydrogel

133. Nurse-initiated analgesia protocols (NIAP) include the following:
  a. nonpharmacologic intervention
  b. nonopioid
  c. opioids
  d. all of the above

134. Which of the following is true regarding pain management in infants and children?
  a. opioids are contraindicated
  b. infants are less sensitive to pain than adults
  c. pretreatment with local anesthetics prior to procedures, such as lumbar puncture or suturing of a laceration, is recommended
  d. sedation before a painful procedure or imaging with midazolam or propofol is not recommended

135. The Emergency Severity Index (ESI) triage system:
  a. has 5 numerical categories (1 to 5) for patient evaluation
  b. patients are triaged by acuity and expected resource consumption
  c. both A and B
  d. neither A nor B

136. Which of the following is NOT true regarding application of restraints to an aggressive patient?
  a. annual physical restraint training is mandatory
  b. any patient death within 24 hours of being restrained must be reported
  c. once restraints are applied, the patient's condition must be assessed and recorded every 2 hours
  d. reasons for restraints must be documented and duration of application specified

137. Disaster preparation and prevention measures include:
    a. disaster-related supply inventory
    b. plan for housing, food, and water for staff
    c. establish communication protocol for notifying public health and law enforcement
    d. all of the above

138. Organ donation after cardiac death:
    a. is against federal law
    b. requires the consent of the legal next of kin or an advanced directive from the donor
    c. end-of-life care and organ harvesting should be directed by the transplant surgeon
    d. Unlike brain death donations, notification of the local organ procurement organization (OPO) is unnecessary

139. Which of the following is NOT true for peripherally inserted central catheters (PICC) for venous access?
    a. requires a non-coring needle such as a Huber for administering fluids or withdrawing blood
    b. may be single or multilumen
    c. does not require surgery for removal
    d. requires frequent heparin flushing and injection cap changes

140. A chronically anemic patient is receiving a packed red blood cell (PRBC) transfusion. He suddenly develops fever and chills, tachypnea and dyspnea, and tightness in the chest. His urine flow is diminished and dark in color. What is the probable diagnosis and appropriate measures to take?
    a. air embolus; stop infusion, administer oxygen, and turn patient on left side
    b. hemolytic transfusion reaction; stop transfusion, send the untransfused blood and a patient blood sample to the blood bank, monitor UOP and collect sample for the lab
    c. pyrogenic transfusion reaction; stop transfusion and switch to leukocyte-poor PRBCs
    d. circulatory overload; stop transfusion, consider diuretics

141. The best method of limiting absorption in an adult who has ingested an unknown toxic substance is:
    a. induced emesis with syrup of ipecac
    b. gastric lavage
    c. administer activated charcoal
    d. administer activated charcoal plus a cathartic

142. A young unidentified man is brought to the emergency department comatose with poor respiratory function. He has pinpoint pupils. Needle scarring is noted on his arms and legs and he appears underweight and malnourished. What are appropriate emergency care methods to treat him?
    a. endotracheal intubation with oxygen
    b. activated charcoal and cathartic by nasogastric tube
    c. naloxone 0.2 mg intravenously
    d. all of the above

143. An elderly patient has recently taken a large dose of imipramine (*Tofranil*) in an apparent suicide attempt. He is confused and disoriented, hypotensive, and tachycardic with flushed skin and wide pupils. While being brought in by paramedics, he has a seizure. An ECG shows a sinus tachycardia with a prolonged QRS complex and QT-interval and T-wave abnormalities. Which of the following pharmacologic agents would NOT be appropriate?
  a. lorazepam (Ativan)
  b. sodium bicarbonate
  c. phenytoin (Dilantin)
  d. activated charcoal and sorbitol

144. Heat stroke differs from heat exhaustion in that:
  a. heat stroke occurs suddenly; heat exhaustion does not
  b. heat exhaustion occurs mostly in infants and elderly persons
  c. heat exhaustion has up to a 70% mortality rate
  d. heat exhaustion may be treated with ice water immersion

145. Frostbite:
  a. may be superficial, affecting the skin and subcutaneous tissue, or deep, affecting bone and tendons
  b. affected areas may become mottled with blistering
  c. both A and B
  d. neither A nor B

146. A mountain climber is rescued by helicopter several days after an incapacitating fall near the mountain top. His core body temperature in the emergency department is 78°F (28.8°C). Which of the following warming techniques would be most efficient?
  a. warmed humidified oxygen
  b. warmed intravenous fluids
  c. Bair Hugger warming blanket
  d. continuous arteriovenous rewarming (CAVR)

147. A 40-year-old man is rescued from a house fire and brought to the emergency department by paramedics. He is quite lethargic, breathing is rapid and shallow, and heart rate is regular but increased and blood pressure is moderately low. A carboxyhemoglobin (COHb) level is 40%. An endotracheal tube is placed. Which of the following would be the best treatment?
  a. hyperbaric oxygen at 3 atm for 46 minutes; repeat in 6 hours if full CNS activity not restored
  b. hyperbaric oxygen at 6 atm for 1 hour; repeat in 4 hours if full CNS activity not restored
  c. 100% oxygen until the COHb falls below 10%
  d. 60% oxygen until the COHb falls below 10%

148. A 30-year-old adult has extensive full thickness burns on the upper chest (neck to nipples) and the left anterior thigh and lower leg. There are no other injuries.
By the rule of nines, how much of the total body surface area (TBSA) is involved and what should be the disposition of the patient?
  a. 12%; outpatient treatment
  b. 20%; admit to community hospital
  c. 27%; transfer to a burn center
  d. 36%; transfer to a burn center

149. Which of the following is NOT a feature of the shock syndrome?
    a. decreased antidiuretic hormone (ADH) release
    b. increased epinephrine release
    c. increased angiotensin II and aldosterone
    d. increased glucose production

150. Neurogenic shock may be caused by:
    a. spinal cord injury
    b. brain injury
    c. excessive insulin with hypoglycemia
    d. all of the above

151. For patients with hemorrhagic shock due to trauma:
    a. blood pressure should be brought to normal with fluids and banked blood
    b. mean arterial blood pressure (MAP) should be maintained at 40 mm Hg until bleeding controlled
    c. MAP should be maintained above 65 mm Hg at all times
    d. MAP should be maintained above 95 mm Hg

152. Which of the following is NOT recommended for routine hemodynamic monitoring of patients in shock?
    a. pulmonary artery catheter
    b. central venous pressure
    c. pulse oximetry
    d. superior vena cava oxygen saturation (ScvO$_2$)

153. In placing a tourniquet to control arterial bleeding from a lower leg wound:
    a. it should be placed right over the wound
    b. it should be placed as distally as possible
    c. it should be placed distally but at least 5 cm proximal to the wound
    d. it should not be used

154. Acid-base balance in shock patients is characterized by:
    a. respiratory acidosis followed by metabolic alkalosis
    b. respiratory alkalosis
    c. metabolic acidosis
    d. transient respiratory alkalosis followed by metabolic acidosis

155. Which of the following has NOT been shown to improve the survival of patients with septic shock?
    a. colloid rather than crystalloid therapy
    b. antibiotic therapy within 1 hour of diagnosis
    c. keeping the mean arterial pressure at 65 mm Hg or higher
    d. administration of recombinant human activated protein C (rhAPC)

156. Heparin 10 to 100 units/mL: use 1 to 2.5 mL after use and/or every 12 hours. After blood withdrawal or medication administration, flush with saline before heparin flush. No saline flush required before medication administration. These instructions are appropriate for which type venous access?
    a. tunneled catheter
    b. Groshong catheter
    c. implanted port
    d. peripherally inserted central catheter (PICC)

157. Which bone site is least desirable for intraosseous infusion in infants and young children?
    a. sternum
    b. iliac crest
    c. anterior tibia
    d. distal femur

158. A 60-year-old man with type 2 diabetes is taking metformin and a diuretic for hypertension. He ran out of metformin about a week ago and is waiting for his mail order to arrive. He has become lethargic and confused over the past few days with vague abdominal pain, polyuria, and polydipsia. He appears dehydrated. His blood glucose is 900 mg/dL, arterial pH is 7.35, and serum osmolality is 430 mOsm/L; serum ketones 1+ at 1:1 dilution. Serum lactate level is 1.5 mmol/L. What is the most likely diagnosis?
    a. lactic acidosis
    b. diabetic ketoacidosis (DKA)
    c. hyperosmolar hyperglycemia
    d. none of the above

159. A 40-year-old woman with a history of Graves' disease is brought to the emergency department with a fever of 104°F, and she is disoriented and semi-comatose with a Glasgow score of 10. Her ECG shows atrial fibrillation with a ventricular rate of 130. Which of the following drugs should be administered?
    a. beta-blocker
    b. methimazole
    c. iodide
    d. all of the above

160. Which of the following coagulation factors is NOT vitamin K dependent?
    a. prothrombin (factor II)
    b. prothrombin conversion accelerator (factor VII)
    c. antihemophilic factor A (factor VIII)
    d. antihemophilic factor B (factor IX)

161. Which of the following is NOT a feature of the tumor lysis syndrome?
    a. occurs in malignancies with rapid cell lysis
    b. Hypokalemia
    c. hypocalcemia
    d. hyperuricemia

162. All of the following are acute complications of sickle cell anemia EXCEPT:
   a. priapism
   b. chest pain and bilateral pulmonary infiltrates
   c. bone, joint, and spine pain
   d. gastrointestinal bleeding

163. A cancer patient is seen in the emergency department with high fevers and malaise for 2 days. She received chemotherapy about 10 days ago. Her physical exam is not revealing but her temperature is 103°F. A CBC shows a hemoglobin of 10 g/dL, WBC 4000 with 10% polys, 5% bands, 70% lymphs, 10% monos, and 5% other white or unidentified cells. Platelets are 60,000/mm³. Which of the following is NOT immediately appropriate?
   a. blood cultures from different sites
   b. electrolytes, liver and renal function tests
   c. ask if she has been receiving granulocyte colony-stimulating factor (G-CSF)
   d. white blood cell transfusion

164. Which of the following devices is most likely to give accurate intracranial pressure (ICP) readings?
   a. intraventricular
   b. subdural
   c. epidural
   d. intraparenchymal

165. Members of a particular government office are exposed to anthrax spores when an envelope is opened. Terrorist activity is strongly suspected. Which of the following is true?
   a. inhalation anthrax is the most common form
   b. human to human transfer does not occur
   c. inhalation of live bacteria causes the disease
   d. antibiotics are ineffective

166. A patient presents with a history of nausea, vomiting, and diarrhea for several days after a Caribbean cruise. In the emergency department, she is weak, moderately hypotensive, and dehydrated. An ECG shows bradycardia, mild ST depression, and a U wave with some ventricular ectopic beats. What is the most likely electrolyte abnormality?
   a. hypomagnesemia
   b. hyperkalemia
   c. Hypokalemia
   d. hypocalcemia

167. To check orthostatic vital signs, blood pressure and pulse rate should be measured after the patient is:
   a. 1 minute supine, 1 minute sitting, and 1 minute standing
   b. 3 minutes supine, 1 minute sitting and/or standing
   c. 3 minutes prone and 3 minutes standing
   d. none of the above

Copyright © Mometrix Media. You have been licensed one copy of this document for personal use only. Any other reproduction or redistribution is strictly prohibited. All rights reserved.

168. A 7-year-old child is brought to the emergency department after multiple bee stings about 30 minutes previously. He complains of itching, swollen lips, and difficulty breathing. Wheezing and stridor are heard. In addition to giving epinephrine, treatment will include all of the following except:

    a. IV fluids

    b. intravenous corticosteroid

    c. intravenous antihistamine

    d. broad-spectrum antibiotic

169. A chronic renal failure patient is sent to the emergency department because his external arteriovenous fistula is not patent. Possible solution to the problem is:

    a. infuse fibrinolytics

    b. surgically remove clot

    c. repair fistula; insert dual lumen subclavian catheter

    d. all of the above

170. Semen samples for DNA evidence in rape cases:

    a. cannot be collected from clothing

    b. may be collected up to 5 to 7 days after the crime in adults

    c. may be collected up to 2 weeks after in children and adolescents

    d. may not be stored; must be given to the police directly after collection

171. Which of the following is true regarding informed consent?

    a. minors must always have parental consent

    b. nurses should be certain the patient understands the risks, benefits, and alternatives to treatment

    c. parents may refuse life- or limb-saving treatment for their child based on religious grounds

    d. in an emergency when the patient is unable to give consent, only the doctor can decide whether to proceed

172. The Emergency Medical Treatment and Active Labor Act (EMTALA) includes the following provisions EXCEPT:

    a. participating hospitals have emergency departments and receive funding from Health and Human Services (HHS)

    b. any patient who comes to the emergency department requesting examination or treatment must receive an appropriate medical screening exam to determine if an emergency situation exists

    c. to transfer an unstable patient, the receiving hospital must accept him or her and the transferring doctor must sign a form stating that the benefits of the transfer outweigh the risks

    d. verbal patient refusal of examination or treatment absolves the hospital from possible legal penalty

173. Clues to child abuse include the following EXCEPT:

    a. multiple emergency department visits for trauma

    b. multiple fractures in various states of healing

    c. scattered scalding of the head, torso, or upper arms

    d. retinal hemorrhages

174. Regarding statutory disease and specific trauma reporting to health or law enforcement authorities, it is true that
    a. it is uniform in all states.
    b. it does not include suicide, nonlethal gunshot wounds, or certain communicable diseases.
    c. the nurse shares reporting responsibility with the physician.
    d. the nurse cannot report an event or disease without physician permission.

175. In clinical research:
    a. a P value of 0.05 means there is a 95% indication the result is not due to chance
    b. a VII level of evidence is the best possible on a scale of I to VII
    c. a confidence interval of 95% indicates that 95 out of 100 subjects reacted favorably
    d. none of the above

Answer Key and Explanations

1. C: A family member can register the patient into the system, blood tests must be done but can be done after the EKG, and, although nitroglycerin is an appropriate intervention for pain, the low blood pressure may need evaluation before choosing to give nitroglycerin. The appropriate intervention is to place the client on a cardiac monitor, give oxygen to decrease cardiac workload, and obtain an EKG to immediately evaluate the heart. The ED is a controlled setting where a physician should be readily available to look at the client, evaluate the cardiac monitor, and interpret the EKG to determine further interventions.

2. B: The primary assessment is done in a systematic way. Identifying a need and performing an intervention are essential before going on to the next step. Assess the airway and then intervene, assess the breathing and then intervene, and so on until you have performed a complete head-to-toe assessment to identify the immediate illness or injury and provided an immediate emergency intervention. Answer a is incorrect because it neglects the intervention aspect of the assessment. Answers c and d are incorrect because they are not aspects of the primary assessment.

3. C: The goal for any suspected acute coronary syndrome is a time frame of ED door to cath lab or to balloon those arteries to be 90 minutes or less. ST segment deviation in two or more leads usually indicates an acute ischemic event, which requires an angiogram or angioplasty. The nurse may give a report and may order labs and repeat EKGs, but the immediate intervention is to get the client ready for the cardiac cath lab. This may require calling in a cardiac team, undressing the patient completely, and removing jewelry. It may also include any other orders a cardiologist requires for the patient before the procedure. An ED nurse should be prepared for the possibility of this invasive procedure.

4. B: Troponin levels are elevated 3 to 12 hours after an acute onset of MI. Answer a is incorrect because troponin levels have taken the place of enzymes as cardiac biomarkers. However, troponin levels can also elevate in other disease states, including renal failure, making answer c incorrect. Answer d is incorrect because troponin levels actually help to distinguish between unstable angina (UA) and MI. Troponin levels do not elevate in UA.

5. B: A nonsmoking female may not have any risk factors, but a female complaining of chest pain should be evaluated for an acute cardiac problem, like any client with risk factors. Females present with different symptoms when having an MI and may not have classic symptoms, and they may also have an MI without having risk factors. The other answers are all risk factors for cardiac disease and acute cardiac syndromes.

6. C: A cardiac monitor, oxygen, and an IV should be in place for anyone complaining of chest pain and before administering nitroglycerin, especially in an elderly client, who may develop hypotension quickly. When a client does not respond to sublingual nitroglycerin, it indicates possible unstable angina and may require other interventions to relieve the pain.

7. D: The cause of heart failure in the pediatric population is most often a congenital heart defect. When triaging a pediatric patient, it is important to ask about congenital heart defects because often parents do not think to mention those defects that may have been surgically corrected, especially if the ED visit seems unrelated to a heart issue. The other choices may need further evaluation but may be unrelated to symptoms of heart failure.

8. A: The immediate intervention for a pediatric client is to maintain the airway and facilitate breathing. The other selections can be addressed after the airway and breathing are considered. Pediatric patients will compromise for a long time, and then they just stop. It is imperative to ensure that an adequate airway is in place and effective breathing is established before proceeding to the next step of the interventions.

9. C: Cardiomyopathy is a term that covers the diseases that have affected the myocardium and cause the symptoms listed. Dilated cardiomyopathy is the most common type of cardiomyopathies, giving symptoms of edema and heart failure. Other causes of cardiomyopathy may be toxins, acute diseases, infections, and chronic conditions. Often, diuretics are administered to reduce edema and ease breathing. The emergency treatment of a cardiomyopathy is the same as with any cardiac condition. It requires interventions to secure the airway and facilitate breathing and circulation before going on to any other intervention.

10. B: Dysrhythmia of any type causes a decrease in cardiac output. The emergent treatment intervention is directly related to the stability of the client's blood pressure, heart rate, and breathing ability. The other selections are incorrect.

11. C: With non-q-wave MIs, ST depression is usually visible on the ECG, but there are no abnormal q waves. With this type of MI, the coronary occlusion is usually incomplete (in about 70%) and many will re-infarct. Peak CK levels will usually be reached in about 12-13 hours.

12. D: The client should be kept on a nothing-by-mouth (NPO) status when presenting with chest pain until it is certain that surgery is not immediate. A low-salt diet would not be ordered from the ED. The other tasks should be performed as part of the preparation for any patient with chest pain.

13. C: Manifestations of a dissecting aortic aneurysm include a sharp/ripping posterior chest pain with a sudden onset, mediastinal widening on chest x-ray or other radiological studies, syncope, and impaired peripheral pulses or blood pressure differential.

14. B: In the ED, monitoring airway, blood pressure, and oximetry are essential for a client with chest pain. A meal is not usually offered, and an IV line should already be established as the protocol for a client with chest pain. Documentation of insurance is the responsibility of the admissions clerk and not an immediate concern for the ED nurse.

15. A: A client presenting with left-sided heart failure is often in sudden pulmonary edema with shortness of breath. Venous congestion is a symptom of right-sided failure, and heart failure can present with or without pain. There is always shortness of breath or pulmonary congestion when presenting to the ED, which require intervention.

16. C: The act of inspecting is looking for objective data about the client that reinforce the client's complaints. The style of clothing, how the family interacts, and asking questions may also be part of the complete assessment, but the objective data are collected by observation of the physical signs and symptoms the patient shows.

17. B: Hepatic congestion is a result of acute or chronic heart failure. The other answers can contribute to an abnormal liver study, but the abnormal results would be considered a result of heart failure without alcoholism, hepatitis, or medications.

18. A and C: Dopamine increases contractility and cardiac output, which improves oxygenation delivery to the tissues. It decreases cardiac workload. Dopamine is a vesicant. It is about 1/10 as likely as norepinephrine in producing tachycardias.

19. D: Clucks are not recognized cardiac sounds.

20. C: An ineffective breathing pattern would be the appropriate nursing diagnosis from the information given. Shortness of breath is the only symptom revealed. After further work-up, choices a and b may also be appropriate for a nursing care plan, but ineffective breathing pattern applies to shortness of breath.

21. B: The client showing signs and symptoms of a decreased cardiac output would require an intervention that may include IV access, medications, or even pacing the heart rhythm. The other choices appear to be within normal limits for the situations described.

22. D: A heart rate of 130 beats in an adult could be indicative of paroxysmal supraventricular tachycardia and will need investigation, possible and ECG. If SVT is identified the patient may need an intervention, including vagal maneuvers, medications, or cardioversion. Normal heart rates: Newborn 120-160; 1-3 year olds 80-140; 3-5 year olds 80-120; 6- 12 year olds 70-110; 13+ years 55-105; Adults 60-100.

23. B: First-degree atrioventricular block is diagnosed partially by an EKG showing a PR interval of greater than 0.20 seconds.

24. C: A run of three or more PVCs is considered ventricular tachycardia and may need further intervention.

25. A: Immediately begin CPR upon noting VF until a defibrillator is available. Once the process of resuscitation is initiated and other team members arrive with a defibrillator and medications, then clients may require intubation, IV medications including epinephrine, and defibrillation. CPR is the immediate intervention before help arrives.

26. C: Intussusception is a mechanical bowel obstruction most often found in infants and small children. It occurs most often near the ileocecal valve or near a colon tumor or Meckel's diverticulum. It is life threatening and causes compromise to the vascular supply to the gut. It can lead to gangrene and sepsis and requires immediate surgery to correct.

27. C: The National Institute of Health lists the following as common causes of acute gastritis: NSAID and alcohol consumption and bacterial infections such as *H. Pylori*.

28. C: *H. pylori* may be present in 30% to 50% of the population and may be a contributing factor in chronic gastritis. Chronic gastritis can lead to ulcers, hemorrhage, perforation, and obstruction.

29. B: It is important to remember that a low blood pressure in a child is a late sign of shock and is often not seen until the child has lost 25% of his or her body fluids. It is imperative than that fluid replacement is part of the treatment plan for a child who has sustained any trauma, particularly to the abdomen. A child has a higher percent of water compared to body weight and a higher metabolism, which makes maintaining the acid-base balance difficult. Abdominal trauma is common in children and should not be overlooked when a child complains of stomach pain.

- 221 -

Symptoms may appear several hours after the trauma, especially if it is low impact or wasn't reported, as in an injury during gym class or a fall on the playground.

30. B: Pyloric stenosis is the most common obstruction during infancy. It is also known as infantile hypertrophic pyloric stenosis and is diagnosed most often between 3 and 12 weeks of life. Delay in treatment and diagnosis can lead to dehydration, shock, and mortality. The other choices are incorrect.

31. A: Airway and breathing followed by circulation are the most important initial interventions regardless of the type of traumatic injury sustained. Then IV, CT, and other interventions can be initiated, but the ABCs must be addressed first.

32. B: Pancreatitis may cause hypocalcemia due to the release of lipase into the soft tissue. This binds with the calcium and causes a decrease in ionized calcium during this process. The other conditions do not directly relate to hypocalcemia in this way.

33. D: The serum Lipase level is normally 30-210 U/L. An elevation greater than two times the normal value is suspect for pancreatitis and can be used along with other diagnostic tests and clinical information to make a diagnosis. An elevated WBC count would be indicative of infection or inflammation, but not specific to pancreatitis. The WBC count of 5.0 is normal.

34. B: It would be most appropriate to insert an NG tube and attach it to suction. The other choices would not be appropriate for a newly diagnosed client with an acute abdomen.

35. C: Narcotics may be used for pain. Aspirin would not be appropriate due to the gastric irritability that it may cause. Compazine is an antiemetic and is not used for pain.

36. C: The pain of diverticulitis begins as a general discomfort localizing to the LLQ. The other choices are not correct.

37. B: For uncontrolled bleeding, intubation and a Sengstaken-Blakemore tube to create a mechanical tamponade are appropriate. The IV, nasogastric tube, and type and cross match should already have been done or will be done while preparing for this emergency procedure. The ABCs take first priority in the care of the patient, so protecting the airway and stopping the bleeding will be the immediate interventions for a client with uncontrolled bleeding.

38. D: While all of the bacteria listed can cause diarrhea, the history listed regarding the turtle, a known vector of salmonella, may indicate this being the offending bacteria. Symptoms usually appear 12-72 after infection. Neither campylobacter jejuni nor clostridium difficile usually present with bloody diarrhea. Though Yersinia enterocolitica may present with bloody diarrhea, it is usually green and foul.

39. B: Upper gastrointestinal bleeding is a very common emergency and usually requires prompt treatment. This man almost certainly has cirrhosis of the liver and is bleeding from esophageal varices. This is a complication of the portal hypertension that develops in these patients with ultimate rupture of the esophageal veins. Bleeding is often brisk and must be controlled, usually by endoscopic band ligation or sclerotherapy. Bleeding from a gastric or duodenal ulcer is usually less dramatic and results from mucosal damage caused by anti-inflammatory drugs or *Helicobacter pylori* that render the mucosa more sensitive to gastric acid. Erosion into a blood vessel causes the bleeding but it is most often slow and detected by stool occult blood tests. Gastric cancer may also

- 222 -

be a source of upper gastrointestinal bleeding but it is rarely associated with vehement vomiting of blood and the bleeding may be intermittent. Angiodysplasia refers to dilated and tortuous blood vessels. Bleeding is from a lower gastrointestinal venous source, usually in the cecum or ascending colon.

40. A: This woman's signs and symptoms are typical of acute pancreatitis but other causes of acute and severe abdominal pain must be considered. The most likely cause of pancreatitis in this woman without a history of alcoholism would be gallstones, which can result in ductal hypertension and pancreatic enzyme activation. Serum amylase is nearly always markedly elevated as is the lipase, which tends to remain elevated longer. Ultrasound of the abdomen may disclose gallstones and CT reveals pancreatic edema. Acute cholecystitis is a possibility but can usually be ruled out by ultrasonography. Bowel obstruction would be uncommon with no history of prior abdominal surgery leading to adhesions, diminished bowel sounds, and no change in her usual bowel movement pattern. The pain pattern is unusual for appendicitis but anatomic position of the appendix may cause atypical pain. This possibility may usually be ruled out by abdominal CT.

41. A: Ureteral calculi are a quite common cause of acute emergency evaluation, usually causing flank pain with radiation to the back and/or groin. About 75% of these are calcium oxalate or phosphate; less common are struvite, uric acid, or cystine calculi. While KUB or ultrasound may show the stone, helical CT is now the preferred diagnostic method. Additional workup includes CBC, chemistry panel, urinalysis, and straining of urine to catch a passed stone for chemical analysis. Nursing attention should be directed to intravenous hydration with input and output recording and narcotic or narcotic plus NSAID (e.g., ketorolac) administration for pain. Some patients may be discharged with analgesics and instructions for hydration and calculus capture. Testicular torsion is most common in adolescents and usually presents with testicular and groin pain with abdominal radiation; increasing pain by lifting the scrotum to the level of the pubic symphysis causes exacerbation of the pain (Prehn sign). Cystitis may be infectious or drug–induced, but cystitis usually causes dysuria and pyuria and shows positive urine cultures.

42. C: This woman with lupus may already have compromised renal function and treatment with a nephrotoxic agent such as an aminoglycoside may provoke acute renal failure (ARF). In this situation, the urine output diminishes to less than 0.3 mL/kg/h for 24 hours; sometimes the patient is anuric. The serum creatinine rises sharply to 3 times normal or greater than 4 mg/dL, indicating a diminution in glomerular filtration by 75%. The ECG findings strongly suggest hyperkalemia, a characteristic accompaniment of ARF. Hyponatremia, hypocalcemia, and hyperphosphatemia, along with volume overload, are also characteristic fluid and electrolyte abnormalities of ARF. Immediate intravenous calcium will stabilize the myocardial cell membranes for a short time, decreasing the likelihood of arrhythmia, while glucose and insulin drive the potassium from the extracellular to the intracellular fluid with an onset of action of 5 to 30 minutes and lasting up to 4 hours. An oral or rectal cation exchange resin (*Kayexalate*) and emergency dialysis are longer term methods of hyperkalemic treatment.

43. B: Flank pain and bruising may indicate an injury to the kidney. It would be appropriate to get a urinalysis to test for blood and a CBC to determine how much bleeding may be taking place. The other choices may or may not be necessary for the complaint of flank pain.

44. C: It is always the best practice to undress a client, provide privacy with a gown and sheet, and directly observe for traumatic injury. Genitourinary injuries are very important and can be a source for bleeding.

45. B: The symptoms described would indicate a kidney stone; flank pain is the hallmark for renal calculi. An MI is not a genitourinary emergency. Ovulation would cause pelvic pain. Torsion would not cause flank pain. Testicular torsion causes scrotal pain.

46. C: Acute renal failure is the result of an increase in nitrogenous waste products due to infection, sepsis, shock, or other significant medical emergency.

47. D: A decrease in renal blood flow and ischemia are indications that acute renal failure can follow. Renal calculi, trauma, or a newly diagnosed mass can all lead to renal failure as can a cardiac arrest, sepsis, or any acute medical condition that caused a decrease in blood flow to vital organs for a short time.

48. A: The first year of life for boys is when they are the most susceptible to torsion of the testicle.

49. C: The incomplete ossification of the ribs allows the kidneys to be targets when a child suffers trauma. The kidney of a child is not three times larger than that of an adult but is larger in percentage of body size than that of an adult. The other choices are incorrect.

50. B: Dysuria is the most common symptom of a UTI. The fever may or may not be from the urinary tract, and cloudy urine may indicate dehydration. A fruity odor to the urine may indicate the presence of sugar or diabetes.

51. D: Preterm labor and preeclampsia are complications of pyelonephritis that may be serious to both mother and child.

52. B: After the ABCs are checked, the next things to be done with a client complaining of flank pain would be a urine test to detect blood, an IV for fluids, and medications for pain. The client would be kept NPO in case the flank pain is a kidney stone requiring surgery. Observation should be accompanied by offering pain control.

53. D: Testicular torsion needs surgical intervention within six hours to preserve the testicle. The other choices are not so critical.

54. B: The classic "duck waddle" indicates the client's attempt to avoid touching the scrotum while walking. The other conditions would not cause this type of gait.

55. D: Abruptio placenta is the most critical condition and is the cause of 15% of fetal deaths. Mother and infant may suffer blood loss and shock.

56. C: Vaginal bleeding and uterine tenderness are the hallmark signs of abruptio placenta. Dark vaginal bleeding and uterine pain warrant an ultrasound, IV fluids, and an immediate Cesarean section (C-section).

57. D: The other choices may be appropriate at some point, but the initial and most important step in resuscitation is to establish an adequate airway.

58. B: A ruptured ectopic pregnancy may cause maternal death due to blood loss, shock, and subsequent cardiac arrest of the mother.

59. C: High blood pressure, proteinuria, and edema are the positive symptoms for preeclampsia and eclampsia.

60. B: Seizures and coma may be the result of eclampsia.

61. A: The other choices are not likely.

62. B: It is important to dry the infant under a heat source while assessing and establishing the airway. The other steps will be done after the airway is established.

63. C: A female with DUB who has required a D&C to stop the bleeding would return for a fever because of the risk of sepsis. The other choices are not correct instructions.

64. D: Bacterial vaginitis symptoms are thin white secretions with a foul fishy odor. Candida vaginitis symptoms include white curdy discharge without an odor. Trichomonas vaginitis displays with a green or grayish discharge that is frothy in appearance.

65. C: The client with PID would need pain medications and antibiotics.

66. A: Dysrhythmias offer the most emergent condition requiring interventions.

67. B: Schizophrenia is a functional psychosis.

68. A: The other choices are not correct.

69. D: Several major nursing and medical organizations now support the policy of allowing family members to witness procedures on and resuscitation of their child. This is thought of as an extension of family-centered care, which is desirable for pediatric emergencies. Team members should be made aware of this policy in advance in order to facilitate procedures and avoid any unpleasant confrontations that may emerge due to parenteral concern or stress. A nursing team member should be assigned to the family to explain the medical situation and reassure them, if possible. There should be a specific space assigned to the family members to observe the procedure without getting in the way of diagnostic, surgical, or resuscitative activity. If possible, parents should be allowed to touch the child if it does not impede medical procedures.

70. C: Clinical depression is a very common illness with a suicide risk of 5% to 12% for men and 10% to 25% for women. Suicide is most often seen in young adults (increasingly in teenagers) and elderly patients. The emergency nurse must maintain a high index of suspicion of depression because it may be masked by other factors: drug or alcohol abuse, self-mutilation, anger, and aggression. Brain imaging, electroencephalography, and blood testing may be required to rule out underlying metabolic or neurologic disease. While antidepressant drugs have played a major role in the treatment of this condition, they may take several weeks to show an effect and some patients do not appear to be helped at all. Careful examination for suicidal ideation is mandatory in these patients and psychiatric consultation and hospitalization may be required for those whose safety is in doubt.

71. A: This patient's history and symptoms strongly suggest a panic attack. This ailment frequently masquerades as an acute medical illness and is responsible for many emergency department visits. Careful questioning, examination, and appropriate laboratory analysis usually detects the condition. Some patients make multiple emergency department visits without significant findings. Typically,

the pulse and respiratory rate are increased but blood pressure and temperature are normal. Because chest pain and dyspnea are two of the most common symptoms of panic attack, it is necessary to eliminate underlying disease with chest (or other) x-ray, ECG, and blood tests, including arterial blood gases, serum electrolytes, thyroid tests, glucose for possible hypoglycemia, and urine toxicology for stimulatory drugs, such as cocaine or amphetamines, that the patient may deny using. Once panic attack is diagnosed, intravenous benzodiazepines, such as lorazepam (*Ativan*), may be given. Reassurance of the patient is valuable. Referral to a professional mental health expert is also useful.

72. D: While this child may indeed have been a victim of a fall, the combination of comatose state, retinal hemorrhages, and a subdural hematoma indicate the possibility of the "shaken baby syndrome" in which violent shaking of the child leads to acceleration-deceleration injury to the brain. Coma, retinal hemorrhages, and subdural hematoma are common injuries. Child abuse is a major cause of infant morbidity and mortality and should be considered in cases in which a child has a history of frequent emergency department visits for trauma or scattered bruises and/or healed fractures that defy other explanation. Posterior or lateral rib fractures may be caused by overzealous squeezing of the infant and fractures of several bones in various stages of healing are particularly suspicious for child abuse. Localized burns without scatter or satellite burns, often attributed to spilled hot liquids, are also suspect. Even if there is only a remote possibility of abuse, most state laws require health care professionals to report the possibility to the appropriate social agency.

73. C: Domestic violence, nearly always perpetrated against women, is a major problem confronted by the emergency nurse. Screening for possible cases should include answers A, B and D. Interestingly, victims of intimate partner violence often present with a medical ailment, not trauma. These include back, abdominal, or pelvic pain, headaches, urinary infections, sexually transmitted disease, or symptoms consistent with posttraumatic stress disorder (PTSD). Sometimes evidence of old trauma such as healing fractures or cosmetically concealed bruises may point toward the presence of domestic violence. Many victims will deny it but sometimes compassionate questioning in a private setting will elicit a positive response. The nurse may then offer advice, refer to a social agency or shelter, or ask for a consultation by the hospital social worker.

74. B: The V/Q ratio is a measure of the volume of ventilation and pulmonary blood flow. A normal value is 0.8. Elevated V/Q values indicate dead space ventilation in which alveoli are ventilated but perfusion is impaired. Examples are pulmonary embolus, hypotension, or low cardiac output as in cardiogenic shock. In each of these there is diminution of the pulmonary blood flow. A low V/Q ratio indicates shunting of the alveolar blood supply when the alveoli are perfused but not ventilated. Examples include pneumonia, atelectasis, acute respiratory distress syndrome, pulmonary hemorrhage, or pneumothorax. Other causes of impaired oxygenation are diffusion abnormalities, which block capillary-alveolar gas exchange as in pulmonary edema or pulmonary fibrosis; and poor oxygen-carrying capacity of the red blood cells as in sepsis, or carbon monoxide or cyanide poisoning.

75. D: Mechanical ventilation requires diligent observation of the patient and ventilator by the emergency nurse. Modern ventilators usually come with alarms that indicate high or low airway pressure. High pressure may be caused by endotracheal tube obstruction with sputum or kinks or inadvertent endobronchial displacement. The airway should be suctioned and tube placement checked. A chest x-ray is frequently helpful in determining the cause. Lung collapse, worsening of the underlying disease, and bronchospasm are also causes of elevated pressure. Leaks around the endotracheal tube cuffs will cause low airway pressure. Auto-positive end-expiratory pressure

(auto-PEEP) is caused by premature inspiratory delivery before full expiration (as in asthma or COPD patients) and may lead to increased pressure and lung damage.

76. D: Establish an adequate airway. The other choices would follow.

77. B: ARDS is sudden, progressive, and severe, even leading to death.

78. C: Decreasing respiratory effort and aspiration may be possible under the influence of alcohol.

79. C: The other choices may be given, but for different reasons than respiratory issues.

80. D: A Replogle is not for breathing.

81. D: The spiral CT provides definitive diagnosis for a PE. V/Q scans and pulmonary angiograms can confirm a diagnosis of a PE. D-dimers will be elevated with a PE but can also be elevated for other reasons, and are often elevated in renal patients on dialysis.

82: D: The child in status asthmaticus would need to be treated first as this patient has the most life threatening airway emergency.

83. D: Bronchiolitis affects children under the age of two.

84. D: All of the choices are examples of patient care management tasks.

85. B: A barking cough is the hallmark symptom of croup.

86. C: Although anxiety is a part of any respiratory illness because of the fear of not catching a breath, it is most often associated with hyperventilation.

87. B: "Body packer" is the street term for the person assigned to smuggle drugs by placing them into body cavities.

88. C: PCP causes rhabdomyolysis and renal failure, sometimes requiring dialysis as an intervention.

89. A: When a client presents with paint around the nose and mouth or an odor of solvent on the clothing and hair, it is suspicious for huffing an inhalant.

90. B: Shock is a response to an illness or injury where there is a decrease in tissue perfusion. In distributive shock (including anaphylactic and neurogenic) there is initially an increased cardiac output.

91. B: Increased cardiac output is the opposite of what happens with hypovolemia.

92. D: The ED is required by law to report abuse cases and must never keep abuse quiet. It is not a breach of confidentiality when reporting a case of suspected abuse.

93. C: No drug has proved effective in the clinical management or prevention of ARDS. The following are therapies that are commonly used but per ARDS network there is insufficient evidence that they decrease mortality rates: corticosteroids (may increase mortality rates in some

patient populations, though this is the most common given), nitrous oxide, inhaled surfactant, and anti-inflammatory medications. Treatment of the underlying condition is the only proven treatment, especially identifying and treating with appropriate antibiotics any infection, as sepsis is most common etiology for ARDS, but prophylactic antibiotics are not indicated. Conservative fluid management is indicated to reduce days on the ventilator, but does not reduce overall mortality. Pharmacologic preventive care: enoxaparin, sucralfate, and enteral nutrition support within 24 hours of ICU admission or intubation.

94. C: This patient is agitated and possibly paranoid following a cocaine overdose. The first action, attempting to calm the patient has failed, probably due to the patient's psychological state. The patient may be able to be extubated, but first giving the patient the benzodiazepines and then seeing if the patient were more calm would be the safer choice, as the patient may hyperventilate even without the ventilator depending upon the patient's psychological state. Giving the benzodiazepine would also help the patient relax and the heart rate decrease which would be safer for the patient as well. Changing the tidal volume would not be appropriate at this time.

95. C: Priapism, a prolonged and painful erection not associated with sexual desire, is an occasional reason for emergency evaluation. It is usually caused by obstruction to the venous drainage of the corpora cavernosae with accumulation of deoxygenated blood leading to swelling and pain. Urinary obstruction occurs in 50% of cases, which requires catheterization, but this is not necessarily helpful diagnostically. Ultrasound of the penis or CT of the abdomen or spine may reveal other disease but the initial test in an African American male should be for sickle cell anemia. This is a common cause of priapism because of the relative inability of the abnormal red blood cells to traverse small blood vessels, leading to obstruction and swelling. If positive, oxygen administration and even transfusion may help. Dorsal nerve block with lidocaine 1% (without epinephrine), systemic vasodilators, and
needle aspiration of the corpora, followed by phenylephrine injection, are additional treatments.

96. D: Vaginal discharge and/or painful urination are a common female complaint, especially after recent sexual intercourse. While many such patients are seen in the gynecologist's office, the emergency department is often the medical facility of first and last resort for much of the population. The differential diagnosis includes urinary tract infection (cystitis), and vaginal infection with *Chlamydia, Gonococcus, Trichomonas, Gardnerella*, or *Mycoplasma.* While the character of the discharge may offer a clue (e.g., the greenish-yellow discharge of *Trichomonas* or the fishy–smelling, thin discharge associated with bacterial vaginosis), definite microbiological testing is required. In this patient urine tests for cystitis, most frequently caused by *E. coli*, and vaginal swab testing for *Chlamydia* and gonorrhea are indicated. Additional tests for pregnancy, HIV, HPV, and VDRL may be warranted in a female with a sexually transmitted disease.

97. B: The HELLP syndrome (hemolysis, elevated liver enzymes, and low platelets) is a severe form of preeclampsia in pregnant women and may be life-threatening to both mother and fetus. HELLP usually affects multigravida mothers while the usual form of preeclampsia is more common in primigravidas. It occurs in it up to 12% of women with preeclampsia-eclampsia. Respiratory distress, hypotension, and tachycardia may develop secondary to anemia and blood loss from coagulopathies. Numerous medical conditions must be ruled out and emergency cesarean section to save the fetus is often required. Delivery usually reverses the physiologic changes but not invariably, and rarely the syndrome develops postpartum. Blood pressure greater than 160/110 mm Hg, proteinuria greater than 5 g per 24 hours, pronounced edema including face and hands, persistent headaches, increased tendon reflexes, and liver symptoms including pain and abnormal

liver function tests are additional features of the HELLP syndrome. The proteinuria and edema are considerably more prominent than that seen in usual preeclampsia.

98. A: This woman's symptoms and clinical finding are typical of an ectopic pregnancy. There is failure of endometrial implantation of the fertilized ovum, which instead begins development in an extrauterine site. The most common sites are the ampulla and isthmus of the fallopian tube, but ectopic pregnancies may be present in many other sites in the female reproductive system or even in the abdominal cavity. It often develops in patients with a history of pelvic infections and becomes symptomatic toward the end of the first trimester. Diagnosis is usually made by an elevated β-hCG level and pelvic ultrasound. Ovarian cysts may present with pain and abdominal swelling but β-hCG levels are not elevated and pelvic examination may reveal a cystic mass. Ultrasound is the usual confirmatory diagnostic method. The normal-sized uterus and ultrasonography rule out normal pregnancy or abruptio placenta (usually occurs in the third trimester). Methotrexate with follow-up β-hCG levels is a nonsurgical treatment for ectopic pregnancy but heavy bleeding or other evidence of rupture usually requires surgical intervention.

99. C: Rhabdomyolysis refers to skeletal muscle destruction accompanied by release of myoglobin into the circulation. It is seen in crush injuries, toxic ingestion, and burns. With the widespread use of statin drugs for hypercholesterolemia, this type of drug may currently be the most common cause. Kidney failure may result from diminished renal blood flow or tubular obstruction. Hyperkalemia and elevated CK are characteristic. Proteinuria and hematuria may be detected on urinalysis but because this is due to myoglobin, few red blood cells will be seen. Muscle aches and tenderness, often severe, are usual presenting symptoms. Treatment includes volume replacement, increasing urine flow with an osmotic diuretic such as mannitol, and alkalinization of the urine with sodium bicarbonate to prevent myoglobin precipitation in the urine.

100. C: Nursing procedures for a sexual assault victim are complex and usually require special training to become a sexual assault nurse examiner (SANE) or sexual assault forensic examiner (SAFE). Providing psychological support and reassuring the victim that she is not responsible play a major role. Evidence collection must be done delicately and thoroughly and specimens (e.g., semen, blood, pubic hair, oral swabs) stored in paper bags or special containers (rape kits); avoid plastic bags because they may enhance bacterial or fungal contamination. Transfer of potential evidence must be recorded as to person and time; there are usually special forms for sexual assault cases that must be submitted along with potential evidence. While hospitals are nearly always required by law to report the incident and turn over the examination report and specimens to law enforcement, the patient may refuse to speak to authorities (around 40% demur according to a recent study).

101. D: Nosebleeds (epistaxis) are quite commonly seen in the emergency setting and are usually divided into anterior and posterior, depending on the anatomic site of the bleeding. Infection, trauma, foreign bodies, or coagulation deficiency may be the cause; however, the most common cause is nose picking. Anterior nosebleeds usually arise in the most vascular portion of the nasal mucosa (Kiesselbach plexus) and are usually acute. Nasal pinching and nose blowing followed by nasal speculum examination is the usual diagnostic procedure. If the bleeding is anterior, topical vasoconstrictors, nasal packing with petrolatum-iodoform gauze (or newer commercial products), or local cauterization with silver nitrate or electricity are appropriate treatments. For posterior nosebleeds, more common in elderly patients and usually more serious, a posterior nasal pack with a *Merocel* nasal sponge or *Nasostat* epistaxis balloon is appropriate. Sometimes surgical ligation of the bleeding vessel is required.

102. B: Ear infections may cause severe and persistent pain, especially in children in the 6-month to 3-year age group and are a frequent cause of emergency department visits. Loss or distortion of the light reflex and bulging of the tympanic membrane are cardinal signs of otitis media, usually caused by bacteria such as *Streptococcus influenza* or *Haemophilus influenza*. Sinusitis and purulent rhinitis may accompany the otitis. Antibiotics to cover these organisms, topical warmed otic analgesics, and antipyretics are the usual treatment modalities. Otitis externa or swimmer's ear also causes otalgia and frequently follows swimming in contaminated water or a foreign body in the ear. Keeping the ear dry and using otic analgesics and antibiotics are indicated. Ear plugs while swimming or ear drying agents after swimming or showering are the usual preventive measures. Myringotomy is a surgical procedure to keep the middle ear draining in chronic otitis media and hopefully prevent such complications as mastoiditis, meningitis, ruptured tympanic membrane, or permanent hearing loss. Labyrinthitis is an infection of the inner ear and usually causes severe vertigo, most commonly in adults.

103. D: Maxillary fractures are divided into three subtypes, lower third (Le Fort I), middle third (Le Fort II), and upper (Le Fort III). Plain radiographs with a Waters view or panoramic imaging have been used for diagnosis but CT has largely supplanted these techniques. This patient's symptoms and clinical findings are typical for a Le Fort II maxillary fracture. This fracture involves the central maxillary, nasal, and ethmoid bones, and nasal rhinorrhea suggests skull fracture with CSF leak. Orbital and zygomatic fractures often are found together after facial trauma. In zygomatic fractures, there is pain in the lateral cheek and an inability to close the mouth. There is swelling and crepitus over the zygomatic arch. Orbital blowout fractures cause a rise in orbital pressure, blowing out the weak orbital floor with prolapse of the orbital contents into the maxillary sinus. Periorbital edema, subluxation of the lens, dysconjugate gaze, and enophthalmos are some of the signs of an orbital blowout, often caused by a baseball or golf ball's impact on the orbit. Mandibular fractures may cause airway obstruction by forcing the tongue posteriorly. Malocclusion is a typical finding. Paresthesias of the lower lip, broken teeth, and sublingual hematoma are also observed in this type fracture.

104. B: Acute angle-closure glaucoma refers to blockage of the anterior chamber angle near the root of the iris. It is more common in Asian and Eskimo patients. Acute blockage of the aqueous humor results in elevated intraocular pressures, and pressures above 60 mm Hg may cause damage to the eye structures and impair circulation to the retina. It is a significant cause of blindness worldwide. Treatment includes topical miotics and beta-blockers, carbonic anhydrase inhibitors, and immediate ophthalmologic consultation. Open-angle glaucoma occurs when there is impaired drainage of the aqueous humor from the anterior chamber with a resultant rise in intraocular pressure, although the drainage angle at Schlemm canal remains open. It is the second leading cause of blindness. Central retinal artery occlusion causes sudden painless blindness; the patient may give a history of transient attacks of amaurosis in the affected eye. Retinal detachment occurs when the retina tears and allows vitreous humor to separate the retina and choroid. The patient usually complains of flashing lights, floaters, or a "curtain effect" due to a diminution in the retinal light perception.

105. C: Hyphemia refers to bleeding in the anterior chamber of the eye. It is usually caused by blunt trauma, which leads to rupture of the blood vessels of the iris and bleeding into the clear aqueous humor. Clotting of the blood may occur, called "eight-ball hyphema." Pain, photophobia, and blurred vision are the usual symptoms. Hyphema is more easily detected in those with light-colored eyes than in those with darker hues. Rebleeding occurs in about 30% of patients up to 14 days after the original bleed. Limitation of activity, hospitalization, and bed rest are all treatments but there is controversy about which is the best. Children and African American patients are a highest risk for

- 230 -

secondary hemorrhage so aminocaproic acid should be given. Patch and eye shield are commonly used. NSAIDs should be avoided to reduce rebleeding. Antibiotics are not needed for hyphema especially if caused by blunt trauma as in this case.

106. D: TMB is jaw pain caused by dysfunction of the temporomandibular joint (TMJ) and the supporting muscles and ligaments. It may be precipitated by injury, such as whiplash, or grinding or clenching of the teeth, stress, or arthritis. Treatment includes ice pack to jaw area for 10 minutes followed by jaw stretching exercises and warm compress for 5 minutes 3 to 4 times daily, avoidance of heavy chewing by eating soft foods and avoiding hard foods, such as raw carrots and nuts, NSAIDs to relieve pain and inflammation, night mouthguard, and referral for dental treatments to improve bite as necessary.

107. D: Dental avulsions are complete displacement of a tooth from its socket. The tooth may be reimplanted if done within 1 to 2 hours after displacement, although only permanent teeth are reimplanted, not primary. Teeth can be transported from accident site to the ED in Hank solution, saline, or milk. Cleanse tooth with sterile NS or Hank solution, handling only the crown and avoiding any disruption of fibers. If tooth has been dry for 20 to 60 minutes, soak tooth in Hank solution for 30 minutes before reimplantation. If tooth has been dry for more than 60 minutes, soak tooth in citric acid for 5 minutes, stannous fluoride 2% for 5 minutes, and doxycycline solution for 5 minutes prior to reimplantation. Remove clot in socket and gently irrigate with NS. Place tooth into socket firmly, cover with gauze, and have patient bite firmly on gauze until splinting can be applied. Apply splinting material and mold packing over implanted tooth and 2 adjacent teeth on both sides (encompasses 5 teeth).

108. D: Usually only superficial horizontal lacerations are sutured in the ED. As this is a vertical laceration through the muscle in a stable patient, they should be transferred, as serious injuries should be referred to ophthalmologists or ocular plastic surgeons. Treatment includes local anesthesia (supra- or infraorbital), wound irrigation with NS prior to suturing, suturing with 6-0 or 7-0 coated or plain nylon suture (to be removed in 3 to 5 days), using care to avoid suturing into globe, and ophthalmic topical antibiotic in place of dressing.

109. D: Headaches, especially migraines, are a very common complaint in emergency department patients. Tension headaches tend to be diffuse with skeletal muscular contraction of the head and neck and be associated with numerous underlying conditions. Vascular migraines are often unilateral with a severe throbbing quality but may become diffuse. About 12% of the US population has experienced migraines and 70% of those have a family history. Classic migraines (about 15%) are preceded by an aura, usually visual (scintillating scotomata, tunnel vision), but almost any neurologic dysfunction may occur (e.g., transient hemiparesis or paresthesias). Nausea, vomiting, and photophobia are common. Common migraines are not preceded by an aura and may be more diffuse. Migraines may be triggered by a variety of specific and nonspecific factors, including environmental (e.g., bright light, heat, sudden changes in barometric pressure), dietary (e.g., alcohol, certain cheeses, chocolate), stress, or cyclical estrogen levels. Those without a history of migraine may require CT or MRI scanning to exclude intracranial disorders, such as bleeding, stroke, or tumor.

110. B: This patient had several transient ischemic attacks prior to his clear-cut signs of a stroke, shown to be nonhemorrhagic in nature. Such strokes may be caused by local thrombosis, especially in arteriosclerotic vessels, or by emboli arising in the carotid artery (usually at the bifurcation of the internal and external vessels) or the heart, most often in atrial fibrillation patients with clots in the atrial appendage. Because this patient arrived in the emergency department within 3 hours

- 231 -

from the onset of symptoms, the current recommendation is to begin fibrinolytic therapy with recombinant tissue plasminogen activator (r-TPA). Some recent studies indicate benefit from this therapy may be achieved up to 4.5 hours after the onset of symptoms. Blood pressure management in stroke patients is tricky. Most would agree with slow reduction if the value is greater than 220 systolic or 120 diastolic or the stroke is hemorrhagic in nature. For patients treated with a fibrinolytic agent, significantly elevated blood pressure should be lowered to prevent reperfusion problems. If noninvasive carotid scanning shows marked stenosis, neurosurgical consultation for endarterectomy or angioplasty with stent placement is reasonable. Subsequent warfarin treatment may be appropriate if atrial fibrillation is present.

111. C: Seizures are caused by abnormal neuronal function in the brain with excessive or over-synchronized neuron discharge. They are usually caused by some underlying anatomic (e.g., brain tumor) or metabolic (e.g., hypoglycemia, hyponatremia) abnormality. Partial seizures begin in a specific body part and are limited to one hemisphere of the brain. There may be loss of consciousness (complex seizure) or not (simple partial seizure). Seizures that begin in one area and progress to others in an orderly fashion are termed Jacksonian. Temporal lobe seizures are characterized by automatism and are often preceded by olfactory or auditory aura. Status epilepticus refers to a succession of tonic-clonic seizures without regaining consciousness in between or a single seizure that lasts more than 30 minutes and does not respond to conventional therapy. It is a medical emergency, and intravenous sedation, oxygen (with or without intubation), and anticonvulsant drugs are given. If these measures fail, anesthesia is sometimes employed. Naloxone, dextrose 50%, or thiamine may be given for suspected opioid overdose, hypoglycemia, and alcohol withdrawal (delirium tremens).

112. D: Cranial nerves originate in the brainstem and are subject to a variety of traumatic, infectious, degenerative, and metabolic abnormalities. They may be motor, sensory, or both. There are 12 pairs, numbered by Roman numerals and/or the anatomic name. The oculomotor nerve (III) innervates most of the extraocular eye muscles and also controls lid elevation and pupillary constriction as well as eye movements. The trochlear (IV) innervates the superior oblique muscle, responsible for downward inner gaze. The abducens (VI) innervates the lateral rectus muscle, responsible for lateral gaze. The facial nerve (VII) is responsible for facial movement such as eye closure or smiling as well as lacrimation, salivation, and taste. Damage to this nerve by infection, trauma, or idiopathic (often called Bell palsy) results in unilateral facial droop, inability to smile or whistle, and diminished eye closure and tear production. Most cases recover.

113. B: The Glasgow Coma Scale is a useful and rapid method of determining level of consciousness in comatose patients, regardless of the cause. The scale is divided into 3 major subgroups: eye opening, best motor response, and best verbal response with point scores for individual responses.

Eye opening	4: Spontaneous. 3: To verbal stimuli. 2: To pain (not of face). 1: No response.
Verbal	5: Oriented. 4: Conversation confused, but can answer questions. 3: Uses inappropriate words. 2: Speech incomprehensible. 1: No response.

Motor	6: Moves on command.
	5: Moves purposefully respond pain.
	4: Withdraws in response to pain.
	3: Decorticate posturing (flexion) in response to pain.
	2: Decerebrate posturing (extension) in response to pain.
	1: No response.

Injuries/conditions are classified according to the total score: 3-8 Coma; ≤ 8 Severe head injury; 9-12 Moderate head injury; 13-15 Mild head injury.

114. A: The anterior blood supply to the brain is derived from the internal carotid arteries, which split off from the common carotids at about the level of the jawbone. The carotid arteries then supply the posterior communicating artery to the circle of Willis and the anterior and middle cerebral arteries. This anterior circulation supplies most of the cerebral hemispheres, the basal ganglia, and the diencephalon. The posterior circulation is formed by the merger of the two vertebral arteries into the basilar, which then divides into the two posterior cerebral arteries. This posterior circulation supplies the occipital lobes, cerebellum, part of the temporal lobes, the spinal cord, and the brainstem. The anterior circulation supplies about 80% of the blood to the brain while the posterior supplies about 20%. Knowledge of the circulatory pathways assists in determining the location of a lesion. For example, an obstruction of the posterior circulation is likely to cause brainstem symptoms (nausea, vertigo and balance, respiratory or cardiac abnormalities), while anterior circulation obstruction is more likely to cause hemiparesis and abnormalities of speech.

115. B: Fever, headache, confusion, and neck stiffness are signs and symptoms of meningitis. This possibility must be addressed quickly, especially in an HIV-positive individual who is subject to numerous opportunistic infections. A lumbar puncture with culture, chemistry, and inspection of the cerebrospinal fluid (CSF) is most likely to rule in or rule out meningitis. Many neurologists would recommend doing a CT scan of the brain first to rule out brain abscess or other mass lesion that might cause herniation of the brain due to rapid decrease in the intracranial pressure. If this is the case, a neurosurgical consultation should be obtained to get CSF because an LP is contraindicated. Blood cultures may be valuable if sepsis accompanies the meningitis, and brain angiography (MRA or intravascular) may be helpful in distinguishing a mass lesion, but the diagnostic procedure of choice is examination of the CSF.

116. C: This woman presents with typical history and symptoms of Guillain-Barré syndrome, an idiopathic ascending paralysis, most often in the age range of 20 to 30 years. It frequently follows a respiratory or gastrointestinal infection, and decreased myelin is found at the spinal nerve roots and peripheral nerves. The paralysis may ascend to the diaphragm and intercostal muscles, requiring intubation and ventilatory support. There were many cases in the 1970s in those receiving influenza immunizations. The disorder is thought to have an autoimmune basis, and plasmapheresis with or without immunoglobulin administration may hasten recovery. It is a leading cause of nontraumatic paraplegia but the disease is relatively rare. Recovered patients may require considerable rehabilitation. Her symptoms and age are inconsistent with a stroke, although one may occur in young people because of an aneurysm rupture or bleeding from an arteriovenous malformation. Viral meningitis does not cause bilateral paraplegia but may be excluded by LP and CSF exam. Myasthenia gravis also occurs in young adults, mostly women, and usually presents with increased fatigue and ocular symptoms such as ptosis and diplopia and weakness in the jaw or facial muscles.

117. A: Increased ICP often follows a traumatic brain injury but may be present in other conditions such as a mass lesion in the brain. It is usually considered a medical emergency because elevated

pressure may diminish cerebral blood supply and also predispose to herniation. Cerebral perfusion pressure is calculated by subtracting the ICP from the mean arterial pressure. A value of 50 mm Hg or greater is required for adequate delivery of oxygen and nutrients. As the ICP rises, there is cerebral vasodilation and increase in systolic pressure in order to compensate. Headache, slurred speech, and a sluggish pupillary light response are characteristic of early increased ICP. In addition, confusion and restlessness, nausea and vomiting, and impaired strength and sensation may occur. As the ICP continues to rise, there is continuing decline in the level of consciousness, diminished brainstem reflexes, motor posturing (flexion or extension), fixated pupil(s), projectile vomiting, and abnormal reflexes, such as the extensor plantar reflex (Babinski sign).

118. B: There are several ICP monitoring devices, including the intraventricular catheter, subarachnoid screw, epi-or subdural sensor and intraparenchymal insertion. The current indication for treatment is an ICP greater than 20 mm Hg for more than 5 minutes. Sedation with midazolam or lorazepam (*Ativan*) and, increasingly, propofol (*Diprivan*) is usually indicated. Bolus mannitol is a preferred treatment because of its osmotic and neuroprotective properties but continuous infusion may be harmful and is not recommended. Hypertonic (not hypotonic) saline 3% to 10% is being used more frequently, especially in children, because it has both osmotic effects and may increase mean arterial pressure (MAP). Hyperventilation, used for many years in the treatment of increased ICP, has now been demoted in priority because it may reduce cerebral blood flow without reducing ICP.

119. A: Direct trauma to the head is a frequent cause of brain hemorrhage with or without skull fracture. An epidural hematoma, bleeding between the skull and the dura mater, may be due to bleeding from the middle meningeal artery with a rapid hematoma formation. This is a true medical emergency because the morbidity and mortality rate is high, more than 50%. The brief lucid period followed by a comatose state is typical but does not always occur. Immediate surgical intervention is preferred for large hematomas while some smaller ones may be managed conservatively. Bleeding into the subdural space, between the dura and arachnoid meningeal layers, may be acute, subacute, or chronic. The bleeding is from ruptured bridging veins in the subdural space. While the acute form produces immediate neurologic signs, and often loss of consciousness, the subacute form (48 hours to 2 weeks postinjury) causes a slower progression of neurologic signs. Intraventricular hemorrhage is less common with acute trauma and is more likely to result from a ruptured aneurysm or arteriovenous malformation in a young person. Cervical spine injury must be ruled out in many cases of head trauma but does not cause cerebral bleeds.

120. D: This young man has sustained what used to be called a concussion but now the preferred terminology is mild traumatic brain injury (MTBI). This may be caused by a direct trauma to the head or an acceleration-deceleration injury. It usually causes a brief period of unconsciousness followed by a variety of physical, cognitive, or emotional symptoms, or sleep disturbance. Most of these patients do not need hospitalization but do require observation for persistent or new neurologic signs and symptoms. No participation in athletics is permitted until all these disappear. Current thinking is that there is some neurochemical and axonal damage that leads to the postconcussive syndrome. Most authorities recommend a period of brain rest after MTBI with a gradual return to work or school and especially athletics.

121. C: Stabilization of a patient with suspected trauma to the cervical spine is a very common emergency requirement after falls and motor vehicle accidents. The ideal team consists of four persons. A leader maintains the head and neck in-line by use of fingers under the mandible. Gross neurologic assessment can be obtained by asking the patient, if alert, to wiggle his fingers and toes and to respond to light touch on arms and legs. One assistant then applies a rigid cervical collar of

the correct size to the neck of the patient. The patient is then straightened and rolled onto a rigid backboard as a unit by two assistants on one side of the patient. The patient is then strapped to the backboard at the shoulders, hips, and proximal to the knees. His head should be stabilized further with head blocks or towel rolls. Many active sports (e.g., bicycling, in-line skating, hockey, football) require helmets that must be removed to ensure stability of the cervical spine. This should be done by two people with one maintaining in-line stability and the other removing the helmet.

122. A: Extremity fractures are among the most common injuries seen in emergency departments. Immobilization is mandatory for most extremity, hand, or foot fractures, but bleeding and neurovascular compromise should be assessed before applying the splint. Open fractures with bone protrusion or bleeding should be initially irrigated with normal saline and covered with a sterile dressing before immobilization. Pressure should be used for bleeding; tourniquets should only be used as a last measure. The Hare splint is one of several types of traction splints but is appropriate only for fractures of the mid-shaft of the femur or proximal tibia. It is often applied by paramedics before transport to the hospital. After immobilization, there should be another check for neurovascular integrity and the extremity should be raised. Local swelling may be treated with ice packs.

123. D: Traumatic amputations usually occur in workers using farm or industrial machinery or in motor vehicle accidents. Many factors influence the success of reimplantation, including the nature of the amputation (a sharp cut has a better prognosis than crush injuries), the availability of a transplant team, age, and time and method of preservation of the amputated part. The optimal method of preservation is to irrigate the amputated part with cold saline, wrap in saline moistened gauze, and seal in a plastic bag. The bag is then placed on water and crushed ice and delivered to the hospital as soon as possible. Muscle can remain viable for up to 12 hours, and bone, tendon, and skin up to 24 hours if kept cold. Under warm conditions, the viability of the part is considerably reduced. Packing the part directly in ice water or ice may cause tissue damage because of freezing of cells or osmotic depletion of intracellular contents.

124. C: Training patients with foot or leg injuries to use axillary crutches properly is a duty that frequently falls to the emergency nurse. In fitting the crutches to the patient, each crutch should be about 2 inches (2 to 3 fingerbreadths) below the axilla with no weight-bearing on the crutch. Each handpiece should be placed so that the patient's elbow is at a 30-degree angle, usually in line with the wrist. In walking with the crutches, the tips should be placed about 6 inches in front and 6 inches to the side. In tall persons, the crutch tips may be placed up to 12 inches to the side. Standing with the weight on the good foot, the crutches and the injured foot should move forward. Then, while bearing weight on the palms of the hands, the good foot moves forward.

125. C: A strain is a weakening or tear in the muscle where it attaches to the tendon. While it may occur with many different traumas to the joint, athletic injuries are perhaps the most common. A third-degree strain causes complete disruption of the muscle or tendon. A snapping noise at the time of injury and an avulsion fracture may be seen on x-ray. Acute treatment for this and lesser strains is compression bandage or splint, cold packs, analgesia, and no weight-bearing for 48 or more hours. First- and second-degree strains also present with pain and minor swelling but symptoms are less severe and no fracture is seen on x-ray. Sprains occur when a joint exceeds its normal range of motion and ligaments are damaged. A first-degree sprain causes pain and swelling around the joint, usually ankle or knee, but is less severe than the symptoms and signs this patient displays. MRI is probably the best diagnostic method for distinguishing sprains from strains.

126. B: A fracture is a break or disruption in a bone, generally divided into closed (no break in the skin) and open (protrusion of the bone through the skin). Fractures may take different anatomic patterns, depending on the bone location, the nature of the trauma and the bone density (may be diminished with osteoporosis). Compression fractures are most common in the spine in which a fracture of one or more vertebral bodies leads to a collapse of the spine at that location. An avulsion fracture reflects a forceful contraction of muscle mass, which pulls a bone fragment to break away at the tendon's insertion site. This type of fracture is often seen with severe joint strains. This patient has a comminuted fracture in which the trauma causes more than two separated portions of the bone. Often, several small bony fragments are seen at the site of the break.

127. C: Rupture of the Achilles tendon is a common athletic injury, often caused by stepping off abruptly on the forefoot with the knee in full extension. An audible snap or pop is often heard with immediate heel pain radiating to the calf. The patient is unable to walk on the leg and may have a foot-ankle deformity with swelling. Thompson sign, a diagnostic maneuver, will be positive if there is a complete rupture. The patient lies supine on an examining table with both feet extending over the edge. Squeezing the calf results normally in plantar motion; with an Achilles tendon rupture, there is little if any foot motion. Tibial or fibular fractures are not uncommon and usually occur with direct trauma or excessive rotational force. They may be open or closed and cause leg swelling, pain and point tenderness, deformity, and sometimes crepitus over the involved bone. Fractures of the calcaneus occur most often in falls with the person landing on his feet. There is pain in the heel along with swelling and point tenderness.

128. B: Shoulder dislocations are most common in children and athletes; 55% to 60% are recurrent. The typical athletic dislocation occurs when the extended arm is abducted and externally rotated. The head of the humerus is pushed in front of the shoulder joint by the force, called an anterior dislocation, which is most common. Less common are posterior dislocations. These may occur during a seizure when the patient falls with the arm abducted and internally rotated. In all cases in adults, there is pain in the shoulder, deformity, and inability to move the arm. Management requires checking of neurovascular elements in the arm and radiographs, followed by reduction and a postreduction radiograph to check for the correct humeral positioning. The shoulder is then immobilized with a sling and swath or a shoulder immobilizer.

129. A: Most explosions involve a rapid release of gas that displaces an equal volume of air that travels after the blast wave. This wave is particularly strong and does the most damage to hollow organs, such as the lungs, ears, gastrointestinal tract. Concussions are common because of the pressure wave generated by the blast. Secondary causes of injury are related to missiles released by the explosion: fragments of shell casing or metal objects inserted into a bomb, such as nails or ball bearings. Tertiary injuries are caused by a rapid displacement of the exposed individual, which causes impact with the ground or adjacent structures. These injuries are similar to those sustained in a motor vehicle accident when the victim is thrown clear and hits the ground. In addition, burns and inhalation of noxious fumes are commonly seen in blast victims.

130. D: The compartment syndrome results from compression of the muscular compartment by swelling or compression-restriction of the extremity after an injury. The forearm and leg are the most common sites. Pain out of proportion to the injury is common despite strong analgesics. Prolonged external pressure, frostbite or snakebite may also cause the compartment syndrome. Impaired mobility of digits, paresthesias, coolness over the area, and pallor may be seen. Pulses may be compromised but occasionally a palpable pulse is present distal to the affected area. Rapid diagnosis is mandatory because impairment of the microcirculation in the area may lead to irreversible tissue damage within 4 to 6 hours. Compartment pressure may be determined with a

syringe, catheter, or special monitoring device. Pressure above 30 to 60 mm Hg is usually an indication for a fasciotomy.

131. A: Dog bites are extraordinarily common, although there appears to be less risk of infection than with human or cat bites. In general, wounds that occur more than 12 hours before treatment, as in this case, should be irrigated but not sutured. Although antibiotics are not always required for simple dog bites, the delay in treatment and the appearance of the wound strongly suggest infection and places the wound at higher risk. Many different antibiotics may suffice but amoxicillin/clavulanate or clindamycin plus trimethoprim/sulfamethoxazole provides good coverage for those who are penicillin allergic. Irrigation under pressure using a syringe or a commercially available pressure device is ideal. Tetanus status should be checked but because the dog is a house pet and under observation (10 days recommended), there is no need to begin antirabies intervention unless the dog shows clear signs of the disorder. If so, the animal should be euthanized and laboratory testing for the virus done.

132. C: Choosing the correct dressing for wound management, especially if secondary or tertiary close is employed, is important to accelerate closure and enhance healing. Gauze can absorb exudate and support debridement if applied and kept moist. However, for wounds with considerable exudate, it is not the first choice. Transparent film permits exchange of oxygen from the environment to the wound but absorbs poorly and would not be the best choice for this type of wound. Hydrogel is useful after debridement of a wound because it maintains moisture; however, it is a poor absorber of exudate and is most useful for deep or necrotic wounds. It often requires a secondary dressing. An absorption dressing would be the best choice for this wound. It can absorb large amounts of exudate, support debridement, maintain moisture, and obliterate dead space in the wound. It is ideal for infected wounds.

133. D: NIAP is a relatively new phenomenon pioneered in Britain and Australia and developing widespread acceptance. It refers to the administration of various analgesic measures, both pharmacologic and nonpharmacologic, by the emergency department nurse prior to physician evaluation. Depending on the particular protocol, the nurse may give patients pain relief that includes physical methods (ice/heat, positioning, and distraction); nonopioid drugs such as aspirin, acetaminophen, or NSAIDs; or opioids, usually oral combinations such as oxycodone or hydrocodone with acetaminophen. Some research protocols have even allowed intravenous morphine to be given by the nurse under specific clinical situations. NIAP has been propelled by busy waiting rooms with many pain patients waiting lengthy periods for physician evaluation. Some potential hazards of NIAP are safety issues, nurse reluctance to use or follow the protocol, patients that leave before being seen, and drug-seeking patients.

134. C: Pain management in infants and children has been controversial in the past but several myths have been debunked, especially that infants are less sensitive to pain because their nervous system has not fully developed, and that opioids, both oral and parenteral, are contraindicated in very young children because they do not metabolize these drugs quickly. In fact, opioid drugs may be used efficaciously at the correct pediatric doses. Analgesia and sedation prior to painful or uncomfortable diagnostic or therapeutic procedures, such as LP, suturing lacerations, x-ray, or CT scanning are recommended. Local vapocoolants given before venipunctures or immunization are helpful, as are sucrose drops, swaddling, maternal breastfeeding, and touching the infant. The Faces pain scale for verbal patients and the Faces, Legs, Activity, Cry, Consolability (FLACC) scale for nonverbal patients are useful adjuncts in assessing the presence and severity of pain.

135. C: The job of triage nurse in the emergency department requires a lot of clinical knowledge and the ability to deal with stressful situations without abandoning professional standards. Because of increasingly crowded emergency departments and longer patient waiting times, the position is crucial to the smooth operation of the facility. While triage systems vary, most require an assessment of acuity: emergent defined as severe and life-threatening; urgent requiring care as soon as possible; and nonurgent in which routine care is needed and physician evaluation is not required immediately. One new system, the ESI, developed by emergency physicians and nurses, takes both acuity and available resources into account to sort patients into 5 possible categories: 1) requires life-saving intervention immediately; 2) high risk, confusion or lethargy, and severe pain or distress; 3) age-specific blood pressure, respiratory rate at critical levels, and oxygen saturation less than 92% are not present; 4) one resource needed; 5) no resource needed.

136. C: The rules regarding use of patient restraints have evolved over the past few years. Nurses and other hospital employees with patient care responsibilities must undergo annual training in their use and under what circumstances they may be applied. In general, the confused and uncooperative or aggressive patient who does not conform to treatment or is a threat to himself or herself or the medical personnel is a possible candidate. Every effort should be made to calm the patient with other methods (conversation, intervention of family members, pharmacologic agents such as olanzapine or haloperidol) before physical restraint is applied. The indication for and duration of restraint must be documented in the patient's record. Once they are applied, the patient should be checked every 15 minutes and observations recorded. Any death within 24 hours of being restrained must be reported to the Centers for Medicare and Medicaid Services (CMS).

137. D: Disaster planning for multiple patients with a variety of injuries is now mandated by federal law and administered by Department of Homeland Security guidelines. These include algorithms for prevention, protection, response, and recovery for both personal and professional duties. It is critical in preparation for any disaster and a large influx of injured or infected patients to ensure adequate disaster-related supplies related to specific types of calamity: fire, flood, earthquake, epidemic, and terrorist attack. Often overlooked are measures to keep the professional staff supplied with places to rest, and food and water, especially in situations where travel or time is limited. Notification protocols for health agencies, law enforcement, hazardous materials teams, EMS, and 911 responders should be in place. Regular disaster drills have become standard practice for emergency and hospital personnel.

138. B: Because of the acute shortage and high demand for organ transplantation, organs from cardiac death patients (declaration of death is based on cessation of cardiopulmonary activity) have become quite common. Like patients with brain death, organ donation from cardiac death patients is allowed by federal law but requires the written consent of the legal next of kin. In some states, advanced permission is recorded on driver's licenses. The local OPO must be notified and the medical examiner's approval may be required by state law. Hastening death in moribund patients is allowed after suitability of the donor and legal consent has been established; this may be done by slow termination of life support. Lethal doses of pharmacologic agents are forbidden. The transplantation team must not participate in the end-of-life care of the donor but the potential donor may be taken to a surgical suite in preparation for the organ removal.

139. A: Central venous access is often required for emergency patients, to replace fluid and electrolytes, for blood product transfusions and blood sample collection, and to monitor hemodynamics (central venous pressure). While arm veins may be used to thread the catheter into the superior vena cava, larger veins such as the subclavian, jugular, or femoral are often preferred for reasons of speed and stability. These catheters may be single or multilumen (e.g., to draw blood

from one channel and administer drugs via another). One advantage is that surgery is unnecessary for removal but they do require frequent heparin flushing and injection cap replacement. They do not require a non-coring needle like that used for totally implanted venous access devices such as a *Port-A-Cath* or *LifePort*.

140. B: Transfusion reactions may be of several types and some of the symptoms may overlap. In nearly every case, the transfusion should be stopped immediately and the line kept open with normal saline or other maintenance fluid. This patient's symptoms and signs strongly suggest a hemolytic transfusion reaction due to ABO incompatibility. Type-specific blood that has been cross-matched is standard for blood and packed cell transfusions, but type O Rh negative (females and males) or type O Rh positive (males) may be given in severe emergencies. Hemolytic transfusion reactions are often severe and may be life-threatening so immediate supportive therapy is required. Pyrogenic reactions are mostly due to recipient antibodies to donor leukocytes and leukocyte-poor blood product is preferred. Air embolus is usually due to catheter manipulation (often by patient) or improper infusion technique. Circulatory overload, by overzealous or too-rapid transfusion, may produce symptoms of pulmonary edema; give diuretic and other appropriate treatment for this immediately.

141. D: One method of reducing absorption of an orally ingested toxic substance is by gastric decontamination. This is appropriate in cases of an unknown substance and even with known drugs or toxins that are not corrosive and for which an antidote is available. Syrup of ipecac has been used for many years to induce emesis and reduce upper gastrointestinal concentration of the toxic substance. It is rarely used now and is contraindicated by many authorities because it may cause numerous complications and no studies have shown that it actually improves clinical outcomes. Gastric lavage is also a traditional method that is used less frequently now; its use is beneficial mostly for large ingestions within the first 60 minutes. Activated charcoal is the preferred substance to administer; it absorbs most poisons (except alcohols or heavy metals) and should not be used for corrosive alkali or acid substances. Because activated charcoal is constipating, mixing a cathartic such as sorbitol or magnesium citrate with activated charcoal will enhance elimination of the poison.

142. D: Opioid overdoses, both oral and parenteral, are among the most common problems seen in emergency departments. This patient has typical findings of chronic opioid abuse. As with most emergency department patients, the ABC of emergency patient care is the primary concern; airway maintenance is critical because respiratory depression is the main deleterious effect of these drugs. Activated charcoal is effective in absorbing opioids and should be used with a cathartic after the airway is secure to overcome the constipating effect of the opioid. Many addicts use both oral and intravenous drugs. Naloxone is an opiate antagonist that acts on the brain to reduce respiratory depression and improve the level of consciousness. Repeat or continuous doses may be needed because the drug has a short half-life. A toxicological screen for the opiate and the frequently observed multi-drug abuse should be done but serum levels are not often helpful because of the large variety of opioid drugs with varying half-lives. Clinical response is the best indicator of effective therapy.

143. C: Overdose of tricyclic antidepressants, often by elderly patients with suicidal intent, is less common now since the advent of SSRI drugs for depression but is still a fairly frequent medical emergency. More common is CNS dysfunction ranging from disorientation and confusion to seizures and frank coma; anticholinergic effects including flushed skin, dry mucous membranes, and mydriasis; and cardiac effects including conduction abnormalities and ventricular tachycardia. Phenytoin is contraindicated for seizures in these patients because it has sodium channel blocking

- *239* -

activity and may worsen arrhythmias. The drugs are very well absorbed by activated charcoal; the combination of activated charcoal with sorbitol to overcome the anticholinergics effects on the bowel is useful. Sodium bicarbonate raises the blood pH and lowers the free drug concentration, improving some of the ECG abnormalities.

144. B: Heat exhaustion occurs mainly in young children and elderly persons, usually because they are unable to replace fluid and electrolyte loss adequately. It often occurs suddenly and is characterized by thirst, malaise, muscle cramping, nausea, and vomiting. If untreated, it may cause hypotension, mild to severe temperature elevations, syncope, and possible progression to heat stroke. Diaphoresis may or may not be present. Treatment is based on removal to a cooler environment, replacement of fluid and electrolyte losses (oral or intravenous), and placement of moist clothing on patient to enhance perspiration. Heat stroke occurs when the physiologic cooling mechanisms become impaired and it is a medical emergency. It occurs in classic form in which the individual is exposed to prolonged elevated environmental temperatures, and in exertional form, mostly seen in athletes or military personnel. Core temperatures greater than 104°F are found but these patients are only modestly fluid depleted. Ice packs may be used; total immersion in ice water is controversial and may cause shivering, which raises the body temperature.

145. C: Frostbite is a common medical emergency and its seriousness depends on exposure time and temperature, protective clothing, wind chill, wet or dry body parts, and contact with metal. Superficial frostbite affects skin and subcutaneous tissue and resembles a superficial burn. It mostly occurs on fingertips and toes, ears, nose, and cheeks. The area affected becomes extremely sensitive to further cold or heat exposure and becomes mottled with blisters, which form within a few hours. Basic treatment is application with warm soaks (104°F to 110°F) and extremity elevation. Deep frostbite occurs with low limb temperature and affects bone, muscle, and tendons. The patient senses a burning sensation followed by warmth and numbness. Edema, blistering, and gray-black mottling leading to necrotic gangrene may occur. Rapid rewarming of the tissue is the treatment of choice. This may be quite painful and potent analgesics may be required.

146. D: There are numerous techniques for rewarming body hypothermia. Treatment choice is largely dependent on core body temperature and may be active or passive. For mild hypothermia (93.2°F to 98.6°F), removing wet clothing, warm environment, and blankets may be satisfactory; warmed humidified oxygen and warmed glucose-containing fluids are an active option. For moderate hypothermia (86°F to 93.2°F), heating blankets (*Bair Hugger* therapy), radiant heating lamps, and hot water bottles may be used in addition to the active methods. Numerous other methods are available, such as peritoneal lavage, gastrointestinal rewarming by irrigation, hemodialysis, and even cardiopulmonary bypass. For severe hypothermia (below 78.8°F), as in the case above, the CAVR method is perhaps the most efficient. A catheter in the femoral artery delivers blood to a countercurrent extracorporeal rewarming chamber and the blood is then returned to the venous cordis. The patient's own heart drives the system as there is no external pump as in a heart-lung machine. Hypotension and ventricular arrhythmias are complications of extreme hypothermia.

147. A: Carbon monoxide poisoning is the most frequent cause of poisoning in the United States and results predominantly from house fires, vehicle exhaust (often with suicidal intent), and defective heating equipment. Hypoxia is due to the marked affinity of CO for hemoglobin (200 times that of oxygen) and impaired delivery of oxygen to the tissues. The cytochrome oxidase system of cellular respiration is also affected by CO. Symptoms are related to the amount of CO inspired and the duration of exposure, measured as the percent attached to hemoglobin. Symptoms range from headaches, nausea, and confusion at 10% to 25% COHb to cardiopulmonary arrest at levels of 60% or greater. The main therapeutic objective is to displace the CO from hemoglobin (and myoglobin)

with high-flow oxygen. The half-life of COHb at room air is 5 to 6 hours, 1 hour with 100% oxygen, and less than 20 minutes with hyperbaric oxygen. Delivery at 3 atm for 46 minutes with repeat in 6 hours if symptoms persist has been found to be most effective.

148. C: Burns are defined by the thickness, partial for the epidermis, full for the dermis and deeper. Often it may take 48 hours or more after the injury to determine the correct level. In addition, the extent of the burn injury is very important for management and can be estimated by a variety of tables or charts. Perhaps the most well known and simplest is the rule of nines, in which specific body areas are assigned percentages of the TBSA: 4.5% for anterior or posterior head; 18% for anterior or posterior thorax; 4.5% for anterior or posterior abdomen or for either upper extremity; and 9% for anterior or posterior leg. Scatter burns are given 1% of TBSA if they are hand size, including fingers of the examiner. Disposition of the patient is based on criteria formulated by the American Burn Association. This patient has a 27% burn area (9% for the leg, 18% for the anterior chest). An adult younger than 40 with 25% or more TBSA involvement should be transferred to a burn center if stable.

149. A: Clinical shock is caused by inadequate perfusion of tissues with resulting hypoxia. Tachycardia, tachypnea, poor peripheral circulation, and diminished urine output are clinical features as blood is shunted from the periphery to the three most vital organs: brain, heart, and lungs. The release of several hormones is increased in response. Epinephrine and norepinephrine are released by the adrenal gland and cause peripheral vasoconstriction, enhancing blood shifting to the critical organs and also stimulating the heart; cortisol is released by the adrenal glands, stimulating hepatic glucose production. Although the glucose level rises, there is also an increase in insulin resistance so that tissues may still be deprived of essential fuel. The increased conversion of renin from the kidney to angiotensin II and adrenal aldosterone enhance renal sodium reabsorption and restoration of fluid to the intravascular space. Decreased renal perfusion leads to increased ADH release from the posterior pituitary gland to maintain intravascular volume; consequently urine output is diminished.

150. D: Most shock syndrome differentiation is based on categories: hypovolemic (blood loss, third spacing of intravascular fluid); septic (sepsis, usually with gram-negative bacteria that release endogenous pyrogens, provoking numerous cytokines and proinflammatory mediators causing vascular insufficiency); cardiogenic (impaired cardiac output, usually due to myocardial infarction); anaphylactic (excessive allergic reaction); and neurogenic (may be caused by brain injury or spinal cord injury). Excessive insulin may also produce a neurogenic shock by sharply causing hypoglycemia. The vasomotor center of the brain is depressed, diminishing sympathetic outflow that controls the vascular response. Unopposed parasympathetic discharge leads to peripheral vasodilation and impaired cardiac performance, resulting in shock.

151. B: In shock resuscitation, the patient response to corrective measures is probably the best index of effective therapy. A minimum MAP of 40 mm Hg is recommended by authorities in those patients who are actively bleeding. Too vigorous administration of intravenous fluids may result in dislodgement of clots, dilution of coagulation factors, venous dilation, and hypothermia. Once bleeding is controlled by surgical or nonsurgical means, higher pressures may be sought with blood and fluid administration. A higher MAP is advised for other shock states: 90 mm Hg for traumatic brain injury without hemorrhage, and greater than 65 mm Hg for most other forms of shock. Massive blood transfusion for shock patients may lead to complications such as coagulopathies, ARDS, or multiorgan failure. Vasopressors, such as dobutamine, dopamine, epinephrine, or norepinephrine, may be required to sustain blood pressure in many forms of shock.

152. A: While observation of the patient's heart and respiratory rates, mental status, and adequacy of peripheral circulation are clinical indicators of shock, several invasive and noninvasive methods for following effectiveness of treatment are available. Pulse oximetry is a simple and noninvasive technique to measure peripheral oxygen saturation but is subject to limitations in estimating circulation and hypoxia, especially with use of vasoactive medications or hypothermia. Central venous pressure is a useful measure of circulating volume, cardiac performance, and vascular tone. Values under the normal range of 4 to 10 cm H_2O indicate a low circulating volume while values above this range may indicate excessive fluid administration, pulmonary edema, or vascular obstruction. $ScvO_2$ is measured from a catheter in the superior vena cava and a value of 70% is used to guide therapy even if clinical signs show improvement. Pulmonary artery catheters (e.g., Swan-Ganz) are not recommended for routine hemodynamic monitoring.

153. C: Acute management of bleeding is an extremely common task in the emergency department and often the emergency department nurse must initially address the problem. Some of the rules of tourniquet placement are: 1) do not place directly over the wound; direct pressure to the wound is preferable; 2) the tourniquet should be placed as distally as possible but 5 cm proximal to the bleeding site; 3) apply it directly to the exposed skin, not over clothing or a dressing; 4) do not apply over a joint; 5) do not apply over a foreign object; 6) release the tourniquet as soon as possible when bleeding is controlled; it may be left in place for up to 2 hours without excessive tissue damage.

154. D: Poor tissue perfusion and hypoxemia in shock states lead to anaerobic metabolism and increase in lactic acid and base deficit. This tissue acidosis stimulates the respiratory centers and is initially compensated by increased respiratory action, which tends to increase oxygenation and buffer the acidosis by diminishing CO_2 levels. Without treatment, the acidosis prevails and is the most common finding in shock patients. If the pH is very low (less than 7.1), sodium bicarbonate should be administered because lethal cardiac arrhythmias may occur; with pH values above this, treatment of the cause of the shock along with ventilation and oxygenation and fluid replacement should improve the acidosis. Persistent or very low pH levels indicate a high risk for complications such as multiorgan failure, ARDS, or DIC.

155. A: Frequently intensive care measures must be initiated in the emergency department because of lack of beds and other logistical or bureaucratic problems. The early goal-directed therapy (EGDT) study for septic patients with elevated lactate levels or refractory hypotension treated in the emergency department for 6 hours prior to ICU admission showed an increased survival over standard treatment (46.5% vs 30.5%). Fluid resuscitation remains a cornerstone of treatment in these patients but the debate of the superiority of colloids vs crystalloids remains unsettled. Many patients receive both (e.g., fresh frozen plasma and normal saline). Antibiotic therapy begun within 1 hour of diagnosis has also lessened mortality. Numerous antibiotic combinations may be satisfactory but adequate gram-negative coverage is essential. Maintaining the MAP at 65 mm Hg or greater and a $ScvO_2$ of at least 70% are two of the EGTD parameters. Administration of rhAPC to septic patients in whom protein C levels are low has shown some decrease in risk and mortality.

156. D: There are several different types of central venous access devices for fluid and electrolyte, blood product, or drug administration and withdrawal of blood samples. The tunneled catheter is surgically threaded into the subclavian vein and then into the superior vena cava or right atrium. The distal end of the catheter emerges below the clavicle with a Dacron cuff for stability. These require withdrawal of 10 mL of blood before aspirating a sample for the lab and a 5 mL flush before medication administration. A Groshong type catheter requires 5 mL saline flushes after use or once per week; no heparin needed. An implanted port requires a 500 unit heparin flush once a month if

not in use and a 10 mL saline flush followed by heparin after blood withdrawal. The instructions in the question are most appropriate for a PICC.

157. A: Intraosseous infusion is a rapid alternative for intravenous administration, especially for infants and children whose veins are not easily accessible or in adults until more traditional venous access is obtained. An 18-gauge needle is used for infants and a 15-gauge needle for older children and adults. The sternum is quite thin in young children and insertion of the needle here is contraindicated; however, it may be used in adults. Preferable sites are the iliac crest, anterior tibia at the tibial tuberosity (best for children), external femoral condyle or medial malleolus. Needles should not be inserted through infected or burned tissue. Manual pressure or an infusion pump is often required if large volumes must be administered quickly. Alternative vascular access should be obtained within 4 hours.

158. C: This patient's history, presentation, and laboratory findings are fairly typical of hyperosmolar hyperglycemia. In contrast to DKA, patients with hyperosmolar hyperglycemia tend to be older, have type 2 diabetes, and often present with neurologic signs and symptoms. Usually the glucose level is above 800 mg/dL and the serum osmolality above 350 mOsm/L, but test for ketones is negative or only slightly positive and the pH is in the normal or only slightly low range. Type 2 diabetic patients have adequate insulin levels to keep them out of ketoacidosis but not enough to overcome the marked hyperglycemia due to increased insulin resistance and increased hepatic gluconeogenesis. Often this syndrome is triggered by stopping medication and exacerbated by osmotic diuresis or diuretics causing dehydration. Mortality may be as high as 60%. Lactic acidosis may be triggered by metformin but he has been off the drug for a while and levels above 4 to 5 mmol/L are usually seen with lactic acidosis.

159. D: This patient has extreme thyrotoxicosis, which usually is caused by underlying Grave disease with cessation of antithyroid medications. Presentation usually involves high fever, tremors, agitation, and delirium or coma. The disorder, often called thyroid storm, is life-threatening and has a 90% mortality rate if left untreated. Often a history is difficult because of the patient's condition but the clinical picture usually is enough to make the diagnosis. Beta-blockers are given to control adrenergic effects and reduce the ventricular rate. Anti-thyroid drugs such as propylthiouracil (PTU) or methimazole are given orally or by nasogastric tube to block further synthesis of thyroid hormone. The onset of action is in about 1 hour but full effect may take 3 to 6 weeks. Iodides may also be given to inhibit hormone release from the thyroid and block the conversion of T4 to T3, but these drugs should be given for at least 1 hour after the antithyroid medications.

160. C: Blood coagulation is complex and consists of a series of reactions, sometimes called the coagulation cascade, that involve tissue and endothelial factors, plasma coagulation factors (proteins), and platelets. In addition, there is a fibrinolytic system that lyses clots. The vitamin K–dependent factors are II, VII, IX, and X (thrombokinase factor). The drug warfarin (*Coumadin*) has been used for many years to inhibit synthesis of these factors in the treatment and prevention of thromboembolic disease (deep vein thrombosis [DVT], pulmonary embolus, emboli from the heart, especially in patients with atrial fibrillation). Factor VIII is not vitamin K dependent and is the missing or dysfunctional factor in hemophilia A, usually a sex-linked inherited disorder but occasionally caused by mutation. Interestingly, factor IX is absent or defective in hemophilia B (less common than hemophilia A) and is vitamin K dependent. Vitamin K administration may reverse deficiency of the dependent factors (usually due to excessive warfarin) but is usually given only if there is significant bleeding.

161. B: Tumor lysis syndrome results from a large breakdown of tumor cells, usually after chemotherapy but occasionally spontaneously. It is most often seen in highly proliferative tumors. Breakdown of cells lead to marked potassium and phosphate release, leading to hyperkalemia and hyperphosphatemia. Hypocalcemia results from the binding of calcium to the phosphate. Elevated uric acid also occurs because of the breakdown of nucleic acids released from the cells. Fatigue, anorexia, muscle and abdominal cramps, dysrhythmias, flank pain, and renal failure may result. Treatment includes vigorous hydration and sodium bicarbonate to alkalinize the urine and protect against uric acid deposits in the kidney. Diuretics may also be used. Allopurinol is given to diminish the hyperuricemia; phosphate-binding agents to diminish the elevated phosphate. Hyperkalemia is treated with intravenous calcium gluconate or chloride, glucose and insulin and sodium bicarbonate to drive potassium into cells, as well as sodium polystyrene sulfonate (*Kayexalate*) to draw potassium into the gastrointestinal tract.

162. D: Sickle cell anemia is an autosomal disorder, found in about 1 out 500 African-Americans, in which red blood cells contain hemoglobin S instead of the normal hemoglobin A. These abnormal red cells have a shortened lifespan (10 to 20 days vs 120 for normal red cells) and a tendency to form a sickle shape, especially when provoked by hypoxia, dehydration, infection, high altitude, or exercise. The sickle cells are less deformable than normal and tend to occlude small blood vessels, causing tissue hypoxia, infarction, and necrosis. These are referred to as sickle crises and cause diffuse, often severe, pain, especially in bones and joints. An acute chest syndrome with dyspnea, pain, fever, and pulmonary infiltrates may also occur. Priapism in males may be caused by occlusion of the venous drainage of the penis. Aplastic crisis, a condition of bone marrow failure, may also occur. Gastrointestinal bleeding may occur because of aspirin or NSAID medication or stress ulceration but is not considered part of the basic disease.

163. D: This patient has fever and neutropenia after chemotherapy. Neutropenia is defined as an absolute neutrophil count (ANC) under $1000/mm^3$, and a severe neutropenia less than $500/mm^3$ is particularly dangerous. These patients must be worked up quickly and antibiotic and possibly additional therapy started as soon as possible since the situation may be life-threatening. While myelosuppressive drugs differ in the length of time between administration and the nadir of the ANC, 10 to 14 days is typical. Multiple cultures from different possible sites of origin for sepsis must be done along with chest x-ray and other imaging as indicated by examination. Broad-spectrum antibiotics, such as ceftazidime or imipenem/cilastatin, should be started after cultures are obtained. She should be asked if she has been receiving G-CSF (*Neupogen, Neulasta*). WBC transfusions are rarely used today since they have a very short shelf life, do not last long in the circulation, and may cause allergic reactions.

164. A: Intracranial pressure monitoring is indicated for traumatic brain injury with an abnormal CT of the brain or with 2 or more high-risk factors: age older than 40, posturing motor response, or systolic blood pressure less than 90. Under normal circumstances, the ICP is between 0 and 15 mm Hg. The brain can compensate to a point for additional volume but when brain compliance is exhausted the ICP rises sharply. Critical is the central perfusion pressure (CPP), which is the difference between the mean arterial pressure (MAP) and the ICP. CPP values below 50 mm Hg indicate hypoperfusion and brain ischemia. Intraventricular placement of a pressure transducer by catheter into the lateral ventricle gives the most accurate pressure readings and allows easy sampling of CSF, but is harder to place and there is a higher risk of infection than with the other devices.

165. B: Anthrax is a gram-positive bacterium that forms spores that may survive for long periods in soil. The disease may occur in 3 forms: 1) inhalation of spores, the least common but most deadly

- 244 -

form; 2) cutaneous, the most common form that produces localized disease, often contracted directly from handling infected animal hides; and 3) gastrointestinal, acquired by eating the spores, usually from infected meat. Aerosolization of spores enhances their use as a biologic weapon. A flu-like syndrome followed by a short period of improvement, then a severe deterioration and death is a typical course of the inhalation type if left untreated. Mediastinitis and meningitis are complications of the inhaled form. Human to human transfer does not occur so that mass isolation is not required. Decontamination of areas of exposure is usually carried out. Antibiotics such as ciprofloxacin (*Cipro*) or doxycycline are effective but treatment should be carried out for 60 days.

166. C: Hypokalemia (potassium lower than 3.5 mEq/L) may result from gastrointestinal or renal loss, or from transfer from extracellular fluid to intracellular fluid. Drugs such as aldosterone, insulin, and beta2-agonists promote the latter. Gastrointestinal loss is the most likely cause in this patient and hypokalemia may be a feature of traveler's gastroenteritis. Renal loss occurs with diuretics or kidney disease and low potassium may be a feature of diabetic ketoacidosis or excess steroids. The ECG findings described are typical of low potassium but do not necessarily correlate with the degree. Potassium administration should be through a large bore or central venous catheter (it is locally irritating) by an infusion pump at 40 mEq/L not to exceed 10 to 20 mEq per hour. For severe hypokalemia, a 5 to 10 mEq bolus may be given but serial potassium and cardiac monitoring is required to avoid hyperkalemia, ventricular dysrhythmias, and death. Low serum magnesium levels may accompany hypokalemia and should be checked.

167. B: Measurement of pulse and blood pressure while the patient is supine for 3 minutes and then sitting and/or standing for 1 minute is a clinical method (orthostatic vital signs) to determine hypovolemia or impaired sympathetic discharge or venoconstriction in patients with syncope. Generally, lying to standing is more sensitive to orthostatic hypotension. Positive results consist of a rise in pulse rate of 30 beats per minute or blood pressure fall of 20 mm Hg on change of position. Development of dizziness or syncope on standing is also considered a positive sign. While the value of this test in predicting hypovolemia is far from perfect, it is simple to perform, and, if positive, may direct further laboratory or clinical investigation.

168. D: The clinical picture of this patient is that of an anaphylactic reaction to bee stings and is potentially life-threatening. The onset of symptoms within 1 hour after exposure to the allergen is particularly worrisome as are the laryngeal and pulmonary signs. The airway must be established with intubation often necessary; high-flow oxygen, cardiac monitoring, and intravenous fluids are basics. Epinephrine given intramuscularly is the most rapidly acting agent and should be given as soon as possible after the diagnosis of anaphylaxis and every 5 to 15 minutes thereafter as needed. Steroids and antihistamines are slower acting than epinephrine but are often given to alleviate itching, angioedema, and hives. IVF will be given as needed. There is no indication for antibiotics in this clinical situation unless further signs and symptoms develop.

169. D: Clotted vascular access devices for chronic renal failure patients undergoing dialysis are not uncommon emergency department cases. Vascular access for these patients may be carried out with a temporary external arteriovenous shunt, or permanent internal arteriovenous fistula or graft. The cephalic vein and radial artery of the forearm are the most often used. Clotting or infection of the access may occur. If a clot impedes smooth vascular flow, it must be lysed with fibrinolytic agents or removed surgically. A temporary dual lumen subclavian catheter may be inserted for 2 to 3 days. If local signs such as swelling, erythema, or tenderness suggest infection, the device is usually removed and cultures and antibiotics prescribed.

170. B: At one time, collection of vaginal semen from rape victims was limited to 48 hours after the crime but, because of increasingly sensitive DNA testing, many jurisdictions have increased this collection period up to 5 to 7 days. In addition, samples for DNA analysis can be collected from clothing and bed linens; the emergency nurse should collect and preserve such items. Potential evidence must be given to the police and appropriate signatures and times from all who handle the evidence must be obtained to preserve chain of custody. Evidence may be stored in a locked closet or cabinet with limited access.

171. B: Issues of informed consent constantly arise in the emergency department because many patients are incompetent to understand the situation; this may be due to mental illness, altered state of consciousness, or age (minors). Generally, minors require parental consent but exceptions are made for emancipated minors, serious or life-threatening emergencies, or, in some states, if the minor is mature enough to understand the treatment and possible consequences. Parents generally cannot withhold consent for lifesaving treatment on religious grounds. Usually, the emergency physician explains the nature and risks of treatment but the nurse should make sure that this is carried out and witness the patient's signature. Handing the patient an informed consent sheet without explanation may not be enough in many legal jurisdictions. In true emergency situations where the patient is unable to give consent, another authorized person such as a close relative may be satisfactory.

172. D: EMTALA was passed by Congress in 1986 as part of COBRA. Its intent was to prevent "patient dumping" and "economic triage" by hospitals participating in Medicare and receiving federal funds. It applies to all patients seeking emergency treatment whether they are Medicare patients or not. Triage refers to the order in which patients are seen by the physician, not whether or not they require medical examination. The patient must receive a medical screening exam before any disposition is made and the lack of insurance or out-of-plan HMO status is not a basis for transfer or discharge of the patient without medical examination. For unstable patients being transferred to another facility, the receiving hospital must accept the transfer and the emergency physician ordering the transfer must sign an approval note outlining the benefits and risks of the transfer. While a patient may refuse examination and treatment, simple verbal refusal may not be legally sufficient and every attempt should be made to obtain a written refusal, including a statement that the benefits and risks have been explained.

173. C: Injuries due to child neglect and/or physical abuse are extremely common in emergency departments. Often the differentiation of a true accident or disease from intentional harm is difficult and falls to the nurse to decide. While cuts and bruises are extremely common in children, multiple bruises, especially on the head, trunk, upper arms, and buttocks, should raise the possibility of abuse. Skeletal trauma suggestive of abuse includes multiple fractures at various stages of healing, posterior or lateral rib or multiple fractures in infants, presence of "grab" marks over a long bone fracture and spiral or oblique fractures. Purposely inflicted burns tend to be discrete and are not widely scattered as in true accidental scalding from spilling of hot liquids. The shaken baby syndrome (with or without direct head trauma) is suggested by multiple retinal hemorrhages. When parental account of the "accident" does not correlate with the physical findings (e.g., multiple fractures from a fall from the couch), or multiple visits for trauma occur, child abuse should be suspected.

174. C: Individual states have statutes concerning conditions and diseases that must be reported by the emergency department to local law enforcement (homicides, suicides, rapes, child or elder abuse) or to the coroner/medical examiner (unexpected death within 48 hours of admission or during surgery). Communicable diseases such as tuberculosis, HIV/AIDS, or unusual or resistant

organisms are reportable to local health authorities and possibly the CDC. Unexpected drug reactions may be reported to the FDA. Since state requirements vary, the list of reportable conditions is kept in the emergency department for quick reference. The nurse shares responsibility for reporting with the physician and may act independently if the situation warrants. Social services may assume responsibility in certain cases.

175. A: New treatments and protocols are carried out on emergency patients quite frequently. Often the medical staff participates in multi-institutional trials with an established protocol and randomization of patients to the current standard treatment or the new treatment under investigation. Sometimes these studies are "double-blind," in which neither the treating physician nor the patient know which group the latter is in until the study is terminated and the "code broken." Results are often compared statistically to evaluate whether the results of a study are due to chance rather than intervention with the new treatment. The lower the P value, the less likely that the result is due to chance; most clinical researchers accept values less than 0.05 (5%) to indicate that the result is not due to chance. Experimental evidence may be ranked on a scale of I to VII, with I being the most reliable (usually from randomized, controlled studies) and VII being the least (clinical opinions, anecdotal reports). A confidence interval, another statistical method, refers to the degree of precision of the results (i.e., how confident the investigator is that the results are correct).

Secret Key #1 - Time is Your Greatest Enemy

Pace Yourself

Wear a watch. At the beginning of the test, check the time (or start a chronometer on your watch to count the minutes), and check the time after every few questions to make sure you are "on schedule."

If you are forced to speed up, do it efficiently. Usually one or more answer choices can be eliminated without too much difficulty. Above all, don't panic. Don't speed up and just begin guessing at random choices. By pacing yourself, and continually monitoring your progress against your watch, you will always know exactly how far ahead or behind you are with your available time. If you find that you are one minute behind on the test, don't skip one question without spending any time on it, just to catch back up. Take 15 fewer seconds on the next four questions, and after four questions you'll have caught back up. Once you catch back up, you can continue working each problem at your normal pace.

Furthermore, don't dwell on the problems that you were rushed on. If a problem was taking up too much time and you made a hurried guess, it must be difficult. The difficult questions are the ones you are most likely to miss anyway, so it isn't a big loss. It is better to end with more time than you need than to run out of time.

Lastly, sometimes it is beneficial to slow down if you are constantly getting ahead of time. You are always more likely to catch a careless mistake by working more slowly than quickly, and among very high-scoring test takers (those who are likely to have lots of time left over), careless errors affect the score more than mastery of material.

Secret Key #2 - Guessing is not Guesswork

You probably know that guessing is a good idea. Unlike other standardized tests, there is no penalty for getting a wrong answer. Even if you have no idea about a question, you still have a 20-25% chance of getting it right.

Most test takers do not understand the impact that proper guessing can have on their score. Unless you score extremely high, guessing will significantly contribute to your final score.

Monkeys Take the Test

What most test takers don't realize is that to insure that 20-25% chance, you have to guess randomly. If you put 20 monkeys in a room to take this test, assuming they answered once per question and behaved themselves, on average they would get 20-25% of the questions correct. Put 20 test takers in the room, and the average will be much lower among guessed questions. Why?
1. The test writers intentionally write deceptive answer choices that "look" right. A test taker has no idea about a question, so he picks the "best looking" answer, which is often wrong. The monkey has no idea what looks good and what doesn't, so it will consistently be right about 20-25% of the time.
2. Test takers will eliminate answer choices from the guessing pool based on a hunch or intuition. Simple but correct answers often get excluded, leaving a 0% chance of being correct. The monkey has no clue, and often gets lucky with the best choice.

This is why the process of elimination endorsed by most test courses is flawed and detrimental to your performance. Test takers don't guess; they make an ignorant stab in the dark that is usually worse than random.

$5 Challenge

Let me introduce one of the most valuable ideas of this course—the $5 challenge:

You only mark your "best guess" if you are willing to bet $5 on it.
You only eliminate choices from guessing if you are willing to bet $5 on it.

Why $5? Five dollars is an amount of money that is small yet not insignificant, and can really add up fast (20 questions could cost you $100). Likewise, each answer choice on one question of the test will have a small impact on your overall score, but it can really add up to a lot of points in the end.

The process of elimination IS valuable. The following shows your chance of guessing it right:

If you eliminate wrong answer choices until only this many remain:	Chance of getting it correct:
1	100%
2	50%
3	33%

However, if you accidentally eliminate the right answer or go on a hunch for an incorrect answer, your chances drop dramatically—to 0%. By guessing among all the answer choices, you are GUARANTEED to have a shot at the right answer.

That's why the $5 test is so valuable. If you give up the advantage and safety of a pure guess, it had better be worth the risk.

What we still haven't covered is how to be sure that whatever guess you make is truly random. Here's the easiest way:

Always pick the first answer choice among those remaining.

Such a technique means that you have decided, **before you see a single test question**, exactly how you are going to guess, and since the order of choices tells you nothing about which one is correct, this guessing technique is perfectly random.

This section is not meant to scare you away from making educated guesses or eliminating choices; you just need to define when a choice is worth eliminating. The $5 test, along with a pre-defined random guessing strategy, is the best way to make sure you reap all of the benefits of guessing.

Secret Key #3 - Practice Smarter, Not Harder

Many test takers delay the test preparation process because they dread the awful amounts of practice time they think necessary to succeed on the test. We have refined an effective method that will take you only a fraction of the time.

There are a number of "obstacles" in the path to success. Among these are answering questions, finishing in time, and mastering test-taking strategies. All must be executed on the day of the test at peak performance, or your score will suffer. The test is a mental marathon that has a large impact on your future.

Just like a marathon runner, it is important to work your way up to the full challenge. So first you just worry about questions, and then time, and finally strategy:

Success Strategy

1. Find a good source for practice tests.
2. If you are willing to make a larger time investment, consider using more than one study guide. Often the different approaches of multiple authors will help you "get" difficult concepts.
3. Take a practice test with no time constraints, with all study helps, "open book." Take your time with questions and focus on applying strategies.
4. Take a practice test with time constraints, with all guides, "open book."
5. Take a final practice test without open material and with time limits.

If you have time to take more practice tests, just repeat step 5. By gradually exposing yourself to the full rigors of the test environment, you will condition your mind to the stress of test day and maximize your success.

Secret Key #4 - Prepare, Don't Procrastinate

Let me state an obvious fact: if you take the test three times, you will probably get three different scores. This is due to the way you feel on test day, the level of preparedness you have, and the version of the test you see. Despite the test writers' claims to the contrary, some versions of the test WILL be easier for you than others.

Since your future depends so much on your score, you should maximize your chances of success. In order to maximize the likelihood of success, you've got to prepare in advance. This means taking practice tests and spending time learning the information and test taking strategies you will need to succeed.

Never go take the actual test as a "practice" test, expecting that you can just take it again if you need to. Take all the practice tests you can on your own, but when you go to take the official test, be prepared, be focused, and do your best the first time!

Secret Key #5 - Test Yourself

Everyone knows that time is money. There is no need to spend too much of your time or too little of your time preparing for the test. You should only spend as much of your precious time preparing as is necessary for you to get the score you need.

Once you have taken a practice test under real conditions of time constraints, then you will know if you are ready for the test or not.

If you have scored extremely high the first time that you take the practice test, then there is not much point in spending countless hours studying. You are already there.

Benchmark your abilities by retaking practice tests and seeing how much you have improved. Once you consistently score high enough to guarantee success, then you are ready.

If you have scored well below where you need, then knuckle down and begin studying in earnest. Check your improvement regularly through the use of practice tests under real conditions. Above all, don't worry, panic, or give up. The key is perseverance!

Then, when you go to take the test, remain confident and remember how well you did on the practice tests. If you can score high enough on a practice test, then you can do the same on the real thing.

General Strategies

The most important thing you can do is to ignore your fears and jump into the test immediately. Do not be overwhelmed by any strange-sounding terms. You have to jump into the test like jumping into a pool—all at once is the easiest way.

Make Predictions

As you read and understand the question, try to guess what the answer will be. Remember that several of the answer choices are wrong, and once you begin reading them, your mind will immediately become cluttered with answer choices designed to throw you off. Your mind is typically the most focused immediately after you have read the question and digested its contents. If you can, try to predict what the correct answer will be. You may be surprised at what you can predict.

Quickly scan the choices and see if your prediction is in the listed answer choices. If it is, then you can be quite confident that you have the right answer. It still won't hurt to check the other answer choices, but most of the time, you've got it!

Answer the Question

It may seem obvious to only pick answer choices that answer the question, but the test writers can create some excellent answer choices that are wrong. Don't pick an answer just because it sounds right, or you believe it to be true. It MUST answer the question. Once you've made your selection, always go back and check it against the question and make sure that you didn't misread the question and that the answer choice does answer the question posed.

Benchmark

After you read the first answer choice, decide if you think it sounds correct or not. If it doesn't, move on to the next answer choice. If it does, mentally mark that answer choice. This doesn't mean that you've definitely selected it as your answer choice, it just means that it's the best you've seen thus far. Go ahead and read the next choice. If the next choice is worse than the one you've already selected, keep going to the next answer choice. If the next choice is better than the choice you've already selected, mentally mark the new answer choice as your best guess.

The first answer choice that you select becomes your standard. Every other answer choice must be benchmarked against that standard. That choice is correct until proven otherwise by another answer choice beating it out. Once you've decided that no other answer choice seems as good, do one final check to ensure that your answer choice answers the question posed.

Valid Information

Don't discount any of the information provided in the question. Every piece of information may be necessary to determine the correct answer. None of the information in the question is there to throw you off (while the answer choices will certainly have information to throw you off). If two seemingly unrelated topics are discussed, don't ignore either. You can be confident there is a relationship, or it wouldn't be included in the question, and you are probably going to have to determine what is that relationship to find the answer.

Avoid "Fact Traps"

Don't get distracted by a choice that is factually true. Your search is for the answer that answers the question. Stay focused and don't fall for an answer that is true but irrelevant. Always go back to the question and make sure you're choosing an answer that actually answers the question and is not just a true statement. An answer can be factually correct, but it MUST answer the question asked. Additionally, two answers can both be seemingly correct, so be sure to read all of the answer choices, and make sure that you get the one that BEST answers the question.

Milk the Question

Some of the questions may throw you completely off. They might deal with a subject you have not been exposed to, or one that you haven't reviewed in years. While your lack of knowledge about the subject will be a hindrance, the question itself can give you many clues that will help you find the correct answer. Read the question carefully and look for clues. Watch particularly for adjectives and nouns describing difficult terms or words that you don't recognize. Regardless of whether you completely understand a word or not, replacing it with a synonym, either provided or one you more familiar with, may help you to understand what the questions are asking. Rather than wracking your mind about specific detailed information concerning a difficult term or word, try to use mental substitutes that are easier to understand.

The Trap of Familiarity

Don't just choose a word because you recognize it. On difficult questions, you may not recognize a number of words in the answer choices. The test writers don't put "make-believe" words on the test, so don't think that just because you only recognize all the words in one answer choice that that answer choice must be correct. If you only recognize words in one answer choice, then focus on that one. Is it correct? Try your best to determine if it is correct. If it is, that's great. If not, eliminate it. Each word and answer choice you eliminate increases your chances of getting the question correct, even if you then have to guess among the unfamiliar choices.

Eliminate Answers

Eliminate choices as soon as you realize they are wrong. But be careful! Make sure you consider all of the possible answer choices. Just because one appears right, doesn't mean that the next one won't be even better! The test writers will usually put more than one good answer choice for every question, so read all of them. Don't worry if you are stuck between two that seem right. By getting down to just two remaining possible choices, your odds are now 50/50. Rather than wasting too much time, play the odds. You are guessing, but guessing wisely because you've been able to knock out some of the answer choices that you know are wrong. If you are eliminating choices and realize that the last answer choice you are left with is also obviously wrong, don't panic. Start over and consider each choice again. There may easily be something that you missed the first time and will realize on the second pass.

Tough Questions

If you are stumped on a problem or it appears too hard or too difficult, don't waste time. Move on! Remember though, if you can quickly check for obviously incorrect answer choices, your chances of guessing correctly are greatly improved. Before you completely give up, at least try to knock out a couple of possible answers. Eliminate what you can and then guess at the remaining answer choices before moving on.

Brainstorm

If you get stuck on a difficult question, spend a few seconds quickly brainstorming. Run through the complete list of possible answer choices. Look at each choice and ask yourself, "Could this answer the question satisfactorily?" Go through each answer choice and consider it independently of the others. By systematically going through all possibilities, you may find something that you would otherwise overlook. Remember though that when you get stuck, it's important to try to keep moving.

Read Carefully

Understand the problem. Read the question and answer choices carefully. Don't miss the question because you misread the terms. You have plenty of time to read each question thoroughly and make sure you understand what is being asked. Yet a happy medium must be attained, so don't waste too much time. You must read carefully, but efficiently.

Face Value

When in doubt, use common sense. Always accept the situation in the problem at face value. Don't read too much into it. These problems will not require you to make huge leaps of logic. The test writers aren't trying to throw you off with a cheap trick. If you have to go beyond creativity and make a leap of logic in order to have an answer choice answer the question, then you should look at the other answer choices. Don't overcomplicate the problem by creating theoretical relationships or explanations that will warp time or space. These are normal problems rooted in reality. It's just that the applicable relationship or explanation may not be readily apparent and you have to figure things out. Use your common sense to interpret anything that isn't clear.

Prefixes

If you're having trouble with a word in the question or answer choices, try dissecting it. Take advantage of every clue that the word might include. Prefixes and suffixes can be a huge help. Usually they allow you to determine a basic meaning. Pre- means before, post- means after, pro - is positive, de- is negative. From these prefixes and suffixes, you can get an idea of the general meaning of the word and try to put it into context. Beware though of any traps. Just because con- is the opposite of pro-, doesn't necessarily mean congress is the opposite of progress!

Hedge Phrases

Watch out for critical hedge phrases, led off with words such as "likely," "may," "can," "sometimes," "often," "almost," "mostly," "usually," "generally," "rarely," and "sometimes." Question writers insert these hedge phrases to cover every possibility. Often an answer choice will be wrong simply because it leaves no room for exception. Unless the situation calls for them, avoid answer choices that have definitive words like "exactly," and "always."

Switchback Words

Stay alert for "switchbacks." These are the words and phrases frequently used to alert you to shifts in thought. The most common switchback word is "but." Others include "although," "however," "nevertheless," "on the other hand," "even though," "while," "in spite of," "despite," and "regardless of."

New Information

Correct answer choices will rarely have completely new information included. Answer choices typically are straightforward reflections of the material asked about and will directly relate to the question. If a new piece of information is included in an answer choice that doesn't even seem to relate to the topic being asked about, then that answer choice is likely incorrect. All of the information needed to answer the question is usually provided for you in the question. You should not have to make guesses that are unsupported or choose answer choices that require unknown information that cannot be reasoned from what is given.

Time Management

On technical questions, don't get lost on the technical terms. Don't spend too much time on any one question. If you don't know what a term means, then odds are you aren't going to get much further since you don't have a dictionary. You should be able to immediately recognize whether or not you know a term. If you don't, work with the other clues that you have—the other answer choices and terms provided—but don't waste too much time trying to figure out a difficult term that you don't know.

Contextual Clues

Look for contextual clues. An answer can be right but not the correct answer. The contextual clues will help you find the answer that is most right and is correct. Understand the context in which a phrase or statement is made. This will help you make important distinctions.

Don't Panic

Panicking will not answer any questions for you; therefore, it isn't helpful. When you first see the question, if your mind goes blank, take a deep breath. Force yourself to mechanically go through the steps of solving the problem using the strategies you've learned.

Pace Yourself

Don't get clock fever. It's easy to be overwhelmed when you're looking at a page full of questions, your mind is full of random thoughts and feeling confused, and the clock is ticking down faster than you would like. Calm down and maintain the pace that you have set for yourself. As long as you are on track by monitoring your pace, you are guaranteed to have enough time for yourself. When you get to the last few minutes of the test, it may seem like you won't have enough time left, but if you only have as many questions as you should have left at that point, then you're right on track!

Answer Selection

The best way to pick an answer choice is to eliminate all of those that are wrong, until only one is left and confirm that is the correct answer. Sometimes though, an answer choice may immediately look right. Be careful! Take a second to make sure that the other choices are not equally obvious. Don't make a hasty mistake. There are only two times that you should stop before checking other answers. First is when you are positive that the answer choice you have selected is correct. Second is when time is almost out and you have to make a quick guess!

Check Your Work

Since you will probably not know every term listed and the answer to every question, it is important that you get credit for the ones that you do know. Don't miss any questions through careless mistakes. If at all possible, try to take a second to look back over your answer selection and make sure you've selected the correct answer choice and haven't made a costly careless mistake (such as marking an answer choice that you didn't mean to mark). The time it takes for this quick double check should more than pay for itself in caught mistakes.

Beware of Directly Quoted Answers

Sometimes an answer choice will repeat word for word a portion of the question or reference section. However, beware of such exact duplication. It may be a trap! More than likely, the correct choice will paraphrase or summarize a point, rather than being exactly the same wording.

Slang

Scientific sounding answers are better than slang ones. An answer choice that begins "To compare the outcomes…" is much more likely to be correct than one that begins "Because some people insisted…"

Extreme Statements

Avoid wild answers that throw out highly controversial ideas that are proclaimed as established fact. An answer choice that states the "process should used in certain situations, if…" is much more likely to be correct than one that states the "process should be discontinued completely." The first is a calm rational statement and doesn't even make a definitive, uncompromising stance, using a hedge word "if" to provide wiggle room, whereas the second choice is a radical idea and far more extreme.

Answer Choice Families

When you have two or more answer choices that are direct opposites or parallels, one of them is usually the correct answer. For instance, if one answer choice states "x increases" and another answer choice states "x decreases" or "y increases," then those two or three answer choices are very similar in construction and fall into the same family of answer choices. A family of answer choices consists of two or three answer choices, very similar in construction, but often with directly opposite meanings. Usually the correct answer choice will be in that family of answer choices. The "odd man out" or answer choice that doesn't seem to fit the parallel construction of the other answer choices is more likely to be incorrect.

Additional Bonus Material

Due to our efforts to try to keep this book to a manageable length, we've created a link that will give you access to all of your additional bonus material.

Please visit http://www.mometrix.com/bonus948/cen to access the information.

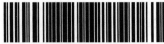

Made in the USA
San Bernardino, CA
08 June 2017